Cognitive-B€
Therapy for
Severe Mental Illness

An Illustrated Guide

Cognitive-Behavior Therapy for Severe Mental Illness

An Illustrated Guide

Jesse H. Wright, M.D., Ph.D.
Professor and Associate Chairman for Academic Affairs, University of Louisville School of Medicine, Louisville, Kentucky

Douglas Turkington, M.D.
Professor of Psychosocial Psychiatry, Department of Neurology, Neurobiology, and Psychiatry, Newcastle University, Royal Victoria Infirmary, Newcastle-upon-Tyne, United Kingdom

David G. Kingdon, M.D.
Professor of Mental Health Care Delivery, Department of Psychiatry, Royal South Hants Hospital and University of Southampton, United Kingdom

Monica Ramirez Basco, Ph.D.
Assistant Professor of Psychology, University of Texas at Arlington; Clinical Associate Professor, Department of Psychiatry, Division of Psychology, University of Texas Southwestern at Dallas, Dallas, Texas

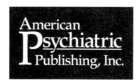

Washington, DC
London, England

To buy 25–99 copies of this or any other APPI title, a 20% discount applies; please contact APPI Customer Service at appi@psych.org or 800-368-5777. To buy 100 or more copies of the same title, please e-mail us at bulksales@psych.org for a price quote.

Copyright © 2009 American Psychiatric Publishing, Inc.
ALL RIGHTS RESERVED

Manufactured in the United States of America on acid-free paper
19 18 17 16 15   7 6 5 4 3
First Edition

Typeset in Adobe's Berling Roman and Frutiger.

American Psychiatric Publishing, Inc.
1000 Wilson Boulevard
Arlington, VA 22209-3901
www.appi.org

Library of Congress Cataloging-in-Publication Data
Cognitive behavior therapy for severe mental illness : an illustrated guide /
Jesse H. Wright ... [et al.].—1st ed.
        p. ; cm.
    Includes bibliographical references and index.
    ISBN 978-1-58562-321-1 (alk. paper)
    1. Cognitive therapy. 2. Mental illness—Treatment. I. Wright, Jesse H.
    [DNLM: 1. Cognitive Therapy—methods. 2. Mental Disorders—therapy.
WM 425.5.C6 C67666 2009]

    RC489.C63C6278 2009
    616.89'1425—dc22

                                                                    2008024612

British Library Cataloguing in Publication Data
A CIP record is available from the British Library.

Contents

Foreword xi

Preface xv

Acknowledgments xix

1 Introduction 1

Why Use CBT for Severe Mental Disorders? 2

The CBT Model for Severe Mental Illnesses 4

Overview of Treatment Methods 12

Efficacy of CBT for Severe Mental Disorders 19

Summary 21

References 22

2 Engaging and Assessing 29

Influences on the Therapeutic Relationship 30

Guidelines for Engaging a Person With
Severe Mental Illness 37

Assessment 45

Indications for CBT 47

Summary 48

References 49

3 Normalizing and Educating...........................51

Normalizing Schizophrenia 51

Normalizing Bipolar Disorder 62

Normalizing Depression 62

The Therapeutic Relationship 63

Education...64

Summary 71

References..72

4 Case Formulation and Treatment Planning 75

Developing the Biopsychosocial Case Conceptualization 76

How to Construct and Use a Mini-Formulation 94

Summary 97

References..98

5 Delusions...99

Treating Delusions: Basic CBT Processes 99

Defining Delusions...................................102

Discussing Delusions 104

Modifying Delusions.................................106

Resistant Delusions 114

Treating Delusions in Mood Disorders 117

Summary 122

References...123

6 Hallucinations......................................125

Impact of Hallucinations..............................125

The CBT Approach to the Hallucinating Patient...........127

Specific CBT Techniques for Hallucinations 132

Summary 141

References...143

7 Depression 145

Hopelessness and Suicidality 146

Low Energy and Lack of Interest.......................160

Low Self-Esteem....................................168

Summary 177

References...177

8 Mania 181

Mania Prevention Plan 182

Summary 208

References 209

9 Interpersonal Problems 211

Common Interpersonal Difficulties 211

Interpersonal Problems in Specific Disorders 222

Summary 235

References 236

10 Impaired Cognitive Functioning .237

Thought Disorder in Schizophrenia 238

Racing Thoughts, Distractibility, and Disorganization in
  Mania and Hypomania 247

Problems With Cognitive Functioning in Depression 251

Summary 254

References 255

11 Negative Symptoms 257

What Are Negative Symptoms? .258

The CBT Conceptualization 259

Demotivation in Schizophrenia .260

Socialization 264

Applying Standard Behavioral Methods 266

Summary 270

References 271

12 Promoting Adherence 273

Types of Nonadherence to Treatment 275

Common Reasons for Nonadherence: Possible Solutions 275

Working With Cognitions 281

Developing a Written Adherence Plan 286

CBT Homework 290

Summary 291

References 292

13 Maintaining Treatment Gains 295

Relapse Prevention. 295

Methods for Continuation and Maintenance CBT 303

Summary 312

References 313

Appendix 1: Worksheets and Checklists 315

Appendix 2: Cognitive-Behavior Therapy Resources 329

Appendix 3: DVD Guide. 335

Index 339

LIST OF LEARNING EXERCISES

▶ **Learning Exercise 2–1.** Identifying and Managing Barriers to Collaborative Therapeutic Relationships 36

▶ **Learning Exercise 3–1.** Normalizing the Diagnosis of Schizophrenia 53

▶ **Learning Exercise 4–1.** Developing a Biopsychosocial Formulation 93

▶ **Learning Exercise 5–1.** Examining the Evidence 109

▶ **Learning Exercise 5–2.** Modifying Delusions 116

▶ **Learning Exercise 6–1.** The Impact of Voices 126

▶ **Learning Exercise 6–2.** Coping With Hallucinations 141

▶ **Learning Exercise 7–1.** Developing an Antisuicide Plan 159

▶ **Learning Exercise 7–2.** Using CBT for Low Energy and Anhedonia. 167

▶ **Learning Exercise 7–3.** Modifying Schemas to Improve Self-Esteem 175

▶ **Learning Exercise 8–1.** A Prevention Plan for Mania 207

▶ **Learning Exercise 9–1.** Advantages and Disadvantages of Assertive Communication 215

▶ **Learning Exercise 9–2.** Emotion Intensity Scale. 228

▶ **Learning Exercise 10–1.** Practicing CBT Methods for Thought Disorder. 246

▶ **Learning Exercise 11–1.** Working With Negative Symptoms 269

▶ **Learning Exercise 12–1.** Developing an Adherence Plan 289

▶ **Learning Exercise 13–1.** Developing a Relapse Prevention Plan 302

LIST OF VIDEO ILLUSTRATIONS

▶ **Video Illustration 1.** Engaging a Patient With Paranoia: Dr. Kingdon and Majir 30

▶ **Video Illustration 2.** Engaging a Patient With Bipolar Disorder: Dr. Basco and Angela 41

▶ **Video Illustration 3.** Engaging a Patient With Chronic Depression: Dr. Wright and Mary 44

▶ **Video Illustration 4.** Normalizing and Educating: Dr. Turkington and Brenda 55

▶ **Video Illustration 5.** Tracing the Origins of Paranoia: Dr. Kingdon and Majir 104

▶ **Video Illustration 6.** Examining the Evidence for Paranoia: Dr. Kingdon and Majir 106

▶ **Video Illustration 7.** Working With a Resistant Delusion: Dr. Kingdon and Majir 115

▶ **Video Illustration 8.** Explaining Hallucinations: Dr. Turkington and Brenda 133

▶ **Video Illustration 9.** Coping With Hallucinations: Dr. Turkington and Brenda 133

▶ **Video Illustration 10.** An Antisuicide Plan: Dr. Wright and Mary. 150

▶ **Video Illustration 11.** Behavioral Intervention for Anhedonia: Dr. Wright and Mary. 163

▶ **Video Illustration 12.** Building Self-Esteem: Dr. Wright and Mary. 171

▶ **Video Illustration 13.** Reducing Grandiosity: Dr. Basco and Angela 204

▶ **Video Illustration 14.** Using an Early Warning System: Dr. Basco and Angela 207

▶ **Video Illustration 15.** Helping With Thought Disorder: Dr. Turkington and Daniel. 243

▶ **Video Illustration 16.** Investigating a Delusion: Dr. Turkington and Daniel. 245

▶ **Video Illustration 17.** Treating Negative Symptoms: Dr. Kingdon and Majir 263

▶ **Video Illustration 18.** Promoting Adherence: Dr. Basco and Angela 280

Foreword

When results of the first randomized controlled study comparing cognitive therapy (also referred to as cognitive-behavior therapy or CBT) with medication for depression appeared in 1977, the positive findings were greeted in many quarters with a certain amount of skepticism. Yet after an outpouring of research and wide dissemination throughout the world, CBT is now recognized as a core empirically supported treatment for psychiatric disorders. And, as evidenced by this exciting new book on CBT for severe mental illness, the reach of cognitive therapy has broadened to include even the most challenging conditions—a range of disorders that were once considered to be largely outside the scope of psychotherapy.

A number of influential research studies have demonstrated, for example, that patients with schizophrenia who are treated with CBT often experience a reduction in delusions, hallucinations, and negative symptoms that goes beyond the results of pharmacotherapy alone. Individuals with bipolar disorder can benefit from CBT methods to lower distress and forestall relapse, and patients with very severe or chronic depression can be helped to regain their previous level of well-being.

Although CBT has the potential to relieve considerable suffering in people with severe mental disorders, only a limited number of clinicians have gained the necessary skills to deliver this specialized form of cognitive therapy. This practical guide, which beautifully describes and illustrates key CBT methods for severe mental illness, is therefore an especially welcome and timely contribution. It provides clinicians with a clear road map for understanding severe mental illness from a cognitive-behavioral perspective, developing a comprehensive treatment plan based on a cognitive formulation, and implementing effective CBT techniques.

As the authors so aptly demonstrate in this book, the basic techniques of CBT are well suited for therapeutic work with patients who have difficult-to-treat disorders. The highly collaborative, empirical, and empowering nature of the therapeutic relationship in cognitive therapy, first described by Aaron Beck in the 1960s, is a cornerstone of the treatment method. In the powerful video illustrations that accompany this book, the authors show how the therapeutic relationship can be greatly enhanced by customizing interventions to match the vulnerabilities and capacities of each patient. For example, David Kingdon demonstrates an extremely sensitive and incremental approach to a man with intense paranoia and social withdrawal. Engaging patients with these types of problems usually requires considerable patience and skill. The pace of engagement is more rapid in the case of hypomania treated by Monica Ramirez Basco—but again, tact, respect for the patient's viewpoints, and sustained relationship-building efforts are required—and deftly demonstrated. In another set of video illustrations, the need for an early emphasis on generating hope in severe and persistent depression is effectively modeled by Jesse Wright. This case demonstrates how a hopeful and action-oriented stance can help forge a healing therapeutic relationship in individuals who have deep despair and suicidal ideation. If it is true that "a picture is worth a thousand words," these videos that show master therapists at work in treating challenging patients are exponentially more valuable. They are immensely rich resources for learning key CBT methods.

Because the principal illnesses (schizophrenia, bipolar disorder, and severe or treatment-resistant depression) that are the focus of this book have significant biological and environmental influences, the authors wisely adopt an integrative model to formulate and plan treatment. Instead of regarding CBT as a competitor to pharmacotherapy, the two approaches are considered partners in reducing symptoms and forestalling relapse. The most obvious way that CBT could assist or augment pharmacotherapy for severe mental illness is to improve adherence—a topic that is covered in detail in the book. Clinicians can learn pragmatic methods for spotting and overcoming barriers to adherence for both medication and CBT. Reported rates of nonadherence to pharmacotherapy are about 50% for many of the severe mental illnesses; utilizing strategies presented in this text can have a significant impact on efforts to decrease this percentage.

Perhaps the most important contribution of CBT in the treatment of severe mental disorders is that it helps patients understand their problems in a healthier, more adaptive manner. If a paranoid patient believes that all his neighbors are spying on him with special listening devices, he is likely to isolate himself and behave in a very secretive manner. He could become paralyzed with behaviors designed for protection, as in the case of Daniel, the young man with schizophrenia shown in one of the video illustrations. Douglas Turkington's treatment of both Daniel and Brenda, another patient with schizophrenia, vividly demonstrate the value of using CBT to help patients modify the meanings they attach to delusional perceptions.

When Dr. Turkington first begins to work with Brenda, she reveals a belief that her voices are coming from the devil—an attribution that is leading to marked distress and that creates an obstacle to visiting with a new granddaughter (the hallucinations are telling her to harm the child). Through a gentle and creative guided discovery process, the therapist is able to help Brenda examine the evidence about her belief that the devil is talking to her and controlling her. As CBT proceeds, Brenda is able to accept a different conceptualization of the problem—including a full awareness of the nature of hallucinations, a normalization of this phenomenon, and an acceptance of her illness. This healthy shift in the meanings attached to her symptoms provides a needed platform for the development of effective coping strategies.

A similar cognitive shift occurs in the treatment of Angela, the patient with bipolar disorder featured in the video illustrations. However, in this case, the therapist, Dr. Basco, helps the patient recognize that grandiosity and risk-taking behavior are part of bipolar disorder, not a product of just "feeling well." Instead of confronting the patient, Dr. Basco shows how to use a collaborative CBT approach to help Angela see for herself that her behavior is part of an illness that needs monitoring and treatment. Again, the change in meanings attached to symptoms sets the stage for devising adaptive coping strategies.

The authors of *Cognitive-Behavior Therapy for Severe Mental Illness: An Illustrated Guide* are experts in their field. Dr. Wright was the founding president of the Academy of Cognitive Therapy, an organization dedicated to disseminating information about cognitive therapy and cognitive therapists worldwide. He is the author of five previous CBT books, including *Cognitive Therapy for Inpatients*, which pioneered efforts to extend CBT methods to patients with severe mental illnesses, and *Learning Cognitive-Behavior Therapy: An Illustrated Guide*, coauthored with Dr. Basco and Dr. Michael Thase.

Drs. Turkington and Kingdon, authors of three important books on CBT for schizophrenia, are among the world's leading authorities on this disorder. Their courageous efforts to advocate CBT for psychotic symptoms began long before this approach gained the favor it has today. They have played a pivotal role in conceptualizing the disorder, developing techniques, studying CBT in randomized controlled trials, and teaching this approach to clinicians throughout the world.

Dr. Basco is renowned for her work in bipolar disorder. Two of her six influential CBT books deal with this severe mental illness. She has also written an accessible and useful self-help workbook for bipolar patients and their families.

In this new book, the authors have crystallized the essence of CBT for severe mental illnesses into practical and easy-to-understand lessons. The video illustrations highlight and deepen understanding of key points. The detailed cases show clinicians how to use CBT for patients who have difficult-to-treat disorders. And the learning exercises provide very stimulating opportunities to build therapeutic skills. As clinicians read this book, they will likely have a renewed appreciation for the daunting task patients have in living with a severe mental disorder. However, clinicians will be better prepared to help these patients overcome symptoms, develop rational beliefs about their illness and about themselves, and achieve well-being.

Judith S. Beck, Ph.D.
Director, Beck Institute for Cognitive Therapy and Research;
Clinical Associate Professor of Psychology in Psychiatry,
University of Pennsylvania, Philadelphia, Pennsylvania

Preface

Our goal in writing this book was to produce a practical how-to guide for using cognitive-behavior therapy (CBT) for some of the most common and difficult-to-treat psychiatric conditions. The book is based on the work we have done together presenting courses and workshops, our previous writings on CBT, and the steady outpouring of outcome research that has documented favorable results when CBT is used in treatment of severe mental illness. Although other texts are available on CBT for several of these psychiatric disorders, we believe that there is a need for a concise guide that wraps into one volume the core methods used for many of the severe mental disorders and that vividly illustrates these techniques. By showing CBT in action, we hope to give you an inside picture of how CBT methods can be used to tackle challenging clinical problems.

The video illustrations in this book were filmed in a naturalistic style without the use of scripted dialogue. We did not use professional actors, but relied on the kind assistance of colleagues who agreed to role-play cases that we believed would illustrate key points. Our intent was to show interventions that are as close as possible to those that actually occur in clinical practice. Thus, the illustrations are not examples of "perfect" technique, but are representations of some of the strengths and weaknesses of typical CBT sessions. The filming was done at clinical sites at the University of Louisville in the United States and the University of Southampton in the United Kingdom with local audiovisual technicians. Variations in video and audio quality are due in part to the facilities and equipment available at each site and ambient noise in the different clinical settings. In order to show many different types of interventions, the length of the videos was kept in a 7- to 12-minute range. In actual practice it could take longer to follow-through with some of these treatment strategies, but we have tried to open a substantial portal into the process of CBT.

Instead of trying to cover the entire range of severe mental disorders, we decided to limit our focus to individual CBT for Axis I conditions of schizophrenia and related psychoses, bipolar disorder, and severe or treatment-resistant depression. We reasoned that it would be more valuable to explain and illustrate individual CBT procedures for these conditions in depth than to try to cover applications for all major psychiatric illnesses and comorbid diagnoses in a more superficial manner. Family, couple, and group methods for delivery of CBT can be quite useful. However, we believed that detailing these methods would be more than could be reasonably handled in a book that gives specific instructions and illustrations for individual CBT of severe mental illness. We do discuss the advantages of asking a significant other to attend some of the CBT sessions and also give an example of a group format for providing long-term maintenance therapy for psychoses (in Chapter 12, "Promoting Adherence," and Chapter 13, "Maintaining Treatment Gains").

Several of the CBT applications that are beyond the scope of this book are substance abuse, borderline personality disorder, other personality disorders, and severe eating disorders. We discuss comorbid substance abuse as a contributing factor to severe mental disorders and urge readers to include substance abuse treatment in the overall plan. Readers interested in gaining further skills on CBT for substance abuse and other conditions not detailed here are referred to Appendix 2 ("Cognitive-Behavior Therapy Resources") for a list of recommended readings.

Although the book features case illustrations for schizophrenia, bipolar disorder, and unipolar depression, we have organized it in a way that presents basic CBT principles for working with many patients who have severe symptoms of Axis I disorders. In Chapter 1 ("Introduction"), we provide a rationale for using CBT along with medication in a comprehensive treatment plan, explain the cognitive-behavioral-biological-sociocultural model, and give an overview of some of the most important treatment methods. The next three chapters describe basic CBT procedures and strategies for working with a variety of severe mental disorders. These critically important processes are covered in Chapter 2, "Engaging and Assessing"; Chapter 3, "Normalizing and Educating"; and Chapter 4, "Case Formulation and Treatment Planning." Although it can be tempting to quickly apply a specific CBT technique to tackle a symptom such as a delusion, a hallucination, or suicidal thinking, we explain that building an effective working relationship, helping patients understand and accept their condition, and developing at least a beginning case conceptualization are fundamental steps to achieving treatment success.

The remainder of the book is devoted to specific problems that are frequently encountered in therapeutic work with severe mental disorders. Chapter 5 ("Delusions") details methods for using CBT to reduce delusional thinking, and Chapter 6 ("Hallucinations") describes ways to effectively cope with hallucinations. Material in these two chapters will be of primary benefit in treatment of schizophrenia and other major psychoses, but the techniques can also be applied for managing psychotic symptoms in mood disorders and other Axis I conditions.

Chapter 7 ("Depression") is geared toward helping clinicians treat hopelessness, suicidality, low energy and interest, and poor self-esteem—problems that are very common in severe or chronic types of depressive illness but also can be frequently encountered in schizophrenia and other major psychiatric illnesses. Chapter 8 ("Mania") is of greatest relevance in treatment of bipolar disorder. The aim of CBT for bipolar disorder is relapse prevention. Methods taught in this chapter, such as symptom monitoring, CBT interventions to promote good sleep, and developing a relapse prevention plan can also be useful in treating a number of other conditions.

Chapter 9 ("Interpersonal Problems") discusses the relationship stresses, strains, and ruptures that so commonly occur in persons with severe mental disorders. If interpersonal problems did not exist before the onset of the illness, the evolution of the syndrome is often accompanied by relationship problems that aggravate the condition and cause much distress. CBT methods are outlined for building support and for coping with dysfunctional and terminated relationships.

Impaired cognitive functioning, especially thought disorder in psychoses, presents special difficulties in CBT of severe mental disorders. Therefore, the content and video illustrations in Chapter 10 ("Impaired Cognitive Functioning") include methods for trying to help patients become better organized in their thinking and to reduce distractibility, flight of ideas, or other major problems with concentration. Another difficulty that can be vexing to both patients and therapists is negative symptoms in schizophrenia. In Chapter 11 ("Negative Symptoms"), we describe some CBT procedures that may be helpful in working with this special challenge.

The last chapters are devoted to two of the most important targets of CBT for severe mental disorders: Chapter 12, "Promoting Adherence," and Chapter 13, "Maintaining Treatment Gains." By the end of treatment, we hope that our patients are armed with knowledge and skills to follow medication regimens, continue to use CBT strategies in daily life, and grow further in their ability to manage symptoms.

The cases presented in the book are either entirely fictitious or are presented as amalgams of types of problems that we have encountered in clinical practice. Where fragments of histories have been blended together in a case illustration, personal identifiers and details of histories and treatment courses have been thoroughly altered to protect confidentiality. We use the convention of writing about cases as if the treatment events actually transpired. This device is used to improve the ease of writing and reading about CBT interventions. To avoid using the cumbersome phrase "he or she" (or "she or he"), we alternate use of personal pronouns when not describing specific cases.

Because worksheets, checklists, and rating scales can be valuable tools in implementing CBT, we describe a number of them throughout the book. These items are also supplied in Appendix 1 ("Worksheets and Checklists") and can be downloaded for free in a full-size page format at the American Psychiatric Publishing Web site (www.appi.org/pdf/62321). Additional CBT resources, such as lists of recommended readings, computer programs, Web sites, and CBT organizations are provided in Appendix 2 ("Cognitive-Behavior Therapy Resources").

Appendix 3 ("DVD Guide") contains a list of videos discussed in the text, along with full instructions on how to play them. We suggest that readers view the video illustrations when they are introduced in the text to use this book to best advantage. The videos are designed to amplify the learning experience for specific topics. Thus, the videos will have the greatest impact if they are viewed in the context of the material that is currently being presented in the text. The videos can be played in personal computers with DVD drives or DVD players.

The development of CBT methods for severe mental disorders has given clinicians, patients, and families new hope for fighting symptoms and improving well-being. If this book is helpful in conveying some of the power of the CBT approach, we will have accomplished our task. We wish you well in your efforts to use CBT for severe mental disorders.

Jesse H. Wright, M.D., Ph.D.
Douglas Turkington, M.D.
David G. Kingdon, M.D.
Monica Ramirez Basco, Ph.D.

Acknowledgments

We want to express our gratitude to the many people who made this book possible. The contributions of our colleagues who depicted the patients in the video illustrations are especially notable: Maged Swalem, M.B. ("Majir"); Virginia Barbrosa, M.D. ("Angela"); Rachelle Felty, L.C.S.W. ("Mary"); Brenda Jackson, R.N. ("Brenda"); and McCray Ashby, M.D. ("Daniel") devoted considerable effort and creativity to the project. The videos of "Majir" were filmed by Nik Martin, Research Nurse, University of Southampton, United Kingdom, and the videos of other patients were filmed by Randy Cissell and Ron Harrison at the University of Louisville. Randy Cissell also assisted with editing the videos and producing the menu and navigation system for the DVD.

Our support team for this book included Maryrose Manshadi and Carol Reed, who helped with manuscript preparation; Ann Schaap, Leslie Pancratz, and Deborah Dobiecz from the Norton Hospital library in Louisville, who provided expert literature retrieval services; and the CBT supervision groups at the University of Louisville and Newcastle University, who offered invaluable advice on the development of CBT methods for severe mental illness. We would also like to thank Ann Eng, Senior Editor in the Books department at American Psychiatric Publishing, for her superb work in preparing this book for publication. Christina Rose Thomas from the University of Texas at Arlington School of Social Work provided very helpful assistance in proofreading and editing. Finally, we want to express our deep appreciation to Robert Hales, M.D., Editor-in-Chief, and John McDuffie, Editorial Director, from American Psychiatric

Publishing, for their belief in our idea to supplement text with video and for their commitment to making CBT training materials widely available to mental health clinicians.

1

Introduction

The originator of cognitive-behavior therapy, Aaron Beck, described a case of successful psychotherapy for delusions in his first publication in psychiatry (Beck 1952). However, most of the early development of cognitive-behavior therapy (CBT) was devoted to methods for mild to moderate depression and anxiety disorders. In the late 1980s and 1990s, interest began to grow in treating more challenging conditions, such as schizophrenia, bipolar disorder, and severe or treatment-resistant depression. Specific CBT methods were detailed for many of the severe mental disorders (Basco and Rush 2005; Chadwick et al. 1996; Fava et al. 1997; Haddock and Slade 1996; Kingdon and Turkington 1994, 2002, 2005; McCullough 2000), treatment programs were developed for inpatients (Stuart et al. 1997; Wright et al. 1993), and outcome studies produced encouraging results (e.g., see DeRubeis et al. 1999; Fava et al. 1997; Lam et al. 2003; Sensky et al. 2000).

In this introductory chapter, we give an overview of the rationale for using CBT with severe mental illness, describe how the CBT model can be adapted for working with these conditions, outline basic methods, and briefly discuss findings of empirical studies. Subsequent chapters detail some of the most useful CBT interventions for helping patients reduce severe symptoms. Video illustrations are provided for many of the key CBT interventions used for patients with complex or demanding clinical problems.

Why Use CBT for Severe Mental Disorders?

Despite major research efforts on understanding the genetics and biological basis of schizophrenia, bipolar disorder, and depression, and over 5 decades of intensive development of new drugs for these conditions, psychopharmacology has not yet provided a full solution for severe mental disorders. Treatment failures, residual symptoms, chronicity, and recurrences are commonplace. For example, the degree of improvement in positive symptoms of schizophrenia with antipsychotic medication is typically less than 20% (Khan et al. 2001); the relapse rate for bipolar disorder treated with mood stabilizers is in the range of 30%–40% in a 1- to 4-year period (Geddes et al. 2004; Ginsberg 2006), and remission rates for treatment of major depression with an adequate dose of an antidepressant range from about 37% to 13%, depending on the number of medications previously tried (Rush et al. 2006). Clearly, there is much room for improvement. Additional treatment methods, such as CBT, are needed to help patients understand and manage their illnesses, reduce symptoms, and solve problems that do not fully respond to medication. Social interventions such as supported employment, case management, and assertive outreach can also play an important role in a comprehensive approach to psychosis and other severe mental disorders.

Some of the potential targets of CBT for severe mental illnesses are listed in Table 1–1. The list of symptoms that can be resistant to pharmacotherapy contains a number of targets for which CBT methods are well established. Suicidality and hopelessness, frequent problems in persons with severe mental disorders, can respond well to CBT (Brown et al. 2005; Rush et al. 1982). Depressive and anxiety symptoms can be treated effectively with CBT, not only in patients with major depression and anxiety disorders, but in patients with schizophrenia as well (Arlow et al. 1997; Hollon et al. 2005; Kingsep et al. 2003; Naeem et al. 2006; Sensky et al. 2000).

Another common problem, sleep disruption, is quite responsive to CBT interventions (Carney et al. 2007; Edinger et al. 2007; Sivertsen et al. 2006), and normalization of sleep patterns is often an important goal in treatment of severe conditions such as mania, chronic depression, and psychosis. Although CBT methods for psychoses are less well known than interventions for mood and anxiety symptoms, there is substantial evidence that cognitive-behavioral interventions can add to the effects of medication in relieving hallucinations, delusions, and negative symptoms (Rector and Beck 2001; Sensky et al. 2000; Tarrier et al. 1993). In fact, the National Institute for Clinical Excellence in the United Kingdom concluded that a course of CBT should be offered to all patients with schizophrenia (National Institute for Clinical Excellence 2002).

Table 1–1. Possible targets of CBT for severe mental illness

Symptoms resistant to medication	Other targets
Anhedonia	Adherence to pharmacotherapy
Anxiety	Empowerment
Delusions	Interpersonal problems
Depression	Isolation
Hallucinations	Motivational problems and
Mania and hypomania	procrastination
Negative symptoms	Relapse prevention
Sleep difficulties	Social skills deficits
Suicidality and hopelessness	Self-esteem
	Substance abuse

Another important target of CBT is adherence to pharmacotherapy. Nonadherence rates are very high in depression, bipolar disorder, and schizophrenia (Akincigil et al. 2007; Kane 1985; Keck et al. 1997) and are primary reasons for poor treatment responses and relapses. For example, Keck and coworkers (1997) found that 51% of patients with bipolar disorder were nonadherent with treatment during a 1-year follow-up period, and Akincigil et al. (2007) reported that 49% of depressed patients in a large study failed to have their prescription for an antidepressant filled in the 16 weeks of acute therapy. Cochran (1986), Kemp et al. (1996), and others have shown that CBT can improve adherence to pharmacotherapy.

The list of targets for CBT (Table 1–1) also includes several social, cultural, and interpersonal problems for which CBT may be able to provide more help than pharmacotherapy alone. Stigma, a formidable social and personal issue, is addressed directly in CBT (Kingdon and Turkington 1991, 2005); interpersonal problems, social skills difficulties, and isolation can be identified and treated (Basco 2006; Roder et al. 2002; Safran and Segal 1990; Vittengl et al. 2004); and CBT methods can be used to help with motivational problems and procrastination (Ramsey 2002; Wright et al. 2006). Comorbid substance abuse, a very common condition in persons with major mental disorders, can be another useful application for CBT methods (Barrowclough et al. 2001; Naeem et al. 2005).

One of the most important goals of all treatments for severe mental illnesses is relapse prevention. CBT strategies aim to teach patients specific skills to fight early signs of symptom return and thereby restrict or stop the progression of symptoms (Basco 2006). Research studies reviewed in the last part of this chapter have found strong evidence for long-term positive effects of CBT in forestalling symptom return in depression. Results of studies on bipolar disorder and schizophrenia have yielded mixed results and may indicate that longer-term or more intensive treatment may be required for reducing the risk of relapse for these conditions. Continuation "booster" CBT, in a manner similar to maintenance pharmacotherapy, may be a useful method of achieving maximum results in the treatment of severe mental disorders (Jarret et al. 2001).

The CBT Model for Severe Mental Illnesses

A Comprehensive Perspective

Because there can be a multitude of influences on symptom development and expression in severe mental disorders, we recommend that clinicians use a broad cognitive-behavioral-biological-sociocultural model (Figure 1–1) to conceptualize and plan treatment (Wright et al. 2006). The main emphasis is on understanding cognitive and behavioral elements of the model, but attention is also paid to possible biological contributors (e.g., genetics, medical illnesses, history of response to medications); interpersonal stressors and supports (e.g., life events, traumas, status of relationships); and sociocultural factors (e.g., gender, ethnicity, religion, and spirituality).

Although CBT, pharmacotherapy, and socially oriented treatments such as interpersonal therapy were developed from different theoretical frameworks and propose different mechanisms of action, there is growing evidence that a comprehensive biopsychosocial approach may have advantages in the treatment of severe mental illness (Wright 2003; Wright et al. 2006). For example, CBT has been shown to have an additive effect to antipsychotic medication in the treatment of schizophrenia (see "Efficacy of CBT for Severe Mental Disorders" section later in this chapter), and a stress-vulnerability conceptualization has been used successfully for helping psychotic patients understand and cope with their symptoms (Kingdon and Turkington 2005). Because there is no evidence that CBT is effective as a stand-alone treatment for schizophrenia or bipolar disorder, a combined approach must be used unless the patient refuses medication. Even in the case of medication refusal, one of the goals of CBT is to promote acceptance of pharmacotherapy.

In treatment of depression, there is no absolute requirement for combining pharmacotherapy with psychotherapy. CBT alone has been shown to be as effective as pharmacotherapy with clinical management (Friedman et al. 2006; Hollon et al. 2005). Yet, when results of multiple studies were evaluated together in a meta-analysis, CBT plus pharmacotherapy was found to be superior to either treatment alone (Friedman et al.

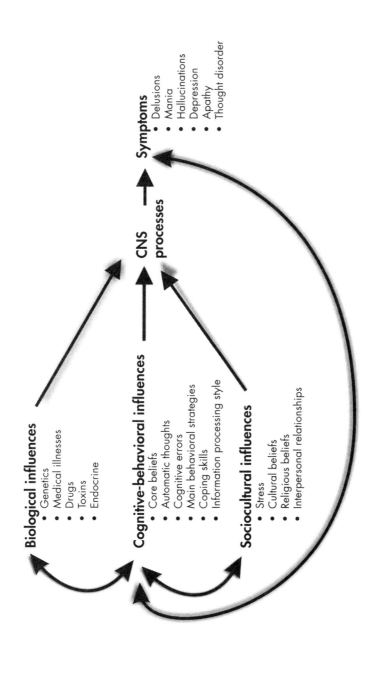

Figure 1–1. Cognitive-behavioral-biological-sociocultural model for severe mental disorders.

Note. CNS=central nervous system.

2006). Thus, studies of schizophrenia, bipolar disorder, and depression indicate that the role of biological factors and pharmacotherapy should be considered when formulating CBT interventions for these conditions.

Another very interesting line of research has demonstrated that CBT has significant effects on brain functioning and other biological processes. CBT can influence electroencephalographic sleep profiles (Thase et al. 1998), thyroid hormone levels (Joffe et al. 1996), and multiple brain pathways for the processing of cognitions and emotion (Brody et al. 1998; Goldapple et al. 2004; Schwartz et al. 1996). One particularly intriguing investigation by Goldapple et al. (2004) of positron emission tomography scans in depressed patients found that CBT modulated cortical and limbic pathways from the "top down" (i.e., cortex changes first, followed by subcortical changes), whereas an antidepressant drug acted from the "bottom up" (i.e., subcortical changes first, followed by cortex changes). This and similar studies indicate that CBT is in many respects a biological therapy and that a multisystem conceptualization for the mechanism of action could include central nervous system and neuroendocrine processes in addition to psychological constructs.

On a more concrete level, the potential influence of genetic background, current physical status (e.g., fitness, weight, metabolic effects of psychotropic medications), and medical illnesses (e.g., endocrine disorders, heart disease, chronic pain) needs to be considered in a comprehensive model for using CBT for severe mental illness. These genetic and medical factors can significantly impact disease progression and treatment response (Kneebone and Dunmore 2000; Lustman et al. 1998).

Consideration of the impact of life stresses, traumas, interpersonal problems, and cultural factors is also essential for developing a full understanding of the patient and planning effective treatment. Environmental factors have emerged as increasingly important risk factors in schizophrenia with migration, living in an urban environment (Krabbendam and van Os 2005), childhood trauma (Read et al. 2005), and use of hallucinogenic drugs (Hall 2006) being implicated. Life events occur more commonly in the period before onset of psychosis than in control populations, although this factor is probably less significant than in affective disorder (Bebbington et al. 1996). Sensitivity to daily hassles (e.g., having to pay bills or having noisy neighbors) has also been implicated (Myin-Germeys et al. 2005). Cultural factors are very relevant: beliefs acceptable in one society may be deemed psychotic in another, whereas attitudes toward minority groups (e.g., racism) may contribute to paranoia and impede social inclusion.

Major life events have been shown to influence the recurrence of episodes in bipolar disorder. For example, several studies have shown an increase in frequency of stressful life events before hospitalization for mania as compared with surgical admission (Ambelas 1979). Hunt et al. (1992) found that the rate of stressful life events in the 3 months preceding a bipolar episode was significantly higher when compared with a 3-month period when no episode occurred. The highest rates of stressful events occurred in the month before relapse. Bidzinska (1984) showed similar findings when comparing patients with nonpsychiatric control subjects, as did Kennedy and coworkers (1983), who also found that bipolar patients before hospitalization had significantly less social support to help them cope with stress. Even developmentally normal and positive life events, such as preparing for college exams (Nusslock et al. 2007) or goal attainment (Johnson et al. 2000), are associated with increased symptoms in bipolar disorder, as are disruptions in daily routines (Malkoff-Schwartz et al. 2000).

Taken together, the results of these studies of life stresses, biological processes, and other influences suggest that a comprehensive approach may provide the best opportunity for understanding patients and designing interventions. The basic features of the cognitive-behavioral-biological-sociocultural model for CBT of severe mental illness are summarized in Table 1-2.

A Working Model for CBT Interventions

After considering a broad range of possible factors in the comprehensive cognitive-behavioral-biological-sociocultural model (see Chapter 4, "Case Formulation and Treatment Planning," for details on forming case concep-

---

Table 1–2. Key elements of the CBT model for severe mental illness

---

Cognitive-behavioral, biological, interpersonal, and sociocultural elements are identified and considered.

An integrative theory and method are used.

CBT is typically used together with medications or other biological treatments.

Interpersonal and sociocultural influences may be addressed directly in the treatment plan.

A stress-vulnerability conceptualization is presented to patients.

The basic CBT model, which details the linkage between events, cognitions, emotions, and behavior, is used to guide treatment interventions.

---

tualizations), therapists need to concentrate on developing the cognitive-behavioral components of the treatment plan. A less complex working CBT model can be used to narrow the focus and provide a template for therapy interventions (Figure 1–2). This working model is purposefully simplified to draw the clinician's attention to the fundamental relationships between: 1) environmental events (or memories of events, delusional perceptions, hallucinations, etc.); 2) cognitive appraisal of the meaning of these events or perceptions; 3) emotional responses; and 4) behaviors. Cognitive appraisal is given a central place in this working model because the meanings attached to events or perceptions are a primary influence on subsequent emotional responses and behavior (Beck et al. 1979; Clark et al. 1999; Wright et al. 2006, 2008).

This working model posits a tightly connected, two-way relationship between cognition and behavior in which behavioral patterns (e.g., avoidance, procrastination, hypervigilance) affect cognitions (e.g., estimates of risk, self-efficacy, or acceptance by others) and vice versa in multiple feedback loops that can perpetuate or deepen symptoms. Thus, both maladaptive cognitions

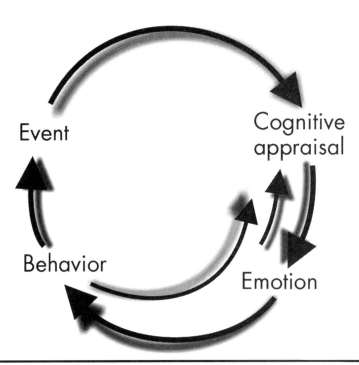

Figure 1–2.   Basic cognitive-behavioral model.

Source.   Reprinted from Wright JH, Basco MR, Thase ME: *Learning Cognitive-Behavior Therapy: An Illustrated Guide.* Washington, DC, American Psychiatric Publishing, 2006, p. 5. Used with permission. Copyright © 2006 American Psychiatric Publishing.

and behavior can be targeted for change. Three cases that will be used throughout this book are briefly introduced here to show how the working CBT model can direct treatment interventions. Comprehensive formulations and video illustrations for these cases are provided in subsequent chapters.

Majir

This 28-year-old man has been diagnosed with paranoid schizophrenia and has been treated extensively with antipsychotic medication. Unfortunately, he still has intense paranoia coupled with marked social isolation and withdrawal. He spends most of his time in his room, occasionally going out to babysit at his sister's house nearby. He feels somewhat comfortable in this safe environment but typically becomes more anxious and delusional when he tries to go elsewhere outdoors or venture to shops or other public places. A reaction to one such trip is outlined in Figure 1–3. As will be shown later in this book and video illustrations, a cognitive-behavioral approach to helping Majir could include gentle questioning about his perceptions when he goes to public places, examining the evidence about his conclusions, and behavioral assignments to try to break out of his pattern of social isolation.

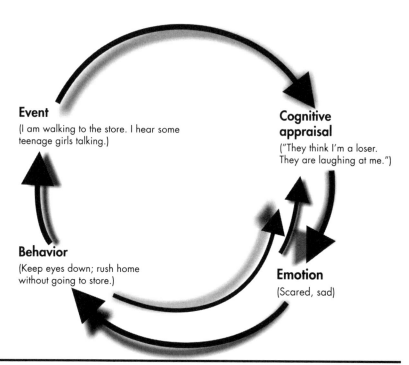

Figure 1–3. Majir's example: basic cognitive-behavioral model.

Angela

This 35-year-old woman with bipolar disorder has been urged to get treatment by her boss because of a series of work problems. She has been irritable, grandiose, and offensive to coworkers and customers. When hypomanic or manic she believes that she is the best at her job in a marketing firm and that others are dull or uncreative. During these times, her inflated self-esteem and insensitive behavior have gotten her into trouble. An example is diagrammed in Figure 1–4. CBT interventions could be directed at helping Angela recognize and modify the cognitive distortions that are part of her hypomanic and manic upswings and also interrupt the spiral of dysfunctional behavior that is endangering her job.

Mary

A patient with severe, chronic depression, Mary is a 44-year-old woman who has had depression for as long as she can remember. Recently her

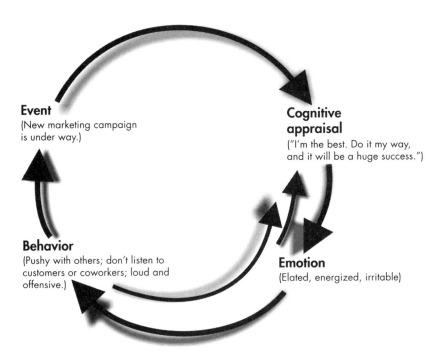

Figure 1–4.   Angela's example: basic cognitive-behavioral model.

depression has intensified as she has encountered financial and relationship problems. Mary was unable to hold a job because of depression but was providing day care for a few small children in her home. All of the children have now grown to attend kindergarten or preschool, so she has lost this source of income in addition to the companionship of the children. Her husband has become more critical and has been making remarks about her not helping with the finances and spending most of her day watching TV.

The CBT interventions for Mary detailed later in this book and in video illustrations address the self-denigrating cognitions, deep hopelessness, suicide risk, and helpless behavior in people with severe, chronic depression (Figure 1–5).

These examples demonstrate how a CBT conceptualization can be applied to understanding symptoms and targeting treatment interventions for a variety of severe mental disorders. Of course, a more complete formulation with consideration of a full range of environmental stressors, underlying schemas, developmental influences if applicable, enduring behavioral strategies, strengths, and other factors will promote effective treatment planning (see Chapter 4, "Case Formulation and Treatment Planning").

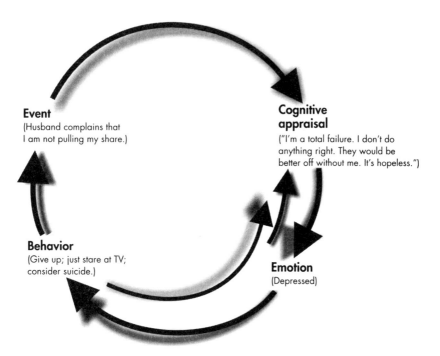

Figure 1–5.   Mary's example: basic cognitive-behavioral model.

However, CBT for severe mental illness also relies on the simple working conceptualizations demonstrated in Figures 1–3 through 1–5. These types of conceptualizations, sometimes called mini-formulations, can provide a rapid and parsimonious way of putting the basic constructs of CBT to work. In Chapter 4, we explain how mini-formulations can be effective tools for helping patients understand and manage their symptoms.

Overview of Treatment Methods

Optimize the Therapeutic Relationship

Some of the commonly used methods or foci for CBT of severe mental illness are listed in Table 1–3. The first entry in this table, "optimize the therapeutic relationship," is perhaps the most important. Patients with severe conditions often have had previous attempts at treatment that have had varying levels of success. They may be wary of starting again or have frank aversion to engaging in treatment. Take, for example, a patient with florid mania who is "on a roll"—euphoric with ideas, plans, and perceived highs from recent experiences. He believes that others are trying to hold him back. He doesn't want to accept the opinion that he has a psychiatric disorder and needs treatment. In another case, a patient with severe depression may be so demoralized by previous treatment failures and chronicity that she has little or no hope that CBT could be helpful. An even more difficult situation for engaging a patient may be encountered when a psychotic patient has delusional beliefs about the

---

Table 1–3.   Common CBT methods for severe mental illness

Optimize the therapeutic relationship

Normalize and destigmatize

Provide psychoeducation

Modify automatic thoughts

Implement behavioral strategies

Modify core beliefs

Address problems with concentration or thought disorder

Enhance adherence

Treat comorbid substance abuse or misuse

Build skills for relapse prevention

---

therapist's intentions. In all of these treatment challenges, the skill of the therapist in promoting a good working relationship is the rate-limiting step for treatment progress.

In treatment of severe mental illness, therapists may need to take more time to develop the relationship and use slowly paced, nonthreatening questioning as a mainstay of early sessions. The collaborative empirical style of relationship advocated for all CBT applications is emphasized, but for many persons with severe problems such as schizophrenia or treatment-resistant depression a modicum of "befriending" is also required (Kingdon and Turkington 2005). This strategy involves relating to the patient in a very kind and supportive manner, demonstrating genuine interest in the details of the patient's daily struggles. The nature of the professional relationship does not include acting as an actual friend, and appropriate boundaries must be maintained. However, the therapist may exert a special effort to encourage a "friendly" tone to the sessions and to forge a cooperative working relationship before attempting to modify delusional beliefs or tackle other difficult-to-treat symptoms. This strategy is demonstrated later in the book in the treatment of Majir, the young man with paranoid schizophrenia.

Normalize and Destigmatize

One of the most troubling aspects of severe mental illness is the stigmatization and alienation that so many of these patients experience. A person with auditory hallucinations may think that he is alone in suffering from voices and that this is a mark of being possessed by some demonic spirit. A woman with recurrent depression and difficulty functioning may think that she is a "loser"—a failure in life—and that her depression is a failure of will. A man with bipolar disorder may conclude that he is incapable of sustaining any type of relationship or work because his wife left him and he lost his job after having two manic episodes.

The normalization strategy in CBT includes attempts to help the patient see that the types of experiences that he is having are shared by many others in the world (e.g., voices and paranoid thoughts are very common even in people who are not diagnosed with mental disorders, mood disorders are found in over 20% of the population) and that stresses (e.g., sleep deprivation, traumas, losses) are well known to trigger symptoms. As the normalization and destigmatization process unfolds, the therapist provides an understanding and accepting view of the patient's problems. The goals of this intervention are to help the patient 1) develop healthy attributions (i.e., meanings attached to illness) about their disorder; 2) minimize self-criticism; 3) adopt a problem-solving attitude; 4) accept a stress-vulnerability conceptualization; and 5) view the therapist as an ally in the fight against symptoms.

Provide Psychoeducation

Education about illnesses and CBT methods is provided throughout therapy, including during the normalization process described above. Usually psychoeducation is done in a conversational style at points in the session that offer good opportunities to explain or illustrate concepts. Thus, education is woven into sessions in a rather seamless and easy-to-digest manner. An overly didactic delivery method is avoided in favor of brief demonstrations and discussions. Depending on the patient's cognitive capacity and level of reality testing, assignments may be suggested for readings, Internet searches, or computer programs for psychoeducation. A patient with bipolar disorder who is currently having low-level symptoms may benefit from reading books such as *An Unquiet Mind* (Jamison 1995). However, a patient with severe paranoia, low motivation, and significant thought disorder probably would not be able to benefit from such psychoeducational homework assignments. Instead, she might look at a simple leaflet (Kingdon and Turkington 2005) or agree to "think about what we've talked about" in between sessions.

Modify Automatic Thoughts

Many of the maladaptive cognitions of persons with severe mental disorders can be conceptualized as automatic thoughts—cognitions that occur rapidly in situations, or in response to memories or other perceptions, and are typically not subjected to rational analysis. Because automatic thoughts are often negatively distorted or have other inaccuracies, they make good targets for CBT interventions. Methods such as thought recording, examining the evidence, and reattribution are used extensively in the treatment of depression and anxiety disorders (Beck et al. 1979; Wright et al. 2008). These techniques also can play an important role in work with schizophrenia and bipolar disorder. For example, a delusional perception can be relabeled as an automatic thought (e.g., "Someone is spying on me from the apartment across the street") and then a series of alternative explanations can be explored (e.g., "The woman on the fourth floor may be looking out the window all the time because she is bored or because she is ill and can't leave her apartment").

Another commonly used method of modifying automatic thoughts is to spot cognitive distortions such as ignoring the evidence, personalizing, magnifying and minimizing, overgeneralizing, and all-or-nothing thinking.

Patients with hypomania or mania are prone to have these errors in thinking (Basco and Rush 2005). Angela, the woman described earlier in this chapter, *ignored the evidence* that she was offending others and that her behavior was endangering her job. She was *magnifying* her job skills and *minimizing* the contributions of others. Angela also was engaging in *all-or-nothing thinking* when she saw herself as the "best" while others were characterized as slow, lazy, or uncreative. These types of cognitive errors played a significant part in the escalation of her symptoms; but as is often the case in CBT, a problem can be turned into an opportunity. Identification of these cognitive errors could help Angela gain better control over her mood swings.

Implement Behavioral Strategies

For Majir, the patient with paranoid schizophrenia, avoidance of social situations, or even walking by himself to a grocery store, was a direct outgrowth of his delusional beliefs. Although his therapist could use cognitive restructuring procedures to try to reduce Majir's paranoid thoughts, he also could utilize behavioral methods such as graded exposure techniques. For example, Majir could be asked if he might feel better about himself if he were able to gradually increase his ability to take walks outside his house or to shop at a market. If they agreed that this would be a good idea, then the therapist could help Majir with stepped exposure to these feared situations. Also, coping strategies, such as breathing training or relaxation exercises, could be taught. Another technique might be to develop a coping card (see Chapter 6, "Hallucinations," section "Coping Cards") for managing the fear that others were talking about him or laughing at him.

Behavioral methods can be particularly helpful for patients with bipolar disorder. A useful technique recommended by Basco and Rush (2005) is the *symptom summary worksheet.* This method involves construction of a list of signs and symptoms that a shift may be beginning toward mania or depression. Then, a specific behavioral plan is made to try to abort the escalation of symptoms. Other behavioral interventions can be employed to enhance sleep hygiene, concentrate attention on task completion (to counter distractibility and hyperactivity), decrease impulsivity, and treat other commonly encountered problems in bipolar disorder.

Chronic, deeply entrenched depression is often treated with activity scheduling and graded task assignments. Mary, the woman with severe anhedonia and social isolation (Figure 1–5), was spending most of her time sitting aimlessly in front of a TV. When her husband criticized her, she spiraled down further and thought of giving up. Because her therapist needed to reverse hopelessness as soon as possible, he suggested practical methods for behavioral activation and scheduling pleasant events as part of the therapy plan. The positive results of this behavioral work are demonstrated later in the book.

Modify Core Beliefs

There can be considerable variability in the importance of modifying schemas or core beliefs in different patients with severe mental disorders. For persons with chronic depression, very low self-esteem, and long-standing patterns of low self-efficacy, schema-level interventions may provide some of the best avenues for reversing symptoms. Also, some patients with psychosis or bipolar disorder who have had developmental problems or traumas that have shaped maladaptive beliefs can be good candidates for schema change methods. However, efforts to modify schemas could be counterproductive in certain patients who are highly delusional, have a pronounced thought disorder, or are having severe problems with concentration. They may not have the cognitive skills, understanding of the CBT process, or capacity to collaborate that are required to benefit from this type of work. Also, there may be little need to focus heavily on schemas in cases where patients have very strong biological or environmental contributors to the illness and marginal evidence of underlying maladaptive beliefs. But even in these situations, beliefs about the illness, or about oneself as a victim of the illness, can be elicited and questioned.

Methods for modifying schemas in treatment-resistant depression utilize the standard techniques first described by Beck and colleagues (1979), but there is a special emphasis on identifying core beliefs that may be involved in hopelessness and treatment stagnation (Wright 2003). In treatment of schizophrenia, schemas about basic trust, dangerousness or risk, acceptance, and self-efficacy may be elicited. Core beliefs about self-image can also be important in bipolar disorder. For all of these conditions, therapists can choose from a broad range of schema change techniques including examining the evidence, listing advantages and disadvantages, and using homework assignments to practice modified schemas in real-world situations.

Address Problems With Concentration or Thought Disorder

With mild to moderate depression or anxiety disorders, problems with cognitive capacity or disordered thought processes rarely interfere with treatment. However, for many persons with severe conditions, therapists need to modify treatment methods to account for difficulties in cognitive processing. Severe thought disorders present a particularly challenging therapeutic dilemma. Traditional CBT methods such as goal and agenda setting can be helpful in this regard, but tightly constructed agendas may not always be well received by persons with schizophrenia or mania who may misperceive the therapist's intent. If they believe that the therapist is trying to manipulate or control them by forcing an agenda, the quality of the relationship and the cooperation with treatment may suffer. Thus, it may work best in these situations to give judicious, well-paced feedback to keep the session and the communication on track instead of attempting to follow a carefully constructed agenda.

An alternative strategy that can be used for patients with thought disorder is to try to identify issues or concerns that are increasing anxiety or derailing their thinking. If these influences can be moderated, the patient may be able to improve focus on other matters. Also, aides for concentration can be used, such as lists and simply constructed coping cards. Finally, behavioral plans to limit the number of current projects or to reduce involvement in various activities can help manic patients and others who have problems with distractibility and impaired concentration.

Enhance Adherence

The procedures described earlier for building a collaborative relationship, normalizing and destigmatizing, and implementing psychoeducation are all very important components of the CBT approach to improving treatment adherence. If the relationship is highly collaborative, and if patients understand their disorders and their treatments, they may be more likely to accept and utilize clinician's recommendations. Also, if patients are empowered to participate in decision making about treatments, they may be more open to discuss negative thoughts about medication or to report variations from a suggested routine.

Some of the specific interventions used to enhance adherence to pharmacotherapy are behavioral methods such as reminder systems, pillboxes, and assessment of barriers to adherence. If barriers can be identified, therapists and patients can work together to devise strategies to overcome these roadblocks to taking medication. Common barriers to adherence can be financial constraints, forgetfulness, negative attitudes or lack of support from family members, and side effects. Behavioral plans to eliminate or cope with barriers can also be very helpful in assisting patients with adherence to homework assignments.

When patients have automatic thoughts or core beliefs that interfere with adherence, these cognitions can be targeted for change. Examples might include thoughts such as "People who take antidepressants are weak"; "I should be able to do this on my own"; and "I'm always the one to get side effects." Patients with psychotic conditions may have suspicious or delusional thoughts about medication, such as "This drug is tainted"; "The doctor isn't telling me the truth"; and "They are trying to poison me." By building an effective treatment relationship, providing psychoeducation, gently exploring dysfunctional cognitions, examining the evidence, and using other core CBT techniques, therapists can help patients gain a rational perspective on the use of medications in the treatment of severe mental illness.

Treat Comorbid Substance Abuse or Misuse

Problems with substance abuse are quite common in persons with severe mental illness. For example, about 47% of persons with schizophrenia and 56% of persons with bipolar disorder have comorbid alcohol or drug abuse (Regier et al. 1990). Thus, treatment of coexisting substance abuse is an important part of the overall treatment plan in CBT for severe mental illness. Barrowclough and coworkers (2001), Naeem and associates (2005), Weiss et al. (2007), and others have described valuable methods for applying CBT in the treatment of substance abuse and misuse. For example, Barrowclough et al. (2001) describe a method of combining CBT, motivational interviewing, and family work for substance abuse in schizophrenia. Several other groups of investigators have reported positive results of developing a "broad spectrum" CBT approach to substance abuse disorders (Baker et al. 2006; Brown et al. 2006; Davidson et al. 2007; Weiss et al. 2007). Because treatment of substance abuse is a very complex topic, deserving a volume unto itself, we do not detail methods for treatment of these problems here. We recommend that readers consult the classic book by Beck and associates (1993), and publications by Barrowclough et al. (2001) and others (Baker et al. 2006; Brown et al. 2006; Davidson et al. 2007; Graham et al. 2003; Haddock et al. 2003; Thase 1997; Weiss et al. 2007) to learn about basic CBT methods for treatment of substance abuse.

Build Skills for Relapse Prevention

One of the goals of CBT is to help patients acquire skills that they can use on their own to maintain treatment gains and to reduce the risk of relapse. In addition to learning basic methods (e.g., identifying automatic thoughts, spotting cognitive errors, using thought change records, scheduling activities, using graded task assignments or desensitization protocols), therapists may employ cognitive and behavioral rehearsal to identify possible triggers for symptom worsening or relapse and then coach patients on methods to effectively manage these stressors. Some examples of these strategies are to 1) develop an antisuicide plan to be used if future adverse circumstances begin to stimulate hopeless thinking, 2) generate a list of early signs of a switch into either mania or depression and an action plan for stopping the progression of symptoms, and 3) articulate a strategy in advance for managing a possible increase in the intensity or frequency of hallucinations.

Efficacy of CBT for Severe Mental Disorders

Schizophrenia

Meta-analyses (Zimmermann et al. 2005) and more than 20 randomized controlled studies have established the efficacy for CBT in schizophrenia in reducing persistent positive symptoms in patients (Turkington et al. 2006b). There is also evidence of benefit for negative symptoms (Sensky et al. 2000), reducing relapse (Gumley et al. 2003), comorbid substance misuse (Haddock et al. 2003), and prodromal symptoms of psychosis (Morrison et al. 2004). Another important finding has been the demonstration of effectiveness and acceptability in clinical practice (Kingdon and Kirschen 2006; Turkington et al. 2006a). Such effects occur over and above that of supportive therapies, but these less specific interventions do appear to have positive effects in their own right. This finding is important to consider therapeutically because it underscores the value of developing a strong therapeutic relationship.

Bipolar Disorder

One of the earliest controlled studies of CBT for bipolar disorder was conducted by Cochran (1986), who tested a 6-week CBT intervention aimed at improving treatment adherence in patients receiving their care in a university-based lithium clinic. She found that the CBT group had better composite adherence scores than patients who received standard clinic care, with the effect still present 6 months after completion of CBT. Lam and coworkers (2000) found CBT effective relative to a medication-only control group. Patients receiving 12–20 sessions of adjunctive CBT had fewer bipolar episodes, showed better coping skills, and were more adherent to pharmacotherapy at posttreatment and at 6-month follow-up than patients receiving medication only. Similarly, Scott et al. (2001) randomly assigned patients to CBT plus pharmacotherapy ($n=21$) or medication alone ($n=21$) and found that the former showed significantly fewer symptoms and improved social functioning after 6 months of CBT. When focusing specifically on patients reporting medication nonadherence, Lam and coworkers (2003) found that those receiving 14 sessions of CBT along with medication had significantly fewer bipolar episodes, fewer days in an episode, and fewer number of hospital admissions. The CBT group also reported higher social functioning and fewer mood symptoms, especially manic symptoms, with the effects showing durability over 18 months. To lower the risk of relapse, Fava et al. (2001) added CBT to pharmacotherapy to reduce residual symptoms. This uncontrolled study showed a significant decrease in residual symptoms and an increase in the number of months to relapse following CBT, compared with baseline levels. A 6-month study of adjunctive CBT versus treatment as usual by Ball and associates (2006) had similar results, with CBT participants showing significantly less severe depression and mania scores, improved attitudes, better self-control, better treatment adherence, and a lower relapse rate.

Most studies of CBT for bipolar disorder have compared it as an adjunct to pharmacotherapy with treatment as usual, without control for attention or nonspecific effects of psychotherapy. When additional psychotherapy was allowed as part of the control condition, thus controlling for attention to some degree, Scott and coworkers (2006) were unable to replicate the superiority of CBT as in other studies. However, these findings might be attributable to other design deficiencies and a 40% dropout rate (Lam 2006). Another study found that a variety of psychotherapies including CBT, interpersonal and social rhythms therapy, and family-focused therapy were highly effective in improving outcomes for bipolar depression compared with treatment as usual (Miklowitz et al. 2007). Patients who were treated with intensive psychotherapy of these three forms were 1.58 times more likely to be clinically well than patients treated in routine care (Miklowitz et al. 2007). Additional research is needed to determine the extent to which the specific clinical methods of CBT account for changes above and beyond the nonspecific effects of psychotherapy, such as the therapeutic alliance.

Severe, Chronic, or Treatment-Resistant Depression

The extensive controlled research on CBT for severe, chronic, or treatment-resistant depression has been evaluated and summarized in several meta-analyses and reviews (DeRubeis et al. 1999; Friedman et al. 2006; Hollon et al. 2005; Wright 2003; Wright et al. 2008). Despite one report that CBT might not be as effective as pharmacotherapy for severe depression (Elkin et al. 1995), a meta-analysis of major studies found that patients with Hamilton Rating Scale for Depression scores of 20 or above fared just as well with CBT as with treatment with antidepressants (DeRubeis et al. 1999). Also, a major study of CBT and interpersonal therapy for severe depression, not included in the earlier meta-analyses, found that both treatments were effective, but CBT had more robust effects than interpersonal therapy (Luty et al. 2007).

Research on chronic or treatment-resistant depression has also demonstrated positive effects for CBT. For example, the Sequenced Treatment Alternatives to Relieve Depression (STAR*D) trial found that a standard form of CBT was as effective as any of the switching and augmenting pharmacological strategies used in this large investigation (Rush et al. 2006). Keller and coworkers (2000) studied the Cognitive Behavioral Analysis System of Psychotherapy (CBASP), a form of CBT for chronic depression that places more emphasis on interpersonal factors than standard CBT. They reported that CBASP was as efficacious as an antidepressant in treating chronic depression, whereas the combination of CBASP and medication yielded superior treatment response and remission rates (Keller et al. 2000). Another group of researchers performed a series of studies that demonstrated solid efficacy for CBT for treatment-resistant or relapsing depression (Fava et al. 1996, 1998, 2002, 2004).

Fava's group primarily uses standard CBT interventions but emphasizes methods for reversing common problems in chronic depression, such as anhedonia or hopelessness (Fava et al. 1996, 1997, 1998, 2002, 2004). Because most clinicians are more familiar with standard cognitive-behavioral procedures and are more likely to use these techniques in clinical practice than CBASP, the strategies for treatment-resistant or chronic depression described in this book are based largely on this more commonly used form of CBT (Fava et al. 1996, 1997, 1998; Wright 2003). Also, findings of a significant advantage for combined CBT and pharmacotherapy (Friedman et al. 2006; Hollon et al. 2005; Keller et al. 2000) lead us to recommend comprehensive therapy with CBT and medication for difficult-to-treat depression.

Summary

Key Points for Clinicians

- CBT can target many symptoms and problems that may be resistant to pharmacotherapy.
- CBT has been shown to be efficacious in the treatment of schizophrenia, bipolar disorder, and severe or treatment-resistant depression.
- A comprehensive and integrative CBT model is used for treatment of severe mental illness.

- Special efforts may be required to establish an effective therapeutic relationship when working with difficult-to-treat patients.
- Normalization, destigmatization, and psychoeducation are important features of CBT for severe mental illness.
- Standard CBT methods such as cognitive restructuring, activity scheduling, and exposure and response prevention can be modified and customized for patients with severe conditions.
- Methods for enhancing treatment adherence are especially useful in working with patients with severe or long-standing psychiatric illnesses.
- Relapse prevention is a major goal of CBT for severe mental disorders.

Concepts and Skills for Patients to Learn

- Mental disorders such as schizophrenia, bipolar disorder, and severe depression are very common, and many of the symptoms of these conditions are experienced by large numbers of people.
- Stress can bring on or aggravate symptoms; thus, learning to cope with stress can improve outcome.
- The best results in treatment of psychiatric disorders occur when patients and therapists work together effectively as a team.
- The thoughts that just pop into our heads (automatic thoughts) can be inaccurate and can lead to much distress; it can help to stop and check on the validity of these thoughts.
- Many coping strategies are available and can be learned to help people solve problems.
- A large number of research studies have shown that CBT is helpful in treatment of significant mental conditions.

References

Akincigil A, Bowblis JR, Levin C, et al: Adherence to antidepressant treatment among privately insured patients diagnosed with depression. Med Care 45:363–369, 2007

Ambelas A: Psychologically stressful events in the precipitation of manic episodes. Br J Psychiatry 135:15–21, 1979

Arlow PB, Moran ME, Bermanzohn PC, et al: Cognitive-behavior therapy for treatment of panic attacks in chronic schizophrenia. J Psychother Pract Res 6:145–150, 1997

Baker A, Bucci S, Lewin T, et al: Cognitive-behavioral therapy for substance abuse disorders in people with psychotic disorders: randomized controlled trial. Br J Psychiatry 188:439–448, 2006

Ball JR, Mitchell PB, Corry JC, et al: A randomized controlled trial of cognitive therapy for bipolar disorder: focus on long-term change. J Clin Psychiatry 67:277–286, 2006

Barrowclough C, Haddock G, Tarrier N, et al: Randomized controlled trial of motivational interviewing, cognitive behavior therapy, and family intervention for patients with comorbid schizophrenia and substance use disorders. Am J Psychiatry 158:1706–1713, 2001

Basco MR: The Bipolar Workbook: Tools for Controlling Your Mood Swings. New York, Guilford, 2006

Basco MR, Rush AJ: Cognitive-Behavioral Therapy for Bipolar Disorder, 2nd Edition. New York, Guilford, 2005

Bebbington P, Wilkins S, Sham P, et al: Life events before psychotic episodes: do clinical and social variables affect the relationship? Soc Psychiatry Psychiatr Epidemiol 31:122–128, 1996

Beck AT: Successful outpatient psychotherapy of a chronic schizophrenic with a delusion based on borrowed guilt. Psychiatry 15:305–312, 1952

Beck AT, Rush AJ, Shaw BF, et al: Cognitive Therapy of Depression. New York, Guilford, 1979

Beck AT, Wright FD, Newman CF, et al: Cognitive Therapy for Substance Abuse. New York, Guilford, 1993

Bidzinska EJ: Stress factors in affective diseases. Br J Psychiatry 144:161–166, 1984

Brody AL, Saxena S, Schwartz JM, et al: FDG-PET predictors of response to behavioral therapy and pharmacotherapy in obsessive compulsive disorder. Psychiatr Res 84:1–6, 1998

Brown GK, Ten Have T, Henriques GR, et al: Cognitive therapy for the prevention of suicide attempts: a randomized controlled trial. JAMA 294:563–570, 2005

Brown SA, Glasner-Edwards SV, Tate SR, et al: Integrated cognitive behavioral therapy versus twelve-step facilitation therapy for substance-dependent adults with depressive disorders. J Psychoactive Drugs 38:449–460, 2006

Carney CE, Segal ZV, Edinger JD, et al: A comparison of rates of residual symptoms following pharmacotherapy or cognitive-behavior therapy for major depressive disorder. J Clin Psychiatry 68:254–260, 2007

Chadwick P, Birchwood, M, Trower P: Cognitive Therapy of Voices, Delusions, and Paranoia. Chichester, England, Wiley, 1996

Clark DA, Beck AT, Alford BA: Scientific Foundations of Cognitive Theory and Therapy of Depression. New York, Wiley, 1999

Cochran SD: Compliance with lithium regimens in the outpatient treatment of bipolar affective disorders. J Compliance Health Care 1:151–169, 1986

Davidson D, Gulliver SB, Longabaugh R, et al: Building better cognitive-behavioral therapy: is broad spectrum treatment more effective than motivational-enhancement therapy for alcohol-dependent patients treated with naltrexone? J Stud Alcohol Drugs 68:238–247, 2007

DeRubeis RJ, Gelfand LA, Tang TZ, et al: Medications versus cognitive behavior therapy for severely depressed outpatients: mega-analysis of four randomized comparisons. Am J Psychiatry 156:1007–1013, 1999

Edinger JD, Wohlgemuth WK, Radtke RA, et al: Dose-response effects of cognitive-behavioral insomnia therapy: a randomized clinical trial. Sleep 30:203–212, 2007

Elkin I, Gibbons RD, Shea MT, et al: Initial severity and differential treatment outcome in the National Institute of Mental Health Treatment of Depression Collaborative Research Program. J Consult Clin Psychol 63:841–847, 1995

Fava GA, Grandi S, Zielezny M, et al: Four-year outcome for cognitive behavioral treatment of residual symptoms in major depression. Am J Psychiatry 153:945–947, 1996

Fava GA, Savron G, Grandi S, et al: Cognitive-behavioral management of drug-resistant major depressive disorder. J Clin Psychiatry 58:278–282, 1997

Fava GA, Rafanelli C, Grandi S, et al: Prevention of recurrent depression with cognitive behavioral therapy. Arch Gen Psychiatry 55:816–820, 1998

Fava GA, Bartolucci G, Rafanelli C, et al: Cognitive-behavioral management of patients with bipolar disorder who relapsed while on lithium prophylaxis. J Clin Psychiatry 62:556–559, 2001

Fava GA, Ruini C, Rafanelli C, et al: Cognitive behavior approach to loss of clinical effect during long-term antidepressant treatment: a pilot study. Am J Psychiatry 159:2094–2095, 2002

Fava GA, Ruini C, Rafanelli C, et al: Six-year outcome of cognitive behavior therapy for prevention of recurrent depression. Am J Psychiatry 161:1872–1876, 2004

Friedman ES, Wright JH, Jarrett RB, et al: Combining cognitive therapy and medication for mood disorders. Psychiatr Ann 36:320–328, 2006

Geddes JR, Burgess S, Hawton K, et al: Long-term lithium therapy for bipolar disorder: systematic review and meta-analysis of randomized controlled trials. Am J Psychiatry 161:217–222, 2004

Ginsberg LD: A retrospective analysis of changing from alternative agents to carbamazepine extended release capsules in bipolar disorder. Ann Clin Psychiatry 18 Suppl 1:31–34, 2006

Goldapple K, Segal E, Garson C, et al: Modulation of cortical-limbic pathways in major depression: treatment-specific effects of cognitive behavior therapy. Arch Gen Psychiatry 61:34–41, 2004

Graham HL, Copello A, Birchwood MJ, et al: Substance Misuse in Psychosis: Approaches to Treatment and Service Delivery. Chichester, England Wiley, 2003

Gumley A, O'Grady M, McNay L, et al: Early intervention for relapse in schizophrenia: results of a 12-month randomized controlled trial of cognitive behavioural therapy. Psychol Med 33:419–431, 2003

Haddock G, Slade PD (eds): Cognitive Behavioral Interventions With Psychotic Disorders. London, Routledge, 1996

Haddock G, Barrowclough C, Tarrier N, et al: Cognitive-behavioral therapy and motivational interviewing for schizophrenia and substance misuse. 18-month outcomes of a randomized controlled trial. Br J Psychiatry 183:418–426, 2003

Hall W: Is cannabis use psychotogenic? Lancet 367:193–195, 2006

Hollon SD, Jarrett RB, Nierenberg AA, et al: Psychotherapy and medication in the treatment of adult and geriatric depression: which monotherapy or combined treatment? J Clin Psychiatry 66:455–468, 2005

Hunt N, Bruce-Jones WD, Silverstone T: Life events and relapse in bipolar affective disorder. J Affect Disord 25:13–20 1992

Jamison KR: An Unquiet Mind. New York, Knopf, 1995

Jarrett RB, Kraft D, Doyle J, et al: Preventing recurrent depression using cognitive therapy with and without a continuation phase: a randomized clinical trial. Arch Gen Psychiatry 58:381–388, 2001

Joffe R, Segal Z, Singer W: Change in thyroid hormone levels following response to cognitive therapy for major depression. Am J Psychiatry 153:411–413, 1996

Johnson SL, Sandrow D, Meyer B, et al: Increases in manic symptoms after life events involving goal attainment. J Abnorm Psychol 109:721–727, 2000

Kane JM: Compliance issues in outpatient treatment. J Clin Psychopharmacol 5(3 Suppl):22S-27S, 1985

Keck PE, McElroy SL, Strakowski SM, et al: Compliance with maintenance therapy in bipolar disorder. Psychopharmacol Bull 33:87–91, 1997

Keller MB, McCullough JP, Klein DN, et al: A comparison of nefazodone, the cognitive behavioral-analysis system of psychotherapy, and their combination for the treatment of chronic depression. N Engl J Med 342:1462–1470, 2000

Kemp R, Hayward P, Applewhaite G, et al: Compliance therapy in psychotic patients: randomised controlled trial. BMJ 312:345–349, 1996

Kennedy S, Thompson R, Stancer HD, et al: Life events precipitating mania. Br J Psychiatry 142:398–403, 1983

Khan A, Khan SR, Leventhal RM, et al: Symptom reductions and suicide risk among patients treated with placebo in antipsychotic clinical trials: an analysis of the Food and Drug Administration database. Am J Psychiatry 158:1449–1454, 2001

Kingdon D, Kirschen H: Who does not get referred for cognitive behavior therapy in an area where availability has not been limited? Psychiatr Serv 57:1792–1794, 2006

Kingdon D, Turkington D: The use of cognitive behavior therapy with a normalizing rationale in schizophrenia: preliminary report. J Nerv Ment Dis 179:207–211, 1991

Kingdon D, Turkington D: Cognitive Behavior Therapy of Schizophrenia. New York, Guilford, 1994

Kingdon DG, Turkington D: A Case Study Guide to Cognitive Therapy of Psychosis. Chichester, England, Wiley, 2002

Kingdon DG, Turkington D: Cognitive Therapy of Schizophrenia. New York, Guilford, 2005

Kingsep P, Nathan P, Castle D: Cognitive behavioural group treatment for social anxiety in schizophrenia. Schizophr Res 63:121–129, 2003

Kneebone II, Dunmore E: Psychological management of post-stroke depression. Br J Clin Psychol 39(Pt 1):53–65, 2000

Krabbendam L, van Os J: Schizophrenia and urbanicity: a major environmental influence—conditional on genetic risk. Schizophr Bull 31:795–799, 2005

Lam D: What can we conclude from studies on psychotherapy in bipolar disorder? Invited commentary on....Cognitive-behavioural therapy for severe and recurrent bipolar disorders. Br J Psychiatry 188:321–322, 2006

Lam DH, Bright J, Jones S, et al: Cognitive therapy for bipolar illness—a pilot study of relapse prevention. Cognit Ther Res 24:503–520, 2000

Lam DH, Watkins ER, Hayward P, et al: A randomized controlled study of cognitive therapy for relapse prevention for bipolar affective disorder: outcome of the first year. Arch Gen Psychiatry 60:145–152, 2003

Lustman PJ, Freedland KE, Griffith LS, et al: Predicting response to cognitive behavior therapy of depression in type 2 diabetes. Gen Hosp Psychiatry 20: 302–306, 1998

Luty SE, Carter JD, McKensie JM, et al: Randomised controlled trial of interpersonal psychotherapy and cognitive-behavioral therapy for depression. Br J Psychiatry 190:496–502, 2007

Malkoff-Schwartz S, Frank E, Anderson BP, et al: Social rhythm disruption and stressful life events in the onset of bipolar and unipolar episodes. Psychol Med 30:1005–1016, 2000

McCullough JP Jr: Treatment for Chronic Depression: Cognitive Behavioral Analysis System of Psychotherapy. New York, Guilford, 2000

Miklowitz DJ, Otto MW, Frank E, et al: Psychosocial treatments for bipolar depression: a 1-year randomized trial from the Systematic Treatment Enhancement Program. Arch Gen Psychiatry 64:419–426, 2007

Morrison AP, French P, Walford L, et al: Cognitive therapy for the prevention of psychosis in people at ultra-high risk: randomised controlled trial. Br J Psychiatry 185:291–297, 2004

Myin-Germeys I, Delespaul P, van Os J: Behavioral sensitization to daily life stress in psychosis, Psychol Med 5:733–741, 2005

Naeem F, Kingdon D, Turkington D: Cognitive behavior therapy for schizophrenia in patients with mild to moderate substance misuse problems. Cogn Behav Ther 35:207–215, 2005

Naeem F, Kingdon D, Turkington D: Cognitive behavior therapy for schizophrenia: relationship between anxiety symptoms and therapy. Psychol Psychother 79:153–164, 2006

National Institute for Clinical Excellence: Clinical Guideline: 1. Schizophrenia. December 2002. Available at: http://www.nice.org.uk/nicemedia/pdf/CG1NICEguideline.pdf. Accessed May 22, 2008.

Nusslock R, Abramson LY, Harmon-Jones E, et al: A goal-striving life event and the onset of hypomanic and depressive episodes and symptoms: perspective from the behavioral approach system (BAS) dysregulation theory. J Abnorm Psychol 116:105–115, 2007

Ramsey RJ: A cognitive therapy approach for treating chronic procrastination and avoidance: behavioral activation interventions. J Group Psychother Psychodrama Sociom 55:79–92, 2002

Read J, van Os J, Morrison AP, et al: Childhood trauma, psychosis and schizophrenia: a literature review with theoretical and clinical implications. Acta Psychiatr Scand 112:330–350, 2005

Rector NA, Beck AT: Cognitive behavioral therapy for schizophrenia: an empirical review. J Nerv Ment Dis 189:278–287, 2001

Regier DA, Farmer ME, Rae DS, et al: Comorbidity of mental disorders with alcohol and other drug abuse: results from the Epidemiologic Catchment Area (ECA) Study. JAMA 264:2511–2518, 1990

Roder V, Brenner HD, Müller D: Development of specific social skills training programmes for schizophrenia patients: results of a multicentre study. Acta Psychiatr Scand 105:363–371, 2002

Rush AJ, Beck AT, Kovacs M, et al: Comparison of the effects of cognitive therapy and pharmacotherapy on hopelessness and self-concept. Am J Psychiatry 139:862–866, 1982

Rush AJ, Trivedi MH, Wisniewski SR, et al: Acute and longer-term outcomes in depressed outpatients requiring one of several treatment steps: a STAR*D report. Am J Psychiatry 163:1905–1917, 2006

Safran J, Segal Z: Interpersonal Processes in Cognitive Therapy. New York, Basic Books, 1990

Schwartz JM, Stoessel PW, Baxter LR Jr, et al: Systematic changes in cerebral glucose metabolic rate after successful behavior modification treatment of obsessive-compulsive disorder. Arch Gen Psychiatry 53:109–113, 1996

Scott J, Garland A, Moorhead S: A pilot study of cognitive therapy in bipolar disorders. Psychol Med 31:459–467, 2001

Scott J, Paykel E, Morriss R, et al: Cognitive-behavioural therapy for severe and recurrent bipolar disorders. Br J Psychiatry 188:313–320, 2006

Sensky T, Turkington D, Kingdon D, et al: A randomized controlled trial of cognitive-behavioral therapy for persistent symptoms in schizophrenia resistant to medication. Arch Gen Psychiatry 57:165–172, 2000

Sivertsen B, Omvik S, Pallesen S, et al: Cognitive behavioral therapy vs zopiclone for treatment of chronic primary insomnia in older adults: a randomized controlled trial. JAMA 295:2851–2858, 2006

Stuart S, Wright JH, Thase ME, et al: Cognitive therapy with inpatients. Gen Hosp Psychiatry 19:42–50, 1997

Tarrier N, Beckett R, Harwoods S, et al: A trial of two cognitive-behavioral methods of treating drug-resistant residual psychotic symptoms in schizophrenic patients, I: outcome. Br J Psychiatry 162:524–532, 1993

Thase ME: Cognitive-behavioral therapy for substance abuse disorders, in American Psychiatric Press Review of Psychiatry, Vol 16. Edited by Dickstein LJ, Riba MB, Oldham JM. Washington, DC, American Psychiatric Press, 1997, pp 45–71

Thase ME, Fasiczka AL, Berman SR, et al. Electroencephalographic sleep profiles before and after cognitive behavior therapy of depression. Arch Gen Psychiatry 55:138–144, 1998

Turkington D, Kingdon D, Rathod S, et al: Outcomes of an effectiveness trial of cognitive-behavioural intervention by mental health nurses in schizophrenia. Br J Psychiatry 189:36–40, 2006a

Turkington D, Kingdon D, Weiden PJ: Cognitive behavior therapy for schizophrenia. Am J Psychiatry 163:365–373, 2006b

Vittengl JR, Clark LA, Jarrett RB: Improvement in social-interpersonal functioning after cognitive therapy for recurrent depression. Psychol Med 34:643–658, 2004

Weiss RD, Griffin ML, Kolodziej ME, et al: A randomized trial of integrated group therapy versus group drug counseling for patients with bipolar disorder and substance dependence. Am J Psychiatry 164:100–107, 2007

Wright JH: Cognitive-behavior therapy for chronic depression. Psychiatr Ann 33:777–784, 2003

Wright JH, Thase ME, Beck AT, et al (eds): Cognitive Therapy With Inpatients: Developing a Cognitive Milieu. New York, Guilford, 1993

Wright JH, Basco MR, Thase ME: Learning Cognitive-Behavior Therapy: An Illustrated Guide. Washington, DC, American Psychiatric Publishing, 2006

Wright JH, Thase ME, Beck AT: Cognitive therapy, in The American Psychiatric Publishing Textbook of Psychiatry, 5th Edition. Edited by Hales RE, Yudofsky SC, Gabbard GO. Washington, DC, American Psychiatric Publishing, 2008, pp 1211–1256

Zimmermann G, Favrod J, Trieu VH, et al: The effect of cognitive behavioral treatment on the positive symptoms of schizophrenia spectrum disorders: a meta-analysis. Schizophr Res 77:1–9, 2005

2

Engaging and Assessing

Engagement and maintenance of the patient relationship is fundamental to any psychotherapeutic intervention (Wright et al. 2006). If the patient is disengaged and can't be reached, progress in psychotherapy is impossible. Some patients with severe mental illness who have difficulties engaging may walk out, refuse to talk to you, or only allow very superficial conversation. But, a collaborative CBT approach can help even the most paranoid or cognitively impaired patients work with you to meet the broad goals that they have for their lives. Building a therapeutic relationship with persons with severe mental illness often involves a step-by-step process. Initially, there may be a relatively superficial working relationship. However, continued efforts to promote collaboration can progressively allow for more interaction, disclosure, and change.

This chapter concentrates primarily on helping clinicians build skills in engaging patients with schizophrenia and other psychoses. These illnesses are often associated with major barriers to therapeutic engagement, and clinicians who have not had specialized training in CBT for psychotic disorders may not be familiar with the modifications in CBT methods that can promote good working relationships. We also provide guidance and illustrations for enhancing the engagement process in treatment of bipolar disorder and severe or chronic depression. At the end of the chapter, general recommendations are given for assessing patients with difficult-to-treat conditions, and indications and limits of CBT for severe mental illness are discussed. We begin with an illustration of the beginning stages of engagement with a patient with paranoid schizophrenia.

▶ **Video Illustration 1.** Engaging a Patient With
Paranoia: Dr. Kingdon and Majir

The first video illustration shows an initial interview with Majir, who has reluctantly come to the session. The therapist begins by acknowledging the problem: "I know it has been difficult for you, so thanks for coming in." Open questioning about "what the concerns have been" is used to develop conversation without Majir needing, at this stage, to accept that there is anything wrong with him. This questioning strategy allows Majir, a young man with paranoia, to discuss his current situation and interests, and the concerns his family has about him. This nonthreatening and collaborative method of engaging the patient enables a meaningful conversation to develop and allows the therapist to gather information relevant to the assessment. The video illustration concludes with Dr. Kingdon assuring Majir that the topics chosen will be those he is prepared to discuss and will be taken at his pace.

Influences on the Therapeutic Relationship

In building an effective CBT relationship, the therapist may need to identify and address a variety of possible influences that can present obstacles to collaboration. Four broad categories of potential influences are outlined here: 1) symptomatic and behavioral issues, 2) personal circumstances, 3) sociocultural issues, and 4) service issues.

Symptomatic and Behavioral Issues

Symptoms of severe mental illness can seriously interfere with all relationships, including the therapeutic relationship (Table 2–1). Some symptoms interfere directly and others more indirectly. Paranoid beliefs held by patients can interfere directly in their relationships because of patients' perceptions of malevolence or bad intentions of other people toward them. These beliefs need to be considered in attempts to engage the patient and to use the therapeutic process to reduce paranoia. If a therapeutic relationship can be developed, this positive step can break the all-or-nothing belief prevalent in paranoia that "everyone is against me."

Hostility and risk for aggression is a special concern in the engagement process. When severely agitated or threatening patients are encountered, it is wise to think of safety first and to gain assistance from inpatient staff or others and use appropriate medication before proceeding with attempts to begin CBT. With catatonia, another symptom of psychosis, communication may seem to be impossible. But in practice, gentle per-

Table 2–1. Symptoms and behavior that can impair engagement in therapy

Paranoia	Grandiosity
Hostility and threatening behavior	Impulsivity
Catatonia	Social withdrawal
Hallucinations	Thought disorder
Lack of insight	Cognitive impairment
Somatic delusions	Substance misuse
Hopelessness	Preexisting relationship difficulties
Low energy and interest	

sistence may be worthwhile, and over time the patient may begin to engage in meaningful discussions.

Hallucinations can be seriously distracting and can have a marked influence on communication in the therapeutic relationship. Commands from voices may specifically instruct the individual, saying, for example, "Don't talk to that doctor"; "You can't trust her"; or "They are part of the plot." Lack of insight can often be understood in the context of delusional thinking. For example, patients who do not believe that they have any psychological issues and have high delusional conviction in these ideas will be difficult to engage. Delusional beliefs that can interfere may include "I'm a greater psychiatrist than you, so why should I have anything to do with you?" or "Like all the other sinners, you don't believe I am Christ." If patients are experiencing somatic delusions, they will believe that they really require physical health care and may need some persuading that a psychological approach is anything but a distraction from their goals.

Hopelessness is a very common impediment to engagement with patients with chronic depression and other psychiatric disorders. Methods for addressing hopelessness with a depressed patient are demonstrated later in the chapter in Video Illustration 3 and are discussed in more detail in Chapter 7 ("Depression"). Low energy can also decrease the patient's ability to engage in therapy. Patients can be too tired to devote much effort to the therapeutic process and may require CBT interventions for improving energy and interest outlined in Chapter 7. Symptoms of mania (e.g., grandiosity and impulsivity) that can affect the therapeutic relationship are discussed in Chapter 8 ("Mania").

Socially withdrawn patients or those with severe social anxiety may be particularly difficult to engage. They may communicate minimally in sessions. Or, they may be overwhelmed by a new social situation and withdraw further, be unable to complete therapeutic interviews, or have an increase in psychotic symptoms. Thought disorder, another frequently occurring symptom in psychoses, can lead to misunderstandings and communication difficulties that interfere with the process of developing a working relationship. Cognitive impairment (e.g., poor concentration, attention, and memory) can also have negative effects on forming an effective working relationship and thus may require adaptations in the style of interaction. Methods for overcoming difficulties with thought disorder and cognitive impairment are demonstrated in Chapter 10 ("Impaired Cognitive Functioning").

Substance misuse is a very common influencing factor. The direct chemical effects of alcohol or drugs of abuse are a major issue if the patient is currently intoxicated. In emergency room or crisis intervention settings, detoxification may be required before meaningful work can begin. Also, the patient's desire to seek out substances for use can limit engagement. Denial or attempts to hide substance abuse can create a barrier between therapist and patient.

If the patient has had premorbid relationship difficulties arising from past or current interactions with family, friends, colleagues, or authorities, these patterns may be carried over into the therapeutic relationship. Particular difficulties may be encountered if the patient has a comorbid personality disorder (e.g., borderline, antisocial, dependent, or schizoid). When a significant personality disorder is present, relationship building may take longer and be fraught with habitual maladaptive behavioral strategies such as splitting, manipulation, or excessive dependency.

Personal Circumstances

Personal circumstances and experiences can also be relevant to the engagement process. The first episode of illness can be very confusing, and perplexity from the onset of frightening symptoms such as voices, visions, and fears can interfere with attempts to build a working relationship. Initial contacts with the patient may be flavored by prejudice and stigma about mental health services—"they just lock you up and drug you." Also, a lengthy illness history may have included negative experiences of mental health services, and these memories can cloud the patient's view of fresh attempts to engage in treatment.

Traumatic events (e.g., assault, abuse, bereavement, relationship breakups, negative implications of manic excesses) may lead to shock, numbness, and difficulties in engaging. Barriers to forming good therapeutic relationships can be especially hard to surmount when patients have been hurt badly and have become very distrustful and wary of others. A very gentle and gradual process of engagement may be required in these situations. Some patients may be largely uncommunicative during initial sessions. This behavior can be related to a number of personal factors. Examples include marked distrust related to previous trauma, teenage angst or rebellion, and legal difficulties.

Noncollaboration can also occur because of a general lack of belief that psychiatric services, medication, or psychotherapy can help. Expressing feelings or discussing personal matters may be viewed as wrong or a sign of weakness. In some instances, patients may not want change to occur. They may fear that their problems could only get worse (e.g., their family will abandon them or they will lose financial or accommodation supports if they show any signs of improvement or independence), or they may want a manic high to continue because of the pleasure experienced or increased work output. And for some patients, there is a reluctance to give up psychotic symptoms because they are viewed as positive, protective, or even enjoyable experiences (e.g., voices that are friendly or provide companionship, visual hallucinations with pleasurable sexual content, grandiose delusions).

Sociocultural Issues

There can be profound effects of sociocultural differences on therapy process and outcome. Patients from nonwhite cultural groups are more likely to drop out of studies of CBT for schizophrenia and may do less well when they do complete therapy (Rathod et al. 2005). Yet there have been relatively few attempts to adapt and evaluate CBT that is culturally responsive for individual ethnic groups (Hays and Iwamasa 2006).

Past experiences of discrimination and culturally based misunderstandings can have strong influences on attempts to engage patients in CBT. For example, communication styles that differ cross-culturally could be misread and create a gulf between therapist and patient (e.g., different levels of intensity in emotional expression can convey agitation in some cultures or be a component of normal communication in others). Cross-cultural communication in relationship building can be complex but need not be insurmountable. The open and collaborative approach advocated here is more likely to detect misunderstandings and enable them to be overcome. However, to assist with cross-cultural issues, it still may be useful, with patient consent, to involve members of the patient's local community—or where available, mental health workers with diverse ethnic backgrounds.

When interpreters are needed, therapy can become more demanding and lengthy. Convenience may dictate that family members act as interpreters, but this can present difficulties if there are differences of opinion or disagreements between individuals in the family. In these situations, at least one session with an independent interpreter can be useful. Even then, especially where the cultural group is quite small locally, the independent interpreter may be known to the patient or have connections that compromise confidentiality. We have experienced difficulties where, despite a common language, there are fundamental conflicts between the ethnic group of the patient and that of the interpreter. Despite these potential problems, intense efforts should be made to overcome cultural and language barriers and to provide CBT to the same standard available to other groups of patients.

Attitudes of family and friends also can be very influential. If these people are disbelieving, discouraging, or denigrating toward treatment, these potential negative influences need to be addressed in therapy. Educational sessions with the patient and her family or friends may be very helpful in effectively managing these problems (see Chapter 12, "Promoting Adherence," and Chapter 13, "Maintaining Treatment Gains").

Service Issues

Hospitalization may have been a negative experience and thus may affect current attempts to engage the patient, especially if the patient has just been rehospitalized and detained under a legal warrant. Unfortunate experiences with staff (e.g., perceptions that staff were controlling or didn't care), medication side effects, and disruptions in services or lack of continuity of care are other care delivery issues that can affect attempts to develop new relationships. Even previous attempts at psychotherapeutic intervention may have been problematic because of personality clashes or inept therapy.

There also may be major practical issues that interfere with engaging. The patient may live in a remote area, so establishing regular contact can be very difficult. Financial constraints (e.g., transportation costs, lost wages, lack of insurance coverage for treatment) can affect the ability to access and engage in therapy. And the patient may have medical problems that require treatment and draw attention and resources away from psychosocial interventions.

Medication can benefit engagement by ameliorating symptoms, thereby improving the patient's ability to participate in therapy. But in some instances, medication can negatively influence the building of a therapeutic relationship. For example, if the patient receives high levels of medication and is heavily sedated, contact can become more difficult. Other examples of side effects or adverse reactions that could interfere with engagement are 1) poor concentration from drugs with anticholinergic properties; 2) severe extrapyramidal symptoms (e.g., stiffness, akathisia, dystonia) from antipsychotic medications; and 3) abnormal lab tests (e.g., lowered white blood cell count, elevated liver function studies, or impaired renal function) that could be interpreted as evidence that the doctor shouldn't be trusted. Alternatively, some patients and families see medication or other physical approaches as the only possible solution to their problems and are thereby reluctant to engage in CBT.

Factors That Can Facilitate Engagement

There are some patient characteristics that can contribute to improving engagement, at least initially (Table 2–2). Some of these are simply the converse of negative influences described previously. For example, good experiences with previous services, especially with psychotherapy, are likely to facilitate the interaction. Similarly, support from family and friends, commonality of background and ethnicity between therapist and patient, acceptance of having a problem, positive recommendations from a referral source, and a sincere desire to learn and change may enhance the engagement process.

Table 2–2. Factors that can facilitate engagement in therapy

Previous good relationships with clinicians

Family and friends support treatment

Shared cultural or ethnic background

Patient accepts that he or she has a problem

Positive endorsement of therapy by referral source

Desire to understand educational comments about CBT

Wanting to discuss symptoms

Wanting to change a situation (e.g., get out of hospital)

Patient distressed by persistent hallucinations, depression, or other symptoms

At least a minimal level of insight

Hopefulness

Symptomatic improvement from medication

Good tolerability of medication regimen

When symptoms are responding poorly and distress is persisting, the patient may be motivated to seek further help or to work harder in treatment. For example, abusive hallucinations that are resistant to medication may cause patients to be more accepting of help that comprises specific, practical methods to assist in coping—a hallmark of CBT for hallucinations. "A chink of insight"—a glimmering of doubt about the veracity of a hallucination or delusion—is another factor that can promote engagement. The beginnings of insight can be sufficient for someone with a strong delusional conviction to be prepared to consider discussing his beliefs. Hopelessness can undermine therapy, but if the therapist can instill hope that things could be different, this remoralization process can be transformed into a positive factor for engagement.

Medication effects are another potential influence of considerable importance. If the patient is prescribed medications that relieve upsetting symptoms, improve concentration, reduce thought disorder, or have other salutatory influences, he may be better able to participate in therapy. If the prescribing physician is also the therapist or is part of the therapy team, there may be positive implications for the therapy relationship because of reduced suffering.

> **Learning Exercise 2–1.** Identifying and Managing Barriers to Collaborative Therapeutic Relationships
>
> 1. Think of a patient whom you may have found difficult to engage in therapy.
>
> 2. List the factors, both positive and negative, that may have influenced your efforts to establish a collaborative relationship.
>
> 3. Next, consider how you might account for these factors in improving the therapeutic relationship with this patient.

Factor influencing engagement	Ways to adapt approach to account for this factor
1.	
2.	
3.	
4.	
5.	

Guidelines for Engaging a Person With Severe Mental Illness

Psychosis

It is sensible to obtain referral information and data from hospital records or other collateral sources before the initial assessment contact in order to have advance notice of key elements of the history, potential risks, or other factors that may influence the therapeutic process.

In treating moderate to severe levels of psychosis, it may be important to be flexible in finding a setting for the initial interviews that is acceptable and comfortable for the patient. Although it is often possible for the assessment to take place in an office on a ward or in a clinic, sometimes it may work best for an alternative place to be negotiated with the patient. Examples include the patient's home, a neighborhood coffee shop, or even in the parent's car in the hospital parking lot.

When engagement is proving difficult, going for a walk may help. This effort may involve following the patient if he is agitated, strolling around the ward with him, walking around a park, or going to his hospital bed space rather than using a formal interview room. Asking patients to accept a cup of tea, coffee, or a soft drink can relax the atmosphere. Good practice dictates that you should think about where to sit, how your office is designed and decorated, the impact of your posture (e.g., threatening, relaxed, or sloppy), and your clothing (e.g., particular patient groups could feel distanced or comforted by formality, uniforms, or name badges). Generally our experience in working with psychotic patients is that conveying relaxed competence is the most successful overall therapeutic stance.

Consider the use of language. While it is important to avoid unexplained jargon, it is essential to find a common language with vocabulary appropriate to the person's educational level. A judicious use of technical language can reduce distancing and delusional conviction. Patients can often benefit from learning to use phrases such as "having a touch of the schizophrenias" or "feeling particularly paranoid today"; they can even learn to use terms such as *somatic hallucinations* or *thought broadcasting.* This strategy can help them understand the relevant phenomena and communicate their experiences of them. For example, as the relationship builds, they can be asked, "How have the voices been?" or "Have you had much thought broadcasting when you've been out this week?"

Being accurate and factually correct is also important. Responding affirmatively without qualification (e.g., "Yes, of course you will") to a patient who asks, "Will I get better?" can be perceived as patronizing or dismissive. Some discussion of the positive and negative prognostic indicators is a more credible and engaging approach. Reasonable optimism is usually appropriate for individuals who have sufficient insight to ask questions about prognosis. When patients ask questions about the potential benefits of pharmacotherapy or the risks of side effects, collaboration can be enhanced by providing honest answers that can be easily understood.

Near the beginning of most sessions, a simple agenda can be established with the patient (e.g., "help with voices," "discussing situations in which you hear people talk about you," "working on feeling more comfortable going outside the house"). Some goals for the future can also be set (e.g., "getting a job," "getting out of the hospital," or "understanding what is happening to me"). In CBT with psychosis, the agenda-setting process is often less specific or detailed than in therapeutic work with depression or bipolar disorder (Wright et al. 2006).

As the interview progresses, a nondirective approach using open questions is usual (e.g., "How are you today?" and "Your family doctor has asked me to see you, do you want to tell me what's been happening?"). The interview structure is not aimless but allows patients time to decide what they want to say at their own pace, as shown in Video Illustration 1 with Dr. Kingdon and Majir and in the example below:

> The therapist is beginning work with Seth, a young man who has recently developed a paranoid psychotic illness following misuse of amphetamines. The clinician struggles to engage and set a simple agenda, which the patient resists. However, Seth is prepared to talk about social needs and gradually begins to reach a point at which he will discuss specific experiences.

> Therapist: How having you been doing?
> Seth: Alright. But there's nobody around to go cycling or do anything else.
> Therapist: So your friends aren't around at the moment.
> Seth: No, they're all working and doing other stuff....I don't have that many friends.
> Therapist: OK...Today it would be good if we could try to put together some of the information you gave me last week into some sort of shape that would be useful.
> Seth: Mmm. I'm scared of it all though. I can't talk about it. It makes it worse for weeks after I've talked about it.
> Therapist: Did it make it worse after talking about it last week?
> Seth: No...But talking about those subjects gets to me. It's best if I just forget about it.
> Therapist: If you forget about it, do you think it will go away?
> Seth: If I buried it deep enough.

Therapist: And what would you particularly need to bury?
Seth: All of it...All the thoughts I get.
Therapist: Does that work...burying it?
Seth: Yes.
Therapist: Right...OK...So over the last week, what sort of things have you done?
Seth: Well, I saved up some money and got myself a model car....[discusses other activities]
Therapist: What would you like to do in the future?
Seth: I want to have as much fun as possible...to meet people and be happy.
Therapist: Where would you want to meet people?
Seth: Other countries...I want to be able to cope with other people. But when I try, something bad always comes into my head.
Therapist: So when did that last happen to you? (They then gradually begin to discuss paranoid ideas.)

Providing a rationale for working together is another useful and necessary part of the introductory process. The therapist can provide an explanation of the circumstances of the referral or why the therapist has come to see the patient, giving a simple description of what the therapist is hoping to offer.

People with psychotic illnesses are often familiar with being stigmatized or disbelieved and may expect this even from mental health staff. They are therefore more likely to engage with someone who seems ready and able to take their comments at face value and who avoids jumping to conclusions about whether what they say is right or wrong or whether they are ill or not. To accomplish this task, the therapist needs to demonstrate an intention to listen and to fully understand the patient's experiences and how he has understood them. It is important to give first priority to what the person is ready and wishes to say over what you want to tell them. Also, therapists can facilitate engagement by giving and asking for regular feedback to ensure that there is mutual understanding.

If a patient becomes distressed, therapists need to regulate the flow and depth of conversation to a level that can be readily tolerated. In these circumstances, distress may lead to increased thought disorder, more intrusion of hallucinations, or disengagement. Thus, it is usually most productive to move the conversation to less disturbing areas. Gradual pacing over a number of sessions can enable even quite disturbing material to be handled in a manner that allows gentle exploration without the person being overwhelmed. When disengagement seems to be occurring, movement to social conversation (e.g., about their current circumstances, family, sports) can counteract this. Such conversations also have value in providing information about relevant motivators for the person and modeling ways to participate in social interaction. Talking about nonthreatening, peripheral topics can have an additional benefit of keeping the flow of discussion going when the patient has difficulty verbalizing ideas or lapses into silences—episodes that can be anxiety provoking and promote psychotic intrusions. An aim of sessions with this group of patients is to provide positive, even enjoyable, interview experiences, and by doing so to promote and sustain engagement in the therapeutic relationship.

Bipolar Disorder

The strength, trust, and comfort in the therapeutic alliance play a critical role in the treatment of bipolar disorder at several phases. When patients are actively manic, their need to control and dominate can hinder the development of a therapeutic relationship. Nevertheless, our experience is that even at the height of a manic episode, there can be episodic bursts of insight that can be amplified. Reflecting with the patient on the impact of her behavior on others can have some success, although this may seem transient at the time. Developing a humorous banter with patients is sometimes possible as they crack jokes and make puns. We then have been able to use this type of lighter conversation to avoid confrontation, improve self-reflection, and promote acceptance of medication while getting across key messages about acceptable standards of behavior. Despite behavior that can be intrusive, using an adult-to-adult conversational style can allow the development of a constructive relationship.

Once the manic episode has resolved, more detailed therapeutic work can begin. When patients are initially challenging the accuracy of the diagnosis, their acceptance can be facilitated by their comfort with the clinician. Conversely, their rejection of the diagnosis can be amplified by their mistrust of the messenger. Angela, for example, has been through some difficult times in her life (see Video Illustration 2). She finally feels successful in her work, in her relationships, and in caring for her child. She does not want to hear that her success could be threatened by an illness. The suggestion from her employer that there is something wrong with her dismisses her efforts and accomplishments. After years of struggling, she finally feels superior to others but is being asked to accept an explanation for her behavior that suggests she has an illness. This is a hard pill to swallow. The clinician that attempts to help Angela reconcile her view of success with a diagnosis of bipolar disorder must be sensitive to what this will mean to her and about her. Coming on too strong will push the patient away. Video Illustration 2 provides an example of building a therapeutic alliance that will facilitate the patient's eventual acceptance of her diagnosis.

▶ **Video Illustration 2.**   Engaging a Patient With
Bipolar Disorder: Dr. Basco and Angela

There will be times when a clinician must warn the patient about the
risks of substance abuse, involvement in potentially dangerous activities,
the possibility of making bad decisions, or the emergence of manic symptoms. This information can only be successfully conveyed and well received in the context of a trusting therapeutic relationship. The therapist
must be confident, but not parental or overly supportive, and not encouraging of bad behavior. This balance can be tricky to achieve.

Examining the advantages and disadvantages of each choice of action
is a cognitive-behavioral intervention that can facilitate this process while
building the therapeutic alliance. Allowing the patient to explore the
pros and cons of her choice of actions demonstrates respect for the patient's decision-making abilities. It avoids a power struggle like the type
that patients often have with parents or spouses. This type of intervention addresses the problem behavior, but perhaps more importantly, it
builds rapport.

Another place in the treatment of bipolar disorder where the therapeutic relationship can make or break the situation is when the patient recov-
ers from depression and may appear to be on the verge of hypomania.
People who have had depressive episodes welcome relief. Even more so,
they welcome a bit of hypomania to help them regain their self-confidence,
get things done that have been neglected, and have some fun. A therapist
in this situation might convey concern for the emergence of hypomania in
such a way as to sound discouraging or controlling. If the patient does not
believe that the therapist has her best interest at heart, the feedback will
be rejected and trust will be diminished.

For example, hypomania can manifest as a new or creative idea that
seems risky to the therapist but reasonable to the patient. This potential
warning sign will create a sense of urgency in the therapist to suppress the
patient's plans in an effort to keep her behavior from further stimulating
hypomania. However, implying that the patient's idea is not a good idea
but rather a "manic idea" can be viewed by the patient as insulting. Although the patient may not voice displeasure with the therapist for dismissing her plans, the patient may hesitate before sharing her ideas in the
future. Without the trust that allows self-disclosure, it can be difficult to
monitor patients' symptoms.

To maintain the alliance while evaluating the onset of mania, therapists can use cognitive restructuring methods (see Wright et al. 2006 for
details of these basic CBT techniques) to monitor potentially manic
thoughts, just as these techniques are used to evaluate depressive thoughts.

One example of these techniques might be to evaluate the evidence for and against an idea being a good one rather than a manic one. The discussion of evidence will demonstrate the therapist's willingness to trust the patient and keep an open mind while allowing the patient to more objectively review her ideas. What may ultimately occur, however, is that the patient will conclude that a manic idea is actually a reasonable one. In this case, an experiment will have to be devised to more fully test the patient's thoughts. The therapist's willingness to help devise an experiment models for the patient how to keep an open mind—a process that will serve the therapeutic process well in the future.

Severe or Treatment-Resistant Depression

In some respects, engaging a patient with severe or chronic depression presents fewer challenges than are typically encountered in developing relationships with patients with schizophrenia or bipolar disorder with mania. Persons who have depression usually feel considerable emotional pain, are beset with symptoms that are interfering with their life, and are reaching out for help. Unless they are experiencing psychotic features, their reality testing is largely intact, and they can more readily understand the nature and potential benefits of CBT. Yet, there can be roadblocks to engagement with depressed patients that may require special efforts from the therapist.

Some of the possible constraints to engagement that are especially related to the experience of depression are 1) hopelessness and demoralization, 2) suicidality, 3) low energy and difficulty completing tasks, and 4) impaired ability to concentrate. Also, depression can cause underlying personality traits to flower. When people are more symptomatic with depression, traits such as dependency, procrastination, social avoidance, and obsessiveness may be more pronounced and may influence their ability to collaborate in a therapeutic relationship.

Hopelessness and demoralization may be critically important hurdles to overcome in treating patients with chronic depression. These patients have often been through the mill of treatment options: they have tried large numbers of medications and have had repeated failures in benefiting from previous therapies. Thus, if the therapist cannot kindle a sense of hope or show the patient that CBT may have value, the therapy may flounder or the patient may not return for further visits.

Suicidality, which is commonly associated with hopelessness, is perhaps the single most important issue that influences the engagement process in treatment of depression. The patient's suicidal thoughts and danger of actual suicide can affect therapists profoundly (e.g., worries about patient's risk of suicide, memories of patients who have committed suicide, previous lawsuits related to suicide) and can stimulate counter-transference. In fact, studies of therapist's reactions to patient suicides have found that shock, grief, guilt, self-doubt, anger, and a sense of be-trayal are very common (Hendin et al. 2000, 2006).

Some therapists can be reticent to engage with patients with clear sui-cidal risk because of previous traumatic experiences with suicidal pa-tients (Hendin et al. 2000), or the therapist can shy away from asking detailed questions about suicidal thinking and developing effective strat-egies for managing risk. Patients with repeated suicide attempts, or those with comorbid personality disorders associated with self-inflicted harm, may be particularly difficult to engage for some therapists. Yet, CBT methods have been shown to be very effective in reducing the risk of sui-cide attempts (Brown et al. 2005).

CBT methods for hopelessness and suicidality are detailed in Chapter 7 ("Depression"). We think that it is very important for therapists who work with seriously depressed patients to understand their own cogni-tions and behaviors about patient suicidality and to work on developing rational and effective strategies for engaging these patients. If therapists have significant difficulty in doing this, they may need to consult with colleagues on ways to cope with their fears or seek supervision on treating suicidal patients.

Low energy and poor concentration in severely depressed patients can also interfere with the engagement process. If patients are so exhausted and depleted that they can't expend much effort on therapy, the thera-pist will need to reduce demands for homework; present concepts in small, easily understood lessons; and make other adjustments consistent with the patient's ability to participate in meaningful therapeutic work. Similarly, low levels of concentration will require modifications in the speed, structure, and complexity of the therapy (i.e., slower pace, in-creased structure, less complexity) and the use of learning aids such as di-agrams, therapy notebooks, and simple readings. Generally, therapeutic work with severely depressed patients may require the therapist to be more active and to take more responsibility for the flow of the session than in treatment of milder forms of mood disorders. Later in therapy, as the patient's energy and concentration improve, the therapist can gradu-ally shift increasing levels of responsibility to the patient.

When personality traits are creating impediments to engagement, ther-apists need to devise strategies for understanding these influences and managing them effectively. For example, a patient who obsessively does homework to extremes (e.g., completes 10 or more thought records a day, outlines in detail every element of a reading assignment) may frustrate the therapist because the person doesn't display much emotion or seem to truly grasp the emotional aspects of treatment interventions. Or, a patient with intense dependency may be difficult to engage because this person wants the therapist to do all the work. In each instance, the therapist can address the problem in engagement by formulating strategies to overcome the problem (e.g., negotiate specific limits on time spent in homework assignments, look very carefully for any "mood shifts" and devote much attention to helping an obsessive patient recognize and discuss emotions; be wary of falling into a trap of doing too much for a dependent patient; regularly assign small steps that a dependent patient can take to learn to accept responsibilities). The CBT approach to personality disorders is described in Beck et al. (2003). This book provides very helpful strategies for working with personality traits and formal personality disorders.

Some of the commonly encountered problems in engaging a patient with long-standing depression are shown in Video Illustration 3. In this first session with Mary, a middle-aged woman with pronounced, chronic depression, Dr. Wright demonstrates ways to begin to overcome demoralization and hopelessness and to forge an effective therapeutic relationship. The video begins toward the end of the first session after Mary has supplied the basic history. Dr. Wright notes that Mary doesn't seem very optimistic about treatment. In fact, she appears to be very discouraged and not well engaged in the therapeutic relationship.

> **Video Illustration 3.**   Engaging a Patient With
> Chronic Depression: Dr. Wright and Mary

Mary tells Dr. Wright that she is a "hopeless case" and backs up this conclusion by pointing out that 1) her previous psychiatrist sent her for CBT because "there wasn't anything else the therapist could do"; 2) a host of medications had been of no lasting benefit; and 3) other psychotherapies were "just talk" and "really didn't help at all." These kinds of statements can be very discouraging to therapists. The patient's pessimism can be almost infectious at times, and there is a risk that therapists can be drawn into this style of thinking. If this happens, the therapist may not fully engage in the task of combating the demoralization. A tendency to identify with hopeless thinking may be more common in therapists who are depressed themselves or have a pessimistic worldview.

We recommend that therapists who work with patients with severe or chronic depression develop skills in maintaining appropriate and realistic optimism, persistence in helping patients reverse long-standing maladaptive thinking and behavior, and personal resilience against discouragement or defeatism.

The basic methods of CBT are well suited to remoralizing patients with depression. In Video Illustration 3, Dr. Wright uses Socratic questioning and guided discovery after Mary gives a litany of reasons for concluding that she is a "hopeless case." He points out, "But yet you came (to the session)," and follows this comment with "I have a sense that there is something in you that makes you think that this could turn out....So, is there anything from the other side that makes you think we may have some success?" Although the therapist has to exert a fair amount of effort in helping Mary identify reasons to have some hope that therapy could help, they are eventually able to recognize these three factors: 1) her previous psychiatrist strongly recommended CBT; 2) Mary wants to get better for her children; and 3) she had success in the past with facing serious difficulties (i.e., moved, got a job to support self and young daughter, and went to school after her first husband left her).

Other features of the engagement process demonstrated in this video include goal setting and education on the basics of CBT for depression. If the patient begins to understand how CBT can be different from other approaches that haven't worked, and if there can be some agreement on preliminary goals, there may be a significant shift from a demoralized stance to an engagement in the therapy process. Mary has been depressed since she was a child and has deeply entrenched symptoms. Also, her chronic depression has seemed to impair her skills in managing everyday life tasks and has probably strained her marriage. Thus, it is unlikely that her deep hopelessness and inertia will be vastly changed after only one session. Even at the end of this session, she appears somewhat listless and disaffected. Yet, the process of engagement has begun and the first steps have been taken to reverse a very long-standing illness.

Assessment

Assessment of a patient with severe mental illness for CBT builds on the foundation of a comprehensive psychiatric evaluation, including the history of present illness, medical history and current physical symptoms, family history, personal and social history, risk assessment, evaluation of current social circumstances, and a mental status examination. In addition to the routine elements of the psychiatric evaluation, special attention is paid to detailing specific examples of links between cognitions, emotions, and behaviors that are core elements of the basic CBT model (see Chapter 1, "Introduction"). These observations allow the clinician to develop a cognitive-behavioral formulation (see Chapter 4, "Case Formulation and Treatment Planning"). Where possible, attempts are made from the beginning of the assessment to understand how developmental factors, traumas, and other influences may have played a role in the formation of maladaptive schemas. Review of the family and personal history is very important in this regard. Although CBT focuses primarily on the present, past experiences often shape current cognitive and behavioral responses. Thus, understanding the here and now can often be enhanced by knowledge and examination of the "there and then"—the significant life events that occurred in the patient's past.

An example of assessing the cognitive-behavioral dimensions of a person's history is provided in Video Illustration 3, and in subsequent video segments from the treatment of Mary, the woman with severe, chronic depression. As will be seen in later chapters, Mary's history included growing up in a family with marked negativism. She could never please her mother. As an adult, she continued to receive criticism from her husband. His criticism was escalating as her depression worsened. A typical current scenario evolved as follows: a triggering event of her husband criticizing her was followed by automatic thoughts such as "I do nothing," which was followed by intense sadness, which was followed by negative behavior such as sitting blankly in front of the TV—which was followed by more criticism from her husband. Further assessment revealed that this cycle was being influenced by the underlying schema "I will never succeed." The value of drawing out these types of observations is that they provide good targets for interventions and provide needed guidance for treatment planning.

Another modification of assessment methods for CBT, especially for patients with psychosis, is to obtain a clear understanding of the circumstances in which the patient first started to experience symptoms. This information can be invaluable in helping patients reexamine beliefs that arose in the past and are now affecting their everyday lives. For example, Majir, the man in Video Illustration 1, was found to have experienced a traumatic incident involving sexual themes that appeared to play a direct role in promoting paranoid cognitions and behavior (shown in video illustrations in later chapters). The therapist was able to provide more help to Majir because he recognized the impact of this event and developed a formulation to address it.

The mental status examination is similar to that used in routine clinical practice but an assessment for CBT will—

1. Evaluate the dimensions of delusions, hallucinations, and negative symptoms
   • Degree of conviction, frequency, preoccupation, amount and degree of distress, effect on behavior, belief in internal or externality of causation, and identity of voice

- Adaptive coping strategies, if any, for positive and negative symptoms
2. Identify patient strengths and assets
   - Strengths that can be building blocks for therapy interventions and that can promote improved control of symptoms and/or personal growth
   - Support systems that can be drawn upon in fighting symptoms
3. Evaluate capacity for participating in CBT
   - Learning and memory functioning
   - Concentration
   - Organization of thought
   - Ability to complete homework or other therapy tasks

Based on the work of Safran and Segal (1990), Wright et al. (2006) suggested that seven dimensions be considered in evaluating patients for CBT: 1) chronicity and complexity, 2) optimism about the chances for success in therapy, 3) acceptance of responsibility for change, 4) compatibility with the cognitive-behavioral rationale, 5) ability to access automatic thoughts and accompanying emotions, 6) capacity to engage in a therapeutic alliance, and 7) ability to maintain a problem-oriented focus. Although the "ideal patient" for CBT might have positive features in all seven dimensions, patients with severe mental disorders rarely, if ever, fit this profile. Because research has shown that the usefulness of CBT is not limited to the easy-to-treat patient (see Chapter 1, "Introduction," for a brief review of empirical research), clinicians can offer CBT to a wide variety of individuals and adjust treatment methods to match the assets and liabilities of each patient.

In addition to the seven dimensions identified by Wright et al. (2006), several additional characteristics may indicate a favorable engagement in CBT for persons with severe mental illness, including the following factors: 1) having a glimmer of insight into psychosis—just sufficient to encourage patients to talk about their beliefs; 2) having at least a moderate degree of family support and encouragement of therapy; 3) having a sense of humor or having a capacity for humor that can be developed; 4) having spiritual or cultural beliefs that do not aggravate or promote symptom development but encourage hope and positive relations with others.

Indications for CBT

Since the early 1990s, the indications for CBT have rapidly extended into the area of severe mental illnesses that previously were believed to be beyond the scope of CBT. However, CBT may not be acceptable to some patients with severe mental illness, and effective use of CBT procedures may not be possible with some patients who have pronounced symptoms that place insurmountable barriers to treatment implementation. Generally, there are no absolute contraindications to CBT for severe mental disorders except for 1) medical or neurological disorders (e.g., dementia or delirium) that are too extreme to allow for participation in psychotherapy; 2) risk of aggression or assault that cannot be safely managed; and 3) mental retardation that is too severe to allow meaningful work in CBT. Also, psychotic or floridly manic patients with very high levels of agitation or thought disorganization may not be reachable with CBT methods until psychopharmacological treatment is successful in reducing symptoms. Other factors that can work against success with CBT include severe antisocial personality disorder and an extensive history of criminal behavior. And of course, there are patients who only want medication and eschew a psychotherapeutic approach to their problems.

Despite these limitations, many patients with severe mental illness appreciate the collaborative nature of CBT, engage in treatment, and benefit from the pragmatic methods used in this approach. Because research has supported a greatly expanded terrain for CBT applications, this treatment approach is now an accepted component of therapeutic interventions for schizophrenia and related psychoses, bipolar disorder, and severe or treatment-resistant depression.

Summary

Key Points for Clinicians

- Engagement is an active process that needs to address both the positive and negative influences on the patient.
- The engagement process needs to be individually tailored to the patient's current presentation, personal characteristics, and past experiences.
- A sound psychiatric assessment with a full personal history helps to form an excellent basis for CBT. The assessment can be enhanced by specific attention to the period when symptoms emerged, a dimensional assessment of delusions and hallucinations, and attention to links between thoughts, feelings, and behavior.
- Indications for CBT for severe mental illness are broad, and there are few absolute exclusions.

Concepts and Skills for Patients to Learn

- Getting help from therapy depends a great deal on the quality of the relationship between the therapist and the patient.
- Patients can assist in building effective therapeutic relationships by openly expressing their thoughts and feelings about their problems and about the treatments.
- Cognitive-behavior therapy encourages teamwork between the therapist and patient. Both take active roles in identifying problems and working toward solutions.

References

Beck AT, Freeman A, Davis DD, et al: Cognitive Therapy of Personality Disorders, 2nd Edition. New York, Guilford, 2003

Brown GK, Ten Have T, Henriques GR, et al: Cognitive therapy for the prevention of suicide attempts: a randomized controlled trial. JAMA 294:563–570, 2005

Hays IA, Iwamasa GY (eds): Culturally Responsive Cognitive-Behavioral Therapy: Assessment, Practice, and Supervision. Washington, DC, American Psychological Association, 2006

Hendin H, Lipschitz A, Maltsberger JT, et al: Therapists' reactions to patients' suicides. Am J Psychiatry 157:2022–2077, 2000

Hendin H, Haas AP, Maltsberger JT, et al: Problems in psychotherapy with suicidal patients. Am J Psychiatry 163:67–72, 2006

Rathod S, Kingdon D, Smith P, et al: Insight into schizophrenia: the effects of cognitive behavioral therapy on the components of insight and association with sociodemographics—data on a previously published randomized controlled trial. Schizophr Res 74:211–219, 2005

Safran J, Segal Z: Interpersonal Processes in Cognitive Therapy. New York, Basic Books, 1990

Wright JH, Basco MR, Thase ME: Learning Cognitive-Behavior Therapy: An Illustrated Guide. Washington, DC, American Psychiatric Publishing, 2006

3

Normalizing and Educating

This chapter explains the crucial CBT technique of normalizing and then details related educational approaches. *Normalizing* has been termed one of the most important CBT techniques in the treatment of schizophrenia (Dudley et al. 2007). This fundamental element of CBT for psychosis forms the basis of a collaborative reality-testing approach. The chapter begins with the use of normalizing in schizophrenia, procedures first described by Kingdon and Turkington (1991). We also illustrate how normalizing methods can be helpful in the treatment of bipolar disorder and unipolar depression. The final section of the chapter discusses the important role of psychoeducation in treatment of severe mental illness and lists valuable educational resources for clinical practice.

Normalizing Schizophrenia

To most clinicians, the concept of recovery in schizophrenia is more of an oxymoron than a clinical possibility. In the patients we treat, disability appears to accrue from ongoing positive symptoms, negative symptoms, cognitive deficits, and repeated relapses. Frequently these problems are compounded by a progressive deterioration in social functioning. These intrinsic causes of disability are further aggravated by stigma and shame linked to the diagnostic label of schizophrenia and its implications. Patient's automatic thoughts about the label of schizophrenia can be very frightening and catastrophic, as illustrated in Table 3–1.

Although there is still considerable stigma from society toward persons with schizophrenia and other severe mental disorders, patient's automatic thoughts can include cognitive errors or distortions that intensify the degree of shame or self-blame. These distortions can be targets for CBT interventions through normalization, psychoeducation, or cognitive restructuring (e.g., examining the evidence, searching for alternative explanations, thought recording).

Normalizing is an excellent antistigma strategy that can be used effectively within a medical model. Normalizing statements depend on a continuum view of psychopathology but do not minimize the distress experienced at the extreme end of the spectrum where our patients' symptoms lie. The basic normalizing statement is "you are not alone." In terms of mental illness, we are saying, "The human brain can easily become depressed, hallucinate, and so forth—this is part of the human condition. We all have a threshold beyond which we can have paranoid thoughts, frightening obsessional thoughts, and the like."

Medically oriented examples are often helpful in making this point. The symptom of wheezing during a chest infection can be discussed.

Table 3–1. Common automatic thoughts about the diagnosis of schizophrenia

Automatic thought	Cognitive errors
"I am mad."	Labeling, magnifying
"I will never get better."	Jumping to conclusions, all-or-nothing thinking
"I can't be trusted."	Disqualifying the positive, magnifying
"I should not be near my children."	Catastrophizing
"I will end up on the streets."	Jumping to conclusions, catastrophizing
"I will never get a job."	Jumping to conclusions, all-or-nothing thinking
"I am two people—a Jekyll and Hyde."	Lack of evidence
"I must be possessed by a demon."	Lack of evidence
"People will be scared of me."	Jumping to conclusions, magnifying

Anyone can wheeze. It is a normal response of the bronchi; but if asthma is present, regular medication is usually needed because symptoms cause distress. A further point in the normalizing explanation is that anxiety and stigma around the diagnosis of asthma can worsen the course of the illness by mechanisms such as hyperventilation and reduced adherence to medical treatments. Of course asthma now carries much less stigma than it once did. Many illnesses such as cancer, diabetes, and heart disease have gradually become normalized and more acceptable over time. But, individual and community stigma for schizophrenia remains very high.

Patients often report stigmatizing and self-condemning automatic thoughts, such as those in Table 3–1, which can increase anxiety, depression, and shame. This type of thinking also can lead to social avoidance. These stigma-driven emotions and behaviors act to exacerbate the anxiety and depression often inherent in the illness of schizophrenia. These affects, when linked to defensive safety behaviors (primarily avoidance), can lead to worsening of positive and negative symptoms, increased problems with medication adherence, and a heightened risk for relapse. Thus, efforts to forestall this stigma-incited downward spiral with normalization strategies are a key part of the CBT approach to schizophrenia.

> **Learning Exercise 3–1.** Normalizing the Diagnosis of Schizophrenia
>
> 1. Try to put yourself in the position of a person who has just received a diagnosis of schizophrenia. How do you feel about being told about the diagnosis? What thoughts are running through your mind?
>
> 2. Record these emotions and thoughts on a piece of paper.
>
> 3. Now write down ideas for what might have helped you accept that you had a mental health problem. Try to identify some normalizing comments that might have helped you collaborate with a clinician.

The normalizing approach to the diagnosis of schizophrenia can be a solution to distress for both patient and clinician (Table 3–2). The goal is to avoid catastrophizing and to understand these main points: 1) virtually everyone faces a significant illness at some point in their life, 2) schizophrenia is a common problem that affects many people in many cultures, 3) the illness is not the patient's or the family's fault, 4) a large number

---

Table 3–2.   Normalizing statements for the diagnosis of
                 schizophrenia

"Many people develop psychotic symptoms and other similar problems."

"The majority of patients with schizophrenia have a good outcome over time." (Harrison et al. 2001)

"Patients who do the best accept help that is available and work closely with their doctors and therapists."

"It is okay to take a pill/shot to help the stress levels come under control. Almost everyone needs pills at some point in life."

"People with schizophrenia usually can develop very meaningful lives with good relationships, lots of interests, and many other positive daily activities."

"John Nash, the Nobel Prize winner who was the subject of the book and movie *A Beautiful Mind*, is a person with schizophrenia. He believes that mental disorders are associated with creativity."

"Schizophrenia is a medical illness like diabetes—the more patients understand the illness and manage the symptoms, the better they do."

---

of persons with this problem can overcome symptoms, and 5) in some cultures a psychotic episode can even be viewed in a positive way.

It can be useful for clinicians to examine their own automatic thoughts about schizophrenia. Could any of these automatic thoughts be distorted? This list of possible maladaptive automatic thoughts may help you identify any of your own cognitions that could impact treatment of schizophrenia (Table 3–3).

In Learning Exercise 3–1, you identified several of the automatic thoughts that you might have if you were diagnosed with this condition. As a follow-up to the learning exercise, take some time to review the examples in Table 3–3 to see if you have other automatic thoughts that could significantly influence your work with schizophrenia patients. If you find any of your thoughts that you would like to change, write them down on a sheet of paper with two columns marked "automatic thoughts" and "rational thoughts." Try to develop the most rational view possible of the diagnosis, prognosis, and what you can do to help.

Hallucinations

The next video illustration shows Dr. Turkington working with Brenda, who experiences distressing hallucinations. Brenda is an African American woman who is age 47. Brenda has a diagnosis of schizophrenia and

Table 3–3. Common automatic thoughts of clinicians about the diagnosis of schizophrenia

"I shouldn't really tell him the diagnosis—it is too negative."

"If I give information about schizophrenia, she might be more likely to commit suicide."

"I won't give prognostic information. It could overstimulate him and hasten a relapse."

"Improved coping is an illusion—the ultimate road is always downhill."

"It is wrong to raise false hopes when the course is inexorable."

has had distressing auditory hallucinations for at least 25 years. In this first interview with Brenda, Dr. Turkington quickly recognizes that she has intense shame about hearing voices. Brenda noted that "my family hid me away when I became ill."

Dr. Turkington's normalization strategy included the following statements:

> Did you know that lots of people at some point in their lives hear voices?
>
> The figures are that approximately 1 person in 50 in the community are voice hearers.
>
> Did you know that some very famous and successful people are voice hearers?
>
> Do you know the famous actor Anthony Hopkins?...He is a voice hearer.

The normalizing statements used here helped Brenda to feel less alone, less ashamed, and more empowered to try to understand and cope better with her voices.

▶ **Video Illustration 4.** Normalizing and Educating: Dr. Turkington and Brenda

The clinician can use a variety of destigmatizing normalizing explanations and can support these comments with readings, Web sites, and other educational opportunities. Dr. Turkington initially asked Brenda to read over a simple pamphlet as a homework exercise. This pamphlet, "What's Happening to Me? A Voice Hearing Pamphlet" (Kingdon and Turkington 2005), is provided in Appendix 1 ("Worksheets and Checklists"). The pamphlet is only two pages long but describes how commonly voices are found in the community and what kinds of stress can worsen them. At the next session, Brenda reported that she had read the information and had learned that other people hear voices too. Brenda was also helped by the realization that quite successful and famous people can have similar experiences. For example, Table 3–4 lists Web sites that cover voice hearing in other people, including Anthony Hopkins. These Web sites can be excellent sources for patients to learn about hallucinations. (Unless otherwise noted, all Web sites, pamphlets, and books suggested in this chapter are listed in Appendix 2, "Cognitive-Behavior Therapy Resources"; the information in this appendix can be downloaded from the American Psychiatric Publishing Web site at www.appi.org/pdf/62321.)

In addition to Web sites on hallucinations (see Table 3–4), several printed resources by Romme and Escher can assist in normalization. The booklet *Understanding Voices: Coping With Auditory Hallucinations and Confusing Realities* (Romme and Escher 1996) can be very educational for patients. Those patients who struggle to accept the symptom can be helped by reading *Accepting Voices: A New Approach to Voice-Hearing Outside the Illness Model* (Romme and Escher 1993). This can be backed up with homework exercises from *Making Sense of Voices: A Guide for Professionals Who Work With Voice Hearers* (Romme and Escher 2000).

Clinicians can also promote normalization by explaining in treatment sessions that there are numerous stresses or other influences that can precipitate hallucinations. For example, a statement might be made that "anybody can hallucinate if they are deprived of sleep long enough" (Oswald 1974). Because there is a close association between the degree of sleep deprivation and severity of auditory hallucinations, many patients will identify with this explanation. This strategy may even lead to an improvement in adherence because a sedative antipsychotic taken at night

---

Table 3–4.   Web sites with valuable information about voice hearing

---

Mind
www.mind.org.uk/Information/Booklets/Other/The+voice+inside.htm
    A practical guide to understanding voice hearing, written by the Hearing Voices Network

Gloucestershire Hearing Voices and Recovery Groups
www.hearingvoices.org.uk/info_resources11.htm
    Over 20 examples of good advice on coping with voice hearing

Making Common Sense of Voices
www.peter-lehmann-publishing.com/articles/others/klafki_making.htm
    A normalizing essay on the subject of voice hearing that could be used as a homework exercise

---

to improve sleep may seem to "make sense." Other causes of hallucinations in the normal population can also be mentioned, including bereavement, sensory deprivation, extreme trauma, hostage situations, solitary confinement, and illegal drug use. Again, patients will often identify with one or more of these explanations and thereby feel more normal and less stigmatized.

Another part of the normalizing explanation is that many people who are coping well with their hallucinations have learned how to switch the voices off and on. Often they can dismiss the voices for a while and tell them to come back at a particular time for a period of discussion. They can learn how to adapt to hearing voices, even to the point of being employed in a regular job. In summary, normalization works by helping voice hearers realize that they are not alone, that voices can be controlled, and that voice hearers need not be fighting a losing battle.

Some examples of clinically useful normalizing explanations for hallucinations are listed in Table 3–5. These types of statements can be backed up by research that has shown that hallucinations are very common following bereavement (Kersting 2004) or in situations of sensory deprivation (Leff 1968).

Normalizing explanations such as the ones in Table 3–5 can be supplemented with educational material on issues such as sleep hygiene, the

---

Table 3–5. Normalizing statements for hallucinations

"People who are deprived of sleep for long periods are prone to hallucinate."

"Following the death of a close relative or friend, hallucinations are very common."

"Sensory deprivation can make people hallucinate within several hours."

"LSD can make almost anyone hallucinate."

"People who have been involved in combat or severe trauma situations can experience hallucinations."

"One person in every group of 50 is a voice hearer....Think about your old school class, your Bible study group, or your local youth club. There is a high chance that someone in one of these groups hears voices."

"Lots of famous people are voice hearers."

"Voices can be controlled."

"Voice hearers often hold down good jobs."

"The human brain hallucinates fairly easily in response to stress."

---

grieving process, and reducing sensory deprivation situations. Psychoeducational methods and materials will be discussed in the section "Education" later in this chapter.

Delusions

There are a number of normalizing statements that can help patients with delusions. The epidemiology of paranoid thinking and delusion emergence has been described by Freeman and coworkers (2006) and Wiles and associates (2006). On the basis of this research, we can inform paranoid patients that the majority of people have occasional paranoid thoughts. Some of the commonly reported paranoia-tinged thoughts from persons without diagnoses of psychoses are listed in Table 3–6.

The normalizing message in CBT for delusions is that there are lots of people out there with persecutory thoughts and beliefs and that there is no need for shame or sadness in relation to this. However, normalization of delusions does not mean that therapists should encourage patients to believe their distorted beliefs. Instead, the therapist teaches patients that the CBT method involves 1) learning that this kind of thinking is very common, 2) accepting delusional thoughts as a product of the mind, 3) not hiding away from these thoughts, 4) checking out the validity of paranoid perceptions, and 5) developing effective coping strategies.

An illustration of a potentially helpful normalizing strategy is to discuss the usefulness of paranoia in certain social situations. An example could be given of being out in a rough area of town at midnight during a community festival in which many of the celebrants had been drinking heavily. In such a situation it would be wise to consider that fights could break out and that an assault could occur. Thus, a certain degree of hypervigilance and caution would be highly appropriate. This type of example can often prepare patients to begin to relate their own paranoid thoughts and beliefs to specific stressors that may have played a role in the emergence of their psychosis.

Another form of normalizing commentary used in CBT for delusions is to explain to patients that people who don't get stuck in their paranoid thoughts tend to be more open about them and are more likely to be able to carry on with their normal day-to-day activities in an effective manner. To make this point come alive, it may be helpful to describe an example. Patients often like to hear how others have learned to accept and cope with psychotic symptoms. An example that we sometimes use is of a very paranoid young man who was too frightened to leave his house. He read the book *Overcoming Paranoid and Suspicious Thoughts* (Freeman et al. 2006) and then contacted another paranoid patient on the Internet. They

---

Table 3–6. Suspiciousness reported by persons who are not psychotic

---

"People are talking about me."

"There is a conspiracy against me."

"That item on the radio/TV might have referred to me."

"I had something to do with that crime/accident."

"That police car is waiting for me."

"I have been singled out for bad treatment."

"That memo that went around the office is mostly about me."

---

shared their histories and beliefs—and drawing strength from each other, they decided to begin to face their fears and visit some local movies, restaurants, and other facilities. They both improved their quality of life and developed new ways of coping.

Homework assignments can also be used in the normalization process for delusions. One suggestion for homework is for patients to visit the Paranoid Thoughts Web site (www.iop.kcl.ac.uk/apps/paranoidthoughts/default. html). This Web site describes ways of coping with paranoid thoughts and gives references for helpful reading material.

Thought Disorder

Normalizing approaches to thought disorder are typically more difficult to apply than those for hallucinations and delusions. Yet, normalization can still be helpful. Stress, poor sleep, and sensory overload can all lead to difficulties in concentrating and communicating clearly. The example can be given of people with jet lag who struggle to make their flight connections or handle a rental car. Also medical residents often have personal experiences of having problems pulling their thoughts together coherently due to prolonged periods of overwork and sleep deprivation. One of us (D.T.) remembers once going to take a history from a pregnant woman at 3 A.M. He was so tired that no words came out at all. They just sat there looking at each other until his thoughts started to flow again and a rudimentary history was taken. It was a real struggle for him to pull his thoughts together and communicate clearly.

Thought disorder can be normalized by using the types of statements listed in Table 3–7.

A young woman with schizophrenia was expressing her thoughts with "knight's move jumps" and occasionally in a word salad (see Chapter 10,

Table 3–7. Normalizing statements for thought disorder

"Anyone who is sleeping badly can have problems making themselves understood."

"Everyone is trying to get their ideas across but sometimes they don't seem to make that much sense. Even some famous politicians or sports stars can have problems communicating clearly."

"The problem can be that we get too anxious and lose our train of thought."

"It can be useful to practice saying what we want to say in just one sentence."

"It is easy to get confused when you are under stress."

"Most people need training and experience to speak in a clear and concise manner."

"Impaired Cognitive Functioning," for more information on these types of disordered thinking). She was very distressed during the word salad episodes. The normalizing explanation used was that communication was more difficult for her when she was sleeping badly and when she was distressed by events in the news. It was pointed out that news stories about terrorism and violence were often stressful to her, and that a combination of stress and lack of sleep would cause many people to have problems in thinking clearly. The patient agreed to take some steps to improve sleep hygiene and also to watch less distressing programs at nighttime. These strategies helped reduce her word salad to the point that she could begin to use specific CBT techniques for thought disorder (such as thought linkage and theme identification as discussed in Chapter 10).

Negative Symptoms

Negative symptoms also have correlates in normal mental life. Following the experience of extreme trauma, the mind often enters a state of shock with numbing of emotions (e.g., alogia and affective blunting). Social withdrawal and reduced self-care with lowered motivation can follow periods of recuperation from physical illness. A disheveled appearance can result from excessive stress and poor time management. It can therefore be possible to normalize negative symptoms and reduce the self-blame and sense of failure that patients with these problems may experience. Normalization can be useful for negative symptoms, but perhaps to a lesser degree than for delusions and hallucinations. For some patients with negative symptoms, normalizing comments can help them accept the problem and assist them with taking realistic steps to move forward.

The normalizing explanations of negative symptoms in Table 3–8 relate to allowing the mind and body to take time out to recuperate following various life events. These types of conceptualizations of negative symptoms can help reduce demoralization and secondary depression. In this way of viewing the problem, the negative symptoms can be seen as having a positive protective function for the recovering self. A discussion with the patient about the meaning of negative symptoms might be followed by a low-level, graded activity-scheduling intervention. The treatment of Martin illustrates this approach:

> Martin had developed negative symptoms of poor self-care, low motivation, and relationship avoidance following an acute psychotic episode 5 years ago. The therapist normalized his experiences by explaining to Martin that he had become exhausted following his acute psychotic episode and that he had needed some time by himself to recover. It was further noted that anyone who experienced an acute schizophrenic episode would need time to gradually get back into life again. This explanation provided a useful alternative to the strategy of earlier clinicians, which seemed (at least in Martin's view) to be always trying to force him to do more. We then explored his prepsychotic interests and hobbies and agreed that we would see if these might still be enjoyable. The next step was to use a mastery and pleasure chart linked to low-level graded activities (see Chapter 7, "Depression").

Table 3–8. Normalizing statements for negative symptoms

Alogia	"Anyone who has been severely stressed can find it difficult to think for a while."
Affective blunting	"When stress overcomes people, it can seem safer to keep feelings hidden."
Social withdrawal	"Following an illness it can be important for people to take some time out to regain strength."
Reduced self-care	"For any of us facing a hard day's work, it can be tough to get out of bed in the morning, wash, dress, and start the day."
Reduced motivation	"Sometimes people take on tasks that are too big and can give up quickly."
Anhedonia	"When recovering from any illness, small tasks are worthwhile and can be enjoyable."

Normalizing Bipolar Disorder

People with bipolar disorder will experience normal fluctuations in mood related to activities and experiences, seasons of the year, level of energy, and the presence or absence of psychosocial stressors. They also contend with mood swings that are outside the normal range. The dilemma for most people with this illness is how to distinguish between the two. Those who are not ready to accept the reality of having a mood-altering illness will downplay the significance of emotional peaks and valleys. They say, "Everyone has ups and down so mine are nothing to worry about." They are right in that everyone has mood swings, but ignoring all but the most extreme changes in mood can be a mistake.

Those who have accepted their diagnosis and are eager to stay within the normal range of mood will sometimes overinterpret normal shifts in affect as indicators of pathology. They might panic a little when they think they are too excited about getting a new job, making a new friend, or overcoming important life hurdles. They hesitate to enjoy accomplishments. On the depressive end, they might not allow themselves to feel normal and reasonable sadness, like grief over a loss, for fear of it leading to major depression.

The challenge of self-monitoring, uncertainty about their experiences, and not always trusting themselves to accurately interpret mood shifts is common and normal across people who share this illness. Therapists can help patients to become familiar with their unique constellation of symptoms of depression and mania so that these patients can become more accurate in their interpretation of mood swings and take action to control symptoms if necessary.

Normalizing Depression

The normalizing messages in treatment of severe or chronic depression have the same themes as with other severe mental disorders—patients are not alone, severe depression is part of a continuum of symptoms that are experienced in everyday life by many people, and symptoms can be treated effectively. Clinicians can point out that depression is one of the most common illnesses in humans. For example, a large, well-designed study found a lifetime risk for any mood disorder to be about 21%, and the risk for unipolar depression to be about 17% (Kessler et al. 2005). Other useful normalizing statements can emphasize the link between medical illnesses and depression, the intensive research effort to better understand depression, and the generally positive results of studies of CBT for this disorder.

For patients with refractory or chronic depression, it may be useful to let them know that chronicity is a frequent occurrence, but sequential pharmacological strategies and intensive CBT methods are available to help work toward recovery. The treatment of Mary, the woman with chronic depression (shown earlier in Video Illustration 3), demonstrates efforts to help a person who has had many previous failures of treatment.

The process of normalizing depression has been helped by the self-revelations of a number of celebrities (e.g., Brooke Shields, Mike Wallace, William Styron, Terry Bradshaw, Kitty Dukakis) that have described their successful fight against this illness. Therapists can make comments about these people in therapy sessions, and suggestions can be made to read books with personal accounts about recovery from depression. Table 3–9 lists books written by celebrities about depression and also provides useful Web sites for learning about this disorder.

The Therapeutic Relationship

The therapeutic relationship for normalizing interventions should be a collaborative one, as in all other aspects of CBT. The clinician should be relaxed and friendly, honest and respectful. Personal disclosure can be used judiciously, but obviously should not transgress normal clinical limits. There should be, for example, no personal disclosure surrounding areas such as psychiatric treatment, business, or sexuality. It can be acceptable, however, to describe to a patient how you have overcome a degree of pho-

---

Table 3–9. Books and Web sites for helping patients to normalize depression

---

Personal accounts of recovery from depression

Brooke Shields: *Down Came the Rain* (Shields 2005)

William Styron: *Darkness Visible: A Memoir of Madness* (Styron 1990)

Web sites with helpful information about depression

Depression and Bipolar Support Alliance (advocacy and support group): www.dbsalliance.org

National Institute of Mental Health (comprehensive series of articles including personal accounts): www.nimh.nih.gov/healthinformation/depressionmenu.cfm

University of Louisville Depression Center (depression screening, personal accounts, treatment options): http://louisville.edu/depression

University of Michigan Depression Center (depression screening and information about treatment): www.umich.edu/depression

---

bia by using CBT-type techniques. One of us (D.T.) sometimes tells patients that he used to be very anxious about giving lectures. He was hypervigilant for anybody who appeared to be sleeping or bored through the lecture. Using basic CBT principles, he realized that he was trying to perform at an unrealistically high standard. He recognized that he needed to relax to deliver the lecture slowly and clearly and to use a variety of interesting teaching materials. He also learned to use some appropriate humor rather than attempt to cram in a vast amount of information that audiences simply could not absorb. By looking at his automatic thoughts, he was able to identify the problem and was able to make adjustments that led to more enjoyable lectures and reduced anxiety levels. This type of story can be useful in bringing clinician and patient together as joint investigators: neither of them is perfect and both are human and willing to work together on the current problem.

Another example of a normalizing personal disclosure is sometimes used by Dr. Turkington to help people with auditory hallucinations. He explains that some doctors while falling asleep will hear the phone ringing, but when they pick up the phone there is nobody there. They have actually hallucinated the ringing of the phone. This is called a hypnagogic hallucination and is considered to be normal. These kinds of experiences are particularly common in doctors who have been frequently awoken at night by the phone ringing when on call. They have been stressed to a degree by their sleep being repeatedly disturbed in this way; and perhaps that is why that particular hallucination comes back to them. Patients can feel encouraged by being trusted with this information and may then disclose more of their own personal material in therapy sessions.

Education

In this section, we highlight commonly used educational methods and give examples of how they may be used to promote normalization or to help educate the patient on other important topics. The primary educational techniques used in CBT are explanations and illustrations given in sessions, readings and other homework assignments, and computer-assisted CBT. The last method is currently being used for depression (Wright et al. 2002, 2005) and other mental disorders, such as anxiety disorders (Kenwright et al. 2001), but is not typically a part of psychoeducation for schizophrenia. Some of the general principles for psychoeducation in CBT are as follows:

1. Pitch the educational effort at a level that matches the patient's ability to comprehend and process information.

2. Clearly explain principles in brief "mini-didactic" sessions that emphasize collaborative learning instead of lecturing.
3. Use diagrams, handouts, or other written aids when possible.
4. Encourage the patient to ask questions to further the learning process.
5. Ask for feedback, including capsule summaries, to check for understanding.
6. Assign targeted reading, Internet searches, or other educational experiences for homework.
7. Consider use of a therapy notebook, if the patient is able to benefit from this device.

Because persons with severe mental illness often have problems with concentration or learning and memory functioning, the therapist may need to pay special attention to the learning process. In addition to the general principles outlined above, it can be helpful to make teaching points at times when there is significant emotional activation about a particular stressor or problem in the patient's life. If the material is emotionally relevant to the patient, memory retention may be increased. For example, an explanation of the role of automatic thoughts in driving emotion may stick with the patient better if it is tied to a specific situation where the patient had significant stress after a triggering event, and modifying the automatic thoughts led to some relief.

Another useful method to enhance learning is to perform an appropriate amount of repetition. The therapist needs to be careful not to bore the patient or insult his intelligence by excessive repetition or dwelling on educational topics for too long. However, cursory explanations or "one shot" educational efforts may not be effective. One useful way to provide repetitive, yet interesting, learning experiences is for the therapist to suggest that the patient work on understanding the same basic concept from multiple angles. After checking for the level of understanding, a variety of different methods such as readings, Internet or library searches, videos, and other educational tools can be used to deepen and consolidate learning.

Schizophrenia

Some common educational initiatives in CBT for schizophrenia are listed in Table 3–10. These methods can help with normalization and skill building. In educating patients with schizophrenia, it is particularly important to choose topics and educational methods that can be readily understood and do not overwhelm the patient.

In Video Illustration 4, Dr. Turkington uses simple and direct explanations about hallucinations that Brenda appears to understand. He then

---

Table 3–10. Examples of psychoeducation in the treatment of
psychoses

Teach the theory and principles of sleep hygiene.

Explain the principles of stress management.

Use educational material about the frequency of psychotic symptoms in
the general population.

Explain the link between severe trauma and psychosis.

Educate patients about the grieving process.

Provide reading material about sensory and sleep deprivation and
psychosis.

Teach coping strategies for voices.

---

suggests that she check on a Web site to learn about the experiences of a
famous voice hearer, Anthony Hopkins. Brenda does not appear to have
a significant amount of thought disorder, and she demonstrates an ability
to follow the therapist's lead in learning about voices. Other patients
with more severe thought disorder, or less cognitive capacity, would
probably not be able to move so quickly or thoroughly in the learning
process. Thus, therapists need to carefully tailor the educational interventions to a level that matches the patient's ability to learn.

Patients who are able to accept or are reassured by the diagnosis of
schizophrenia can be given an explanation of a chemical imbalance in the
brain as part of an overall cognitive-biological-social formulation of the illness (see Chapter 1, "Introduction"). Such patients can be provided with
basic psychoeducational information about dopamine, genetics, and possible perinatal influences. For some patients this type of information can
help in developing a collaborative case formulation (see Chapter 4, "Case
Formulation and Treatment Planning"), improve adherence, and increase
insight. One caveat here is that certain ethnic groups (e.g., African Carib-
bean, Bangladeshi, and some other Asian patients) may be less likely to accept biological education concerning causation (McCabe and Priebe
2004). Such patients are more prone to accept education linked to social
models of causation.

We need also to be cautious about education around the diagnosis of
schizophrenia. Patients who are not willing to accept this diagnostic term
can become more depressed if educational attempts are made to understand the diagnosis (Carroll et al. 1998; Rathod et al. 2005). The clinician
needs to be very sensitive to the patient's initial response to the information

being given and should use a stress-vulnerability explanation if there are signs that the word "schizophrenia" might further increase distress. In these situations, clinicians can attach more emphasis to the role of particular stressors or accumulated stressors that have developed and preceded the onset of the psychosis. The prepsychotic period should therefore be worked through on a systematic basis using inductive questioning. The various stressors can be clearly labeled as they arise, as shown in this case example:

> Therapist: Can you take me back to the time before you decided it was too dangerous to go out?
> Patient: Yes, I lost my job at the farm where I was working.
> Therapist: How did you feel and what went through your mind?
> Patient: That I did not deserve it, and I had no money (angry).
> Therapist: What happened next?
> Patient: My wife left me.
> Therapist: How did you feel when that happened?
> Patient: I felt lonely and sad. She went off with another man.

In this illustration, we are able to educate the patient that there were indeed a number of clear stressors in the period preceding the onset of psychosis. Patients often tend to disqualify the stressful nature of such events, so it is important to teach the patient that anyone going through a sequence of these kinds of events would be distressed. Further inquiry revealed that this man's brother was receiving long-acting antipsychotic medication injections and had been in several psychiatric hospitals. We were thus able to arrive at a stress-vulnerability explanation of the development of symptoms.

Reading assignments can be used for patients with schizophrenia and other psychoses, but the complexity and amount of material should be carefully geared to the patient's capacity to assimilate the content. Table 3–11 lists some useful readings and briefly describes their content.

Many patients with psychotic symptoms jump to conclusions on the basis of inadequate knowledge or evidence. The following questions can stimulate curiosity and encourage the patient to learn facts instead of jumping to conclusions:

- Does either the therapist or the patient really understand how text messages arrive into mobile phones?
- Do either of them really understand the extent and the limitations of the working of satellites?
- Do they know how small a camera can actually be?

These are the types of real-world knowledge deficits that can be corrected by working together and by participating in fact-finding homework exercises.

Table 3–11. Suggested reading assignments for schizophrenia

Publication	Description
Cognitive-Behavioural Therapy of Schizophrenia (Kingdon and Turkington 1994)	A description of normalizing and education strategies.
Overcoming Paranoid and Suspicious Thoughts (Freeman et al. 2006)	A description of how to understand and overcome paranoia.
Accepting Voices (Romme and Escher 1993)	An educational book on how to engage with voices
Back to Life, Back to Normality (Turkington et al. 2008)	A user and caregiver CBT self-help guide for psychosis.
A Beautiful Mind (Nasar 1998)	An inspiring story of recovery from schizophrenia.

Bipolar Disorder

Psychoeducation is a particularly important part of the CBT approach to bipolar disorder. Methods for educating patients with bipolar disorder will be discussed further in Chapter 8, "Mania." Some of the most frequently used methods and targets for psychoeducation are 1) mood diaries to help patients learn about their mood swings, 2) education on sleep hygiene, 3) teaching patients how to identify stressors that may trigger mood swings, 4) education about medications and side effects, and 5) learning stress management techniques and methods of organizing daily life.

Patients also may be taught how to improve interpersonal relationships and to cope better with the relationship problems that are often associated with bipolar disorder. Another common teaching goal of CBT for bipolar disorder is to help patients understand risks involved with behavioral excesses common to mania (e.g., spending sprees, sexual indiscretions, substance abuse, hostility in relationships) and to learn strategies to reduce these risks.

Reading assignments are used frequently in the treatment of bipolar disorder. These assignments can be helpful to both patients and their families. Some of the most useful books for patients and their families are—

• *An Unquiet Mind* (Jamison 1995) and *Brilliant Madness: Living With Manic Depressive Illness* (Duke 1992) include excellent personal accounts of bipolar disorder by persons who have the illness.

- *The Bipolar Survival Guide: What You and Your Family Need to Know* (Miklowitz 2002) describes the diagnosis and treatment of bipolar disorder, including information on medication and side effects.
- *The Bipolar Workbook: Tools for Controlling Your Mood Swings* (Basco 2006) is specifically designed to teach the concepts of CBT and includes many useful self-help exercises to provide education and help build CBT skills.

Depression

Video Illustration 3 (first shown in Chapter 2, "Engaging and Assessing") depicts an educational intervention in the initial session with Mary, the woman with chronic depression. In this illustration, Dr. Wright teaches Mary that depression distorts thinking in a negative direction, but there is still a part of her that has hope and wants to get better. He then helps her identify some reasons to be hopeful that treatment could work and provides some preliminary, general information on how CBT may be different than other treatments. Finally, he asks her to read a brief pamphlet, *Coping With Depression* (Beck et al. 1995), which is easy to understand and seems appropriate to Mary's level of energy, motivation, and concentration.

The educational efforts shown in the video illustration are typical of the work that may be done early in the treatment of a patient with severe or treatment-resistant depression. Some of the common targets of psychoeducation for depression include—

- Understanding that depression is not the fault of the patient;
- Discovering that depression biases thinking in a negative direction and makes it hard for people to recognize or use their strengths;
- Considering the possibility that there might be a genetic vulnerability to severe depression;
- Learning about the potential benefits of exercise or light therapy (in the case of seasonal affective disorder);
- Understanding the negative effects of alcohol and drugs of abuse in recovery from depression; and
- Most importantly, learning basic CBT methods.

As with the other severe mental disorders discussed here, suggested readings can be very useful in educating patients about depression. *Getting Your Life Back: The Complete Guide to Recovery From Depression* (Wright and Basco 2002) includes general information about depression, in addition to a number of self-help exercises to build CBT knowledge and skills. This book also contains psychoeducational material on pharmacotherapy and interpersonal aspects of depression. Other commonly used books include *Feeling Good* (Burns 1999), a CBT self-help guide, and *Mind Over Mood* (Greenberger and Padesky 1995), a CBT workbook.

One of the most interesting and potentially effective methods of psychoeducation is computer-assisted CBT. Two major programs for depression have been tested empirically and are currently available for clinical use (Proudfoot et al. 2004; Wright et al. 2002, 2004, 2005). Each of these programs have goals that go considerably beyond the provision of psychoeducation because they are intended to be used as therapy tools that make treatment more efficient or to reduce the amount of clinician time required to offer effective CBT for depression.

Good Days Ahead: The Multimedia Program for Cognitive Therapy (Wright et al. 2004) has been shown to be effective in the treatment of major depression and to reduce the requirement for therapist time by about one-half. This program includes a number of video and audio-enhanced interactive exercises, mini-didactic sessions by an experienced cognitive-behavior therapist, videos of professional actors who show how CBT can be used in everyday life, and an electronic workbook that is used for homework exercises. In a randomized, controlled trial with drug-free persons with major depression, computer-assisted CBT was more effective than standard CBT in teaching patients CBT concepts (Wright et al. 2005). *Beating the Blues* (Proudfoot et al. 2004) is another multimedia computer program that has been shown to be effective in clinical trials. This program is used primarily in primary care settings in the United Kingdom.

Whether the clinician uses standard "low-tech" methods, or newer computer-assisted CBT programs, psychoeducation is a fundamental component of the CBT approach to depression. Sources for computer programs and other educational resources for depression are listed in Appendix 2, "Cognitive-Behavior Therapy Resources."

CBT

For patients to fully collaborate with treatment and to gain the maximum benefit from CBT, they need to become experts in the basic principles and methods of this approach. It has often been said that one of the primary goals of CBT is to prepare patients to be their own therapists. Thus, by the end of treatment they have acquired the knowledge and skill to continue to use these methods in daily life to reduce symptoms and lower the risk of relapse.

Discussion of educational methods for each of the specific disorders earlier in the chapter provided suggestions for helping patients learn about CBT and gain important skills in using this approach. There are three general phases that patients undergo in learning CBT:

1. In the first phase (early treatment), the main emphasis is on brief explanations from the therapist to socialize the patient to treatment and readings (or computer programs) that convey core concepts.
2. In the second phase (midtreatment), much of the learning comes from participating in CBT methods in sessions (e.g., examining the evidence, activity scheduling, problem solving, identifying and modifying automatic thoughts) plus additional reading and/or computer work and homework assignments.
3. In the third phase (late therapy and termination), the therapist typically reviews and strengthens lessons from earlier in treatment and teaches the patient relapse prevention methods (see Chapter 13, "Maintaining Treatment Gains").

The pace and goals of learning in all phases is customized to fit the diagnosis and severity of symptoms. When patients do learn the core principles and methods of CBT, therapists can complete the treatment with a sense of gratification that their role as teacher has been well served.

Summary

Key Points for Clinicians

- Normalizing improves collaboration and reduces stigma.
- Normalizing and education are mutually helpful strategies that can be easily used by clinicians in their day-to-day work with patients with severe mental illness.
- Normalizing can be safely used in all forms of severe mental illness and is not antagonistic to the medical model or the use of medication.
- Normalizing and educational approaches are based on the stress-vulnerability model of severe mental illness.
- Patients should receive educational information suitable to their level of symptoms and cognitive capacity.

Concepts and Skills for Patients to Learn

- You are not alone: people in the community commonly have hallucinations, paranoid thoughts, mood swings, and periods of depression.
- Many famous and successful people have problems similar to the ones you are experiencing.

- It is possible to understand symptoms and learn how to cope with them.
- The route to improved coping includes learning how to manage stress and build on your strengths.
- Working with your doctors and therapists, you can fight back and get symptoms under control.

References

Basco MR: The Bipolar Workbook: Tools for Controlling Your Mood Swings. New York, Guilford, 2006

Beck AT, Greenberg RC, Beck J: Coping With Depression (booklet). Bala Cynwyd, PA, The Beck Institute, 1995

Burns D: Feeling Good: The New Mood Therapy. New York, Avon Books, 1999

Carroll Z, Clyde S, Fattah I, et al: The effect of an educational intervention on insight and suicidal ideation in schizophrenia. Schizophr Res 29:28–29, 1998

Dudley R, Bryant C, Hammond K et al: Techniques in cognitive behavioural therapy: using normalizing in schizophrenia. Journal of the Norwegian Psychological Association 44:562–572, 2007

Duke P: Brilliant Madness: Living With Manic Depressive Illness. New York, Bantam Books, 1992

Freeman D, Freeman J, Garety P: Overcoming Paranoid and Suspicious Thoughts. London, Robinson, 2006

Greenberger D, Padesky C: Mind Over Mood. New York, Guilford, 1995

Harrison G, Hopper K, Craig T, et al: Recovery from psychotic illness: a 15 and 25 year international follow-up study. Br J Psychiatry 178:506–518, 2001

Jamison K: An Unquiet Mind. New York, Knopf, 1995

Kenwright M, Liness S, Marks I: Reducing demands on clinicians' time by offering computer-aided self help for phobia/panic: feasibility study. Br J Psychiatry 179:456–459, 2001

Kersting A: The psychodynamics of grief hallucinations—a psychopathological phenomenon of normal and pathological grief. Psychopathology 37:50–51, 2004

Kessler RC, Berglund P, Demler MA, et al: Lifetime prevalence and age-of-onset distributions of DSM-IV disorders in the national comorbidity survey replication. Arch Gen Psychiatry 62:593–602, 2005

Kingdon D, Turkington D: Preliminary report: the use of cognitive behaviour therapy and a normalizing rationale in schizophrenia. J Nerv Ment Dis 179:207–211, 1991

Kingdon D, Turkington D: Cognitive-Behavioural Therapy of Schizophrenia. New York, Guilford, 1994

Kingdon DG, Turkington D: Cognitive Therapy of Schizophrenia. New York, Guilford, 2005

Leff JP: Perceptual phenomena and personality in sensory deprivation. Br J Psychiatry 114:1499–1508, 1968

McCabe R, Priebe S: Explanatory models of illness in schizophrenia: comparison of four ethnic groups. Br J Psychiatry 185:25–30, 2004

Miklowitz DJ: The Bipolar Survival Guide: What You and Your Family Need to Know. New York, Guilford, 2002

Nasar SA: A Beautiful Mind. New York, Touchstone, 1998

Oswald I: Sleep, 3rd Edition. Harmondsworth, England, Penguin, 1974

Proudfoot J, Ryden C, Everitt B, et al: Clinical efficacy of computerised cognitive-behavioural therapy for anxiety and depression in primary care: randomised controlled trial. Br J Psychiatry 185:46–54, 2004

Rathod S, Kingdon D, Smith P, et al: Insight into schizophrenia: the effects of cognitive behavioural therapy on the components of insight and association with sociodemographics—data on a previously published randomised controlled trial. Schizophr Res 74:211–219, 2005

Romme M, Escher S: Accepting Voices: A New Approach to Voice-Hearing Outside the Illness Model. London, Mind, 1993

Romme M, Escher S: Understanding Voices: Coping With Auditory Hallucinations and Confusing Realities. London, Handsell, 1996

Romme M, Escher S: Making Sense of Voices: A Guide for Professionals Who Work With Voice Hearers. London, Mind, 2000

Shields B: Down Came the Rain. New York, Hyperion, 2005

Styron W: Darkness Visible: A Memoir of Madness. New York, Random House, 1990

Turkington D, Rathod S, Wilcock S, et al: Back to Life, Back to Normality: Cognitive Therapy, Recovery and Psychosis. Cambridge, England, Cambridge University Press, 2008

Wiles NJ, Zammit S, Bebbington P, et al: Self-reported psychotic symptoms in the general population: results from the longitudinal study of the British National Psychiatric Morbidity Survey. Br J Psychiatry 188:519–526, 2006

Wright JH, Basco MR: Getting Your Life Back: The Complete Guide to Recovery From Depression. New York, Free Press, 2002

Wright JH, Wright AS, Salmon P, et al: Development and initial testing of a multimedia program for computer-assisted cognitive therapy. Am J Psychother 56:76–86, 2002

Wright JH, Wright AS, Beck AT: Good Days Ahead: The Multimedia Program for Cognitive Therapy, Professional Edition. Louisville, KY, Mindstreet, 2004

Wright JH, Wright AS, Albano AM, et al: Computer-assisted cognitive therapy for depression: maintaining efficacy while reducing therapist time. Am J Psychiatry 162:1158–1164, 2005

4

Case Formulation and Treatment Planning

This chapter will describe how to work with patients in constructing biopsychosocial formulations for CBT. A general framework for developing CBT case conceptualizations has been outlined in an earlier book (Wright et al. 2006). This method is based on recommendations from the Academy of Cognitive Therapy (www.academyofct.org). Because details on basic procedures for case conceptualizations in CBT are available elsewhere (Wright et al. 2006), we focus here on providing practical guidance on developing formulations for patients with severe mental disorders. Case examples, based on four of the individuals featured in the video illustrations, are used to demonstrate methods of developing formulations using a timeline and Socratic questioning—a type of case conceptualization produced jointly with the patient. This process often leads to an improvement in insight for the patient and guides the therapist in treatment planning.

We also explain a method for producing mini-formulations for individual symptoms (e.g., delusions, mania, and depression). This procedure is a form of CBT shorthand, in line with the basic CBT model, that allows the patient to focus on some of the most relevant cognitive and behavioral factors that are exacerbating symptoms.

Treatment planning in CBT flows directly from the case formulation. The comprehensive biopsychosocial formulation provides the information needed for developing the full treatment plan, including interventions that address diverse factors that may influence symptom development or recovery (Figure 4–1). The mini-formulation only looks at a small slice of the overall picture but hones in on the cognitive-behavioral elements of the formulation to give the patient a road map for specific interventions that may have a high yield in reducing symptoms. We first describe methods for doing full biopsychosocial case conceptualizations and then provide some illustrations of the mini-formulation technique.

Developing the Biopsychosocial Case Conceptualization

A worksheet for developing biopsychosocial formulations for CBT is shown in Figure 4–2. A blank version of the CBT case formulation worksheet is provided in Appendix 1 ("Worksheets and Checklists") and can be downloaded from the American Psychiatric Publishing Web site (www. appi.org/pdf/62321). Figure 4–2 displays an example from the treatment of Mary, the woman with depression featured in Video Illustration 3.

As can be seen in the case example, the CBT case formulation worksheet details all of the elements from Figure 4–1, including formative influ-

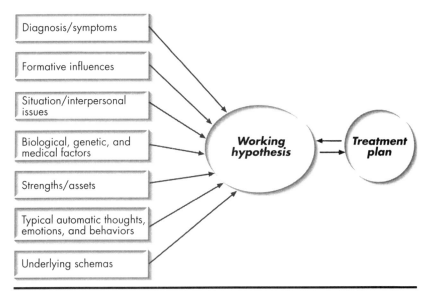

Figure 4–1. Case conceptualization flow chart.

Source. Reprinted from Wright JH, Basco MR, Thase ME: *Learning Cognitive-Behavior Therapy: An Illustrated Guide.* Washington, DC, American Psychiatric Publishing, 2006, p. 51. Used with permission. Copyright © 2006 American Psychiatric Publishing.

ences; situational issues; biological, genetic, and medical factors; strengths and assets; and most importantly, cognitive and behavioral components of the case conceptualization. In Mary's case, there was historical evidence of several developmental influences that may have played a role in subsequent depression—for example, lots of criticism when she was a child, a sense that she could never meet expectations of others, and an unfortunate accident that left her with a slight physical deformity. Her later problems with self-esteem appeared to be rooted, at least in part, in these earlier experiences. Also, Mary experienced a significant loss when her first husband cheated on her and then left her with a small child and limited ability to support herself. The pattern continued to some extent in her current marriage when her husband criticized her for not "pulling her share." There were some added biological contributors. Her mother had experienced depression and Mary had a diagnosis of hypothyroidism—a possible influence on the course of her mood disorder.

On the positive side, Mary had some significant strengths that could be harnessed in her fight against depression. She had a good track record of being able to work productively at several periods in her life. After her first husband left her, she had overcome depression and had worked steadily for several years to provide for her small child. Until recently, she had run a successful day care service out of her home. Mary was also a very loving mother who had excellent relationships with her children. Although her current marriage was strained by depression, it was basically intact; and her husband appeared to be committed to her. Mary's father, who had been somewhat distant when she was a child, was now retired and was expressing an interest in showing more support to Mary and her family.

The middle section of the case formulation worksheet shows three examples of the relationships between events, cognitions, emotions, and behavior, and then lists some underlying schemas or core beliefs. You may remember from Chapter 2 ("Engaging and Assessing") that Mary had some very dysfunctional cognitions about being referred to the cognitive-behavior therapist because her previous psychiatrist had told her that there was "nothing else I can do." The second example shows key cognitions and behaviors related to an incident of criticism from her husband. Methods for helping Mary with the suicidal thoughts stimulated by this argument with her husband are detailed in Chapter 7 ("Depression"). In the third situation, Mary's automatic thoughts about an invitation from a friend lead to dysphoric emotions and further social isolation.

The treatment goals, working hypothesis, and treatment plan are directly related to the biopsychosocial influences articulated in the formulation. Mary decided with her therapist to focus on the treatment goals

Patient Name: Mary

Diagnoses/Symptoms: Major depression, chronic.

Formative Influences: Mary's mother was very critical of her; Mary could never seem to "do anything right." Her father worked two jobs and was "never there." Mary had a bike accident at age 9 that left her with a slight limp. Her first husband was a hypercritical person who cheated on her.

Situational Issues: Current husband is also critical of Mary. Her work providing day care in her home has stopped because young children have grown older and are now attending school full time. Previous psychiatrist has "given up" on Mary.

Biological, Genetic, and Medical Factors: Mother was probably depressed; bike accident left Mary with a minor deformity; has hypothyroidism.

Strengths/Assets: Reasonably intelligent; worked steadily to support young child; although there is marital conflict, marriage is fairly solid; cares deeply for children and has excellent relationships with them; her father is back on the scene and wants to play a bigger role in family; desire to finish school and become a nurse.

Treatment Goals: 1) Break out of pattern of inactivity and social isolation, 2) improve relationship with husband, 3) relieve symptoms of depression.

Event 1	Event 2	Event 3
Psychiatrist refers me for CBT; says there is nothing else she can do.	Husband criticizes me; says I'm not pulling my weight.	I get a call from an old friend from school. She asks me to join a women's bowling league with her.
Automatic Thoughts	**Automatic Thoughts**	**Automatic Thoughts**
"She's given up on me." "Nothing will ever help." "I'm a hopeless case."	"It's true. I'm a drag on the family." "I don't do anything to help." "I'm a loser." "They would be better off with me not around."	"She's been a big success." "She has a great job and all kinds of friends." "I don't know why she asked me to join the league." "I've messed up my life and don't deserve to be around people like that."

Figure 4–2. Case formulation worksheet for Mary.

Emotions	Emotions	Emotions
Depressed A bit angry at my old psychiatrist	Depressed Anxious	Depressed Tense
Behaviors	**Behaviors**	**Behaviors**
Brooding about my fate. Went to appointment with new doctor but didn't expect much. Acting like I have given up—I don't do anything.	Considered suicide; became even more withdrawn and sulky than ever.	Politely told her no. Made an excuse about being too busy.

Schemas: "I'm never good enough." "I will never succeed." "I'm deformed." "I'm a hopeless case."

Working Hypothesis: Mary has repeated patterns of negative automatic thoughts and helpless, self-defeating behavior that are influenced by long-standing, maladaptive core beliefs. Perceived criticism from her mother, a minor physical deformity from a bike accident, and a failed first marriage have played roles in the development of low-self esteem and intense self-criticism. Current stressors, including negative feedback from her husband and loss of her role as an operator of an in-home day care business, are contributing to the problem. Mary's inability to break out of the pattern of inactivity has become part of a vicious cycle, in which lack of positive activity confirms her beliefs that she will never succeed and that she is a hopeless case—in turn, these beliefs make it extremely difficult for her to envision any change in her chronic depressive behavior. Hypothyroidism could influence depression.

Treatment Plan: 1) Tackle hopelessness about treatment and any suicidal thinking first—use guided discovery and other cognitive restructuring methods to generate hope and identify strengths; 2) assess suicidal risk and develop an antisuicide plan; 3) use activity scheduling and graded task assignments to treat low energy and anhedonia; 4) use schema modification methods (e.g., examining the evidence, developing alternative core beliefs, doing homework to practice revised schemas) to modify beliefs that are controlling self-esteem; 5) coordinate evaluation and management of thyroid disease with Mary's primary care doctor; 6) maximize pharmacotherapy regimen for depression; use sequential strategies for treatment resistance.

Figure 4–2. Case formulation worksheet for Mary.

that were set in Video Illustration 3 (as shown in Figure 4–2)—i.e., break
out of a pattern of inactivity and social isolation, improve her relationship
with her husband, and relieve symptoms of depression. The working hypothesis for treatment included the view that core beliefs about inade-
quacy and inability to achieve success were contributing to chronicity.
Also, the behavioral elements of depression (e.g., loss of energy, anhedonia, procrastination, inactivity) were seen as part of a vicious cycle that
was perpetuating her illness. Specific methods for reversing these patterns were detailed in the treatment plan.

Building a Timeline

One of the useful ways to obtain information for effective case formulations is to build a timeline by working backward from the present day. In
the session, this timeline can be drawn on a whiteboard, if available, and
then transferred to paper for further development as homework. The
family can also be engaged in helping with the CBT formulation process.
They can assist the patient by giving perspectives and adding information
for various periods on the time line.

   The process of creating a timeline is illustrated in the case of Brenda,
a woman with a long history of psychosis (Figure 4–3). Brenda was introduced in Chapter 3 ("Normalizing and Educating"), when Dr. Turkington
demonstrated procedures for normalizing symptoms, and you will learn
more about her in Chapter 6 ("Hallucinations"), where she appears in
video illustrations of CBT methods for coping with voices:

> Brenda is a 47-year-old African American woman who reports a history
> of hallucinations for at least 25 years. The voices began when she was 22
> and in nursing school. She is not sure how it all started, but she had stress
> from studying, wasn't sleeping well, had trouble concentrating, and began
> to hear voices telling her, "You're stupid"; "Give up"; "Quit." The voices
> would also call her names. At first she tried not to believe them because
> she didn't see herself as stupid. But the voices became insistent, and she
> had increasing trouble handling her schoolwork. She became convinced
> the voices were from the devil. They were definitely male, but she had
> never heard these voices before and couldn't recognize them as belonging
> to anyone she had known. Brenda had to drop out of school and go back
> home to live with her parents. She was treated with haloperidol at this
> time and eventually improved. But the voices never went away com-
> pletely—they were sometimes reduced to whispers.
>   She claimed a solid family upbringing. Brenda was the fourth of seven
> children and described her parents as loving. They were very religious (Bap-
> tist) and went to church "all the time." There was no history in the family of
> psychosis or other mental disorder except for one aunt who received long-
> acting injections of antipsychotics and was repeatedly hospitalized. The

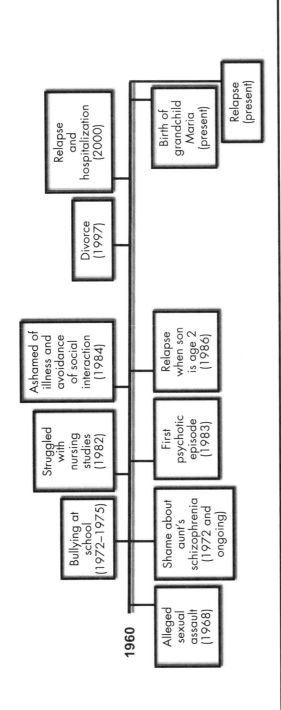

Figure 4–3.   Long-term timeline for Brenda (47 years).

aunt was always spoken about in hushed tones. Brenda once told her parents that a babysitter had "been sexy" with her, but she was not believed and no action was taken. During her school years, Brenda had been the victim of bullying. She was called "fatso" and only had a limited circle of friends. There was no history of any substance abuse in Brenda or her family.

After Brenda returned home from a hospitalization at age 22, her parents treated the problem as if it were shameful. Brenda was "hidden"— they kept her illness a big secret. They watched her very carefully because they "didn't know what to expect."

Brenda did better after about a year of being back at home. Subsequently, she was able to work intermittently as an aide in a nursing home for older persons. She worked the second shift, which suited her because she could stay away from others. Brenda met her husband at about age 24. She became pregnant "pretty quickly" and eventually married him. Things were going fairly well until her first child, Stacy, a male, was about 2 years old. At that time, he became very hard to manage. He was "into everything." Also, Brenda got a new supervisor at work who pressed her to work harder and made her work extra shifts. It was at this time that the voices came back very strongly and were very disturbing. They told her, "Hit him [the baby Stacy]"; "Slap him"; "Choke him." She didn't want to obey the voices, but she was tormented by them. Her husband offered little help. He told her it was her job to "deal with it." Brenda never hurt Stacy or anyone else. Nevertheless, the voices scared her so much that she asked her mother to take Stacy. Her mother did this for about 2 years (during which time Brenda would visit with Stacy about three times a week). After the voices calmed, she took Stacy back home. Brenda and Stacy have appeared to have a good relationship. He is an only child.

During the next 20 years, Brenda went through a divorce, worked part-time, continued to have intermittent hallucinations, and received ongoing treatment with supportive therapy at a community mental health center and with various antipsychotic medications. There was one additional hospitalization at about age 40, but none since then. Brenda has been diagnosed with schizophrenia, and she is aware of this diagnosis. Her recent treatment has consisted of risperidone and a visit with a therapist (nonspecific therapy) two times a month. Brenda admits that she sometimes misses doses of her medication.

The current consultation with Dr. Turkington has been prompted by another relapse of hallucinations. Brenda believes the voices have worsened with the birth of her first grandchild, a girl named Maria, about 5 weeks ago. Brenda desperately wants to be with her grandchild and assist in her care, but the voices tell Brenda, "You're stupid"; "You're no good"; "You're bad-bad-bad"; "Hurt Maria." Also, her sleeping is much worse than usual.

Brenda currently lives by herself. She is on disability, but is able to manage her finances well. She is active in her local Baptist church. When asked about what makes the voices worse, she lists "when it is quiet, nighttime, drinking lots of coffee." Things that she think may make the voices better are doing an activity with a friend at church, singing, playing a CD and singing along with it, visiting her mother, a good night's sleep, some TV shows ("The Price is Right"). Activities that don't seem to make any difference (in intensity of voices) are prayer and being at Stacy's and seeing Maria.

Brenda wants help so that she doesn't hurt her grandchild and so that she can be a part of the family.

Socratic Questioning to Establish a Timeline

An example was given in Chapter 3 ("Normalizing and Educating") of examining the antecedents of the emergence of a severe mental disorder (schizophrenia). This process involves asking a series of questions about the various stressors that were taking place and the patient's thoughts, feelings, and behaviors in the lead up to the emergence of illness. Some examples of questions that may help in establishing these relationships are provided in Table 4–1.

Table 4–1. Inductive questioning to establish a timeline

Can you remember when you last felt really well?

OK…let's take it from there; what was happening in your life at that time?

What age were you and where were you living?

Were there any particular problems going on?

How did your depression/mood swings/voices/delusions first start?

What was happening at that time?

What was going through your mind?

In an examination of the antecedents of the psychosis, manic episode, or depression, we work forward in time from the point where patients last felt really well up to the point of symptom emergence. The line of questioning described in Table 4–1 can be expanded by asking further questions about school or work, relationships, and leisure pursuits. When stressors or other important influences are identified, it is often helpful to ask patients to describe what was going through their mind at that time (automatic thoughts). Other exercises can be used to aid recall and capture automatic thoughts. These might include role-play or imagery as illustrated in the following dialogue:

> Dr. Turkington: OK, you were mentioning that you were a bit stressed during your school years. Just close your eyes for a couple of minutes and imagine yourself back in the classroom. How do you feel and what is going through your mind?
>
> Brenda: Nervous…I am never good enough at my studies, and two of the girls are calling me "fat and stupid."
>
> Dr. Turkington: That sounds unpleasant….What do you do to cope?
>
> Brenda: I can't tell anyone. I don't think anyone will believe me. My confidence is totally gone.
>
> Dr. Turkington: How do you feel, and what are you thinking?
>
> Brenda: Very sad…that I am not as good as the others.

Having discussed possible antecedents of an illness episode, we often find significant environmental stressors that may have precipitated symptoms. Patients have often never realized that incremental stress can trigger psychosis, mood swings, or severe depression in vulnerable people. If the patient is interested in learning about the degree of vulnerability, we can then begin from the time of birth and work forward to further develop the timeline. Linking up the timeline, examining the antecedents, and assessing biological and social influences leads to the full biopsychosocial formulation. Some other questions to add detail to the formulation are listed in Table 4–2.

If there is a sign of significant distress in working though any specific points in the timeline, efforts should be devoted to relieving emotional pain associated with these particular areas. Using CBT techniques, we can often help the patient to take a more balanced view of upsetting situations and get things back in perspective, as demonstrated in the following example:

> Dr. Turkington: You are telling me that when you were 8 years old you had a problem with the babysitter "being sexy." How did you feel then? It is obviously upsetting for you to remember it now.
>
> Brenda: I felt guilty and sad.
>
> Dr. Turkington: What was going through your mind?
>
> Brenda: That it was my fault…that I did something wrong.
>
> Dr. Turkington: How could it have been your fault? You were only a child. Surely if a child is badly treated by a babysitter, it is the adult's fault.

The Cross-Sectional View: Obtaining Examples of Current Cognitions and Behaviors

One of the most important components of the full biopsychosocial formulation method recommended by the Academy of Cognitive Therapy (www.academyofct.org) and Wright et al. (2006) is to elicit several ex-

---

Table 4–2. Questions to assess vulnerability to severe mental illnesses

---

Do you know anything about your birth? Was your mother ill beforehand or was it a difficult birth? These questions are searching for any evidence of maternal viral infection or hypoxic brain damage at birth in relation to a diagnosis of schizophrenia.

Did you suffer any major losses in childhood such as the early death of a parent, sibling, or loved relative? This question aims to identify any key loss experiences that might predispose an individual to depression or other conditions in later life.

Did you have any episodes of bad treatment during childhood such as beatings or sexual assault from an adult? Childhood abuse has been shown to be a predisposing factor for the subsequent development of adult psychosis, particularly hallucinations (Read et al. 2005) and other psychiatric conditions.

Have you always been the type of person who has been fascinated by the occult, magic, and unusual religions? This question is attempting to look for any personality predisposition from schizotypal personality traits.

Have you always been a negativistic or perfectionistic type of person? These traits can predispose to depression.

During your adolescent years were you the subject of extreme bullying? It has been shown that repeated bullying adversely affects self-esteem and can also predispose someone to psychosis.

---

amples of typical relationships among events, cognitions, emotions, and behaviors in the "here and now." These examples can be used as parts of mini-formulations to choose specific treatment methods (as described later in the chapter). The Academy of Cognitive Therapy uses the term *cross-sectional* to describe this part of the formulation because the focus is on current thinking and behavior. The Academy uses the term *longitudinal* to describe the parts of the formulation that consider developmental factors and other long-standing influences.

In helping Brenda develop the cross-sectional component of her formulation, we outlined the following example:

> Event: I hear a voice saying, "Hurt Maria."
> Automatic Thoughts: I might harm the baby. I'm not safe to be with her.
>   It must be the devil talking to me.
> Emotions: Anxiety, abdominal churning, fast breathing
> Behaviors: Run out of son's house.

Once we have access to the patient's typical automatic thoughts, emotions, and behaviors, we can begin to discuss the best way forward. It is vital that the patient be agreeable to the next step so that interventions are not attempted before the patient is ready. For Brenda, one of the early targets for therapy was to revise her maladaptive appraisal of the meaning of the hallucinations (i.e., coming from the devil). Then work could begin on developing coping skills.

Identifying Schemas

In talking with patients about their childhood and adolescence, it is important to attempt to identify core beliefs (schemas) that may be related to illness expression. Beliefs that are laid down in this period of life can play an influential role in psychiatric illnesses because they direct patients' appraisal of situations and their patterns of automatic thoughts and behavior (Clark et al. 1999). Some core beliefs about the self that may be discovered in talking with patients with severe mental illnesses are "I'm not good enough"; "People cannot be trusted"; "I am worthless"; "I am unlovable"; "I am a failure."

Key schemas in schizophrenia can include more distorted beliefs, such as "I am evil"; "I am damaged"; "I am deficient." Example of core beliefs that can be found in bipolar disorder include "I am special"; "I am a failure"; "I must be in control."

People with maladaptive core personal beliefs can attempt to compensate with one of these types of schemas: "I must be approved of at all costs" or "I must be successful."

The various beliefs that a person holds about himself regulate self-esteem (Beck et al. 2003). Later in the course of CBT, techniques can be used to modify these beliefs to improve self-confidence and self-efficacy (see Chapter 7, "Depression," for illustrations). In developing a formulation with Brenda, we detected these core beliefs: "Mental illness is your own fault"; "No one will trust someone who is mentally ill"; "I must be in control"; "The world is a very dangerous place"; "You must always protect yourself."

The Working Hypothesis

The working hypothesis pulls together the most important observations from the formulation into a proposed explanation for the development and maintenance of the patient's symptoms. In the early parts of therapy, the working hypothesis may be rudimentary, and significant gaps in knowledge may exist. But, as therapy evolves and the theories are tested with interventions, a more complete picture usually emerges. Brenda appeared to carry a genetic vulnerability to schizophrenia. She also developed a schema of believing that she was stupid and no good due to sexual assault and subsequent bullying. Brenda came to believe that schizophrenia was a shameful thing due to the reactions of her family to her psychosis and the secrecy surrounding her aunt's illness. Triggers for her first psychotic episode may have been overwork, sleep deprivation, and feelings of failure. Exacerbations occurred at times of increased stress, and adherence problems may have played a role in symptom breakthroughs and relapses.

The Treatment Plan

The primary value of performing a case formulation rests in the treatment plan. A comprehensive formulation using CBT principles will typically generate multiple ideas for useful interventions. These interventions should tie directly to cognitive and behavioral theories and lay out a reasonable course of action. If methods chosen are not successful, then therapist and patient can revise the plan and try again. Because Brenda was experiencing so much shame from her illness and was attributing voices to the devil, the first priorities were to normalize symptoms and to work on revising her explanation for symptoms. The full biopsychosocial formulation and treatment plan for Brenda is shown in Figure 4–4.

Additional Examples of Biopsychosocial Formulations

Two more examples of comprehensive case conceptualizations are provided here for patients featured in the video illustrations.

Majir

Dr. Kingdon engages this young man with a paranoid psychosis by gently exploring the nature of his key concerns. Dr. Kingdon then gradually starts to build a formulation. In Video Illustration 1, only a partial understanding of Majir's problems can be developed. But, there appears to be a pattern of inactivity and social withdrawal related to paranoid thoughts about the intentions of others. Also, Majir is able to talk briefly about a possible triggering event when he was a teenager. The formulation shown in Figure 4–5 was developed over several subsequent sessions, some of which will be shown in video illustrations later in the book.

Angela

Dr. Basco illustrates methods for working with bipolar disorder in her treatment of Angela. At the time of referral, which was initiated by her

Patient Name: Brenda

Diagnoses/Symptoms: Schizophrenia. Primary symptoms are auditory hallucinations, delusions, negative symptoms, depression, anxiety.

Formative Influences: Brenda was brought up in a strict Baptist family. There was an alleged sexual assault and bullying during childhood. She struggled with her nursing studies, and at the time of her first psychotic episode her illness was a source of shame for the family. When her son was 2 years old, he became hard to manage, which was very stressful for her.

Situational Issues: New grandchild Maria has been born. The stress of the new role as grandmother has been a trigger for relapse.

Biological, Genetic, and Medical Factors: There is an aunt with suspected schizophrenia. Adherence with antipsychotics is partial. No medical problems.

Strengths/Assets: A kind and friendly woman; no history of violence or aggression to others; no intent to harm; loves family and is highly motivated to spend time with granddaughter, Maria. Has support from family and from local Baptist church.

Treatment Goals: 1) Reduce stigma, 2) develop more functional explanations of psychotic symptoms, 3) cope better with hallucinations, 4) improve adherence, 5) reduce anxiety that she might harm Maria, 6) begin to spend time with Maria again, 7) improve negative core schemas, 8) develop a relapse prevention plan.

Event 1	Event 2	Event 3
Hear a voice saying "Hurt Maria"	Attempt to use a coping strategy	Discuss the voices in CBT session
Automatic Thoughts	**Automatic Thoughts**	**Automatic Thoughts**
"I might harm the baby." "I'm not safe to be with her." "It must be the devil talking to me."	"This is pointless." "Medication is the only thing that ever helped before."	"The psychiatrist is scared of me." "He knows I am evil." "He will call the police and have me locked up."

Figure 4–4. Case formulation worksheet for Brenda.

Emotions	Emotions	Emotions
Anxiety, abdominal churning, fast breathing	Frustration	Anxiety, tension, and sweating
Behaviors	**Behaviors**	**Behaviors**
Run out of son's house.	Stop using the coping method after one attempt.	Talk about something else. Leave and go home as soon as possible.

Schemas: "Mental illness is your own fault." "No one will trust someone who is mentally ill." "I must be in control." "The world is a very dangerous place." "You must always protect yourself."

Working Hypothesis: Brenda is deeply ashamed of her schizophrenia. Her family background (e.g., an undisclosed sexual assault, her illness being "hidden away," and their strong religious faith) contributed to the development of self-blaming schemas and spiritual explanations of voice hearing. Current situational factors (i.e., the birth of baby Maria and the stresses of her new role as grandmother), in addition to partial adherence to medication, have been triggers for relapse. Brenda does not currently have effective coping strategies for hallucinations.

Treatment Plan: 1) Reduce stigma by using psychoeducation and normalizing; 2) use examining the evidence to develop more functional explanations of voice hearing; 3) develop and test different coping strategies; 4) use imagery and role-play to practice the new coping strategies for being with Maria; 5) use CBT methods for adherence, including behavioral reminder strategies; 6) work on schemas to develop less extreme core beliefs; 7) develop a relapse prevention plan; 8) pay careful attention to the therapeutic relationship, check out possible dysfunctional cognitions about the therapist, and routinely ask for feedback.

Figure 4–4. Case formulation worksheet for Brenda.

Patient Name: Majir

Diagnoses/Symptoms: Schizophrenia. Primary symptoms are a paranoid delusional system, negative symptoms, anxiety in social situations, and lack of insight.

Formative Influences: Paranoid trait within personality; only male child in a family with high parental expectations; failure in school exams.

Situational Issues: Parents have become increasingly critical of Majir's social isolation and lack of progress toward independent living. Majir is unemployed and has very limited social relationships.

Biological, Genetic, and Medical Factors: Forceps delivery at time of birth; uncle with suspected schizophrenia; no medical problems.

Strengths/Assets: Intelligent, articulate young man who is, at least to a degree, psychologically minded.

Treatment Goals: 1) Build trust and a therapeutic alliance to facilitate retention in CBT, 2) reduce conviction in delusions and provide alternative explanations, 3) increase social activities, 4) enhance self-esteem.

Event 1	Event 2	Event 3
I was asked for a sexual act after a night out.	Teenagers saw me going for a computer game at the mall.	Father asked me to go out and find a job.
Automatic Thoughts	**Automatic Thoughts**	**Automatic Thoughts**
"People just use me." "This is terrible." "People will be disgusted with me."	"They are looking at me." "They know all about me." "They know I am a piece of shit."	"He knows there is no hope for me." "He thinks I am completely useless."
Emotions	**Emotions**	**Emotions**
Anxiety, panic, sweating hands, fast breathing	Anxiety, tension, fast breathing	Sadness

Figure 4–5. Case formulation worksheet for Majir.

Behaviors	Behaviors	Behaviors
Avoidance of further social contact	Avoidance, return home without the computer game	Hide away and avoid father, give up on doing anything

Schemas: "I am different from other people." "Others know everything about me." "I must be approved of by other people."

Working Hypothesis: Majir has always had a sensitive component in his personality and has had chronic low self-esteem. He has struggled with socializing and has developed a schema that there is something different about him. His family background includes expectations of success and approval. A request for a sexual act by two men he met that he thought were friends appears to have been a critical incident. His extreme sensitivity, hypervigilance, and paranoia are leading to marked avoidance that lowers his self-esteem.

Treatment Plan: 1) Gradual relationship building to foster trust; 2) psychoeducation regarding the ability of others to know what people are thinking; 3) Socratic questioning with discussion of alternative explanations; 4) correction of cognitive distortions and development of rational responding for negative automatic thoughts; 5) homework exercises involving gradual exposure to social situations; 6) schema-focused work in relation to his core beliefs about being different, being a failure, and having others be able to read his mind; 7) later in therapy, revise maladaptive schemas concerning approval and achievement.

Figure 4–5. Case formulation worksheet for Majir.

employer, Angela demonstrated several symptoms of mania. In Video Illustration 2, Dr. Basco uses guided discovery to help Angela begin to come to terms with the possibility that she has bipolar disorder. Although Angela disagrees with the diagnosis at first, she is able to describe current problems at work and mood symptoms that stretch back to age 17 when she first became severely depressed and attempted suicide. Similar previous episodes were discussed during which the patient experienced hyperactivity, poor judgment, and risk taking (e.g., spending sprees, getting married after only knowing the man for 2 weeks). Numerous thoughts were revealed that appeared to be grandiose at first view ("I am the most creative person there"; "They have to do it the way I want to do it"; "They are jealous") and may have contained cognitive distortions. Angela's grandiose thoughts had been affecting her behavior at work (e.g., yelling and screaming at customers and coworkers).

Patient Name: Angela

Diagnoses/Symptoms: Bipolar disorder. Current symptoms are mania, mood-congruent grandiose delusions, decreased need for sleep, hypersexuality, disinhibition, irritability, and hyperactivity. Behavior is potentially damaging to Angela's work and social life.

Formative Influences: Uncle had bipolar disorder and substance use problems. Father was a strong role model of self-confidence. He encouraged her to assert her intelligence in work situations. Family did not believe in mental illness.

Situational Issues: Increased pressure at work to deliver a new contract; some male coworkers play along with provocative behavior.

Biological, Genetic, and Medical Factors: Genetic predisposition to bipolar disorder; lapses in adherence with lithium carbonate due to denial of the illness and pressure from boyfriend; no medical illnesses.

Strengths/Assets: Very capable, optimistic, articulate, and intelligent; appears to have capacity for improved insight; valued employee who is typically very creative and productive at work; good support from boyfriend except for his negative attitudes about medication.

Treatment Goals: 1) Fully recognize signs and symptoms of mania and hypomania, 2) reduce conviction in grandiose delusions, 3) reduce impulsive and potentially damaging behaviors, 4) improve adherence with lithium, 5) develop a relapse prevention plan.

Event 1	Event 2	Event 3
Argument with boss at work	Friendly interactions with male coworkers	Boyfriend unhappy with diagnosis of bipolar disorder
Automatic Thoughts	**Automatic Thoughts**	**Automatic Thoughts**
"He doesn't know his job." "He is jealous." "I know what the customers want." "I am the most creative person there."	"They are in love with me."	"I don't believe it either." "It is a shameful diagnosis."
Emotions	**Emotions**	**Emotions**
Irritated Angry	Excited Euphoric Feeling sexy	Shame Sadness

Figure 4–6.   Case formulation worksheet for Angela.

Behaviors	Behaviors	Behaviors
Pace up and down; shout back; drink more coffee.	Send them suggestive pictures of me; flirt with them.	Skip doses of medication; hide medication from him; act like I'm not taking medicine.

Schemas: "I am special." "People love me and want to like me." "I am competent." "People are jealous of me." "I am at my best at work."

Working Hypothesis: Angela has a robust self-esteem when euthymic or manic and often believes herself to be special. She has a genetic predisposition to bipolar disorder but is ashamed of the diagnosis, in part because her family did not approve of her uncle, who also had bipolar disorder. Denial of illness has kept her from pursuing treatment. She wants to please others and will therefore avoid discussion of her illness with significant others. Current situational factors (e.g., sleep loss from increased work activities, excessive caffeine intake) may have played a role in triggering symptoms.

Treatment Plan: 1) Help Angela adjust to the diagnosis of bipolar disorder using cognitive restructuring (e.g., Socratic questioning, examining the evidence, percentage-of-belief allocation); 2) develop an action plan for reducing risky behavior; 3) teach her to evaluate depressive and grandiose thoughts using cognitive-behavior techniques (e.g., spotting cognitive errors, thought recording, examining the evidence); 4) use CBT methods to improve sleep hygiene; 5) gradually develop a relapse prevention plan; 6) role-play to help Angela to feel more confident in discussing her diagnosis with her boyfriend; 7) later in therapy, work on modifying underlying schemas.

Figure 4–6. Case formulation worksheet for Angela.

In this first session, Dr. Basco is able to build key elements of the case conceptualization and to devise therapy strategies that specifically address Angela's grandiosity and denial of illness. The interventions shown in the video illustrations are drawn from the comprehensive formulation that is shown in the Figure 4–6. This conceptualization was detailed over several early sessions with Angela.

Learning Exercise 4–1. Developing a Biopsychosocial Formulation

Would you be better prepared to help patients develop biopsychosocial formulations if you constructed one for yourself? Let's do this using a timeline.

1. Take any current emotional or behavioral problem
that is minor. We all have one (e.g., nerves about
speaking in public, getting angry at other drivers,
needing to always be in control, perfectionism, or
being a bit of a workaholic).

2. Put this problem at the end of the timeline and
work backward to childhood to see if there are any
roots for this problem in your early years.

3. Put any key factors down on the timeline.

4. Mark when your problem first appeared. Look at
the stressors present at that time. Mark these on the
timeline.

5. Identify any current automatic thoughts or
behaviors that might be perpetuating this problem.

Developing your own biopsychosocial formulation is
usually a very interesting process. It can yield a sense
of balance and perspective.

If this exercise upsets you in any way, then please seek
appropriate support.

How to Construct and Use a Mini-Formulation

The mini-formulation approach involves collaborative work with the patient in using the basic CBT model to understand key relationships between environmental events, thoughts, emotions, and behaviors. Within
the framework of the comprehensive formulation described earlier, patient and therapist function as a team to identify typical patterns of cognitive and behavioral responses that are 1) perpetuating and/or deepening
symptoms, 2) representative of the patient's style of information processing and behavior, and 3) good targets for change. The essence of this approach is to drill down on the most salient cognitive and behavioral
elements of the formulation to help patients understand symptom development and to plan useful interventions.

   In Chapter 1 ("Introduction"), we gave examples of how the basic
CBT model helped explain the symptoms that Majir, Angela, and Mary
were experiencing. The circular diagrams shown in Chapter 1 are one
way of diagramming mini-formulations with patients. We often use this

type of circular diagram early in treatment to help teach patients about the basics of CBT and to get them engaged in planning ways to change. For example, the diagram for Majir (Figure 4–7) showed how an environmental event (walking to a store in the mall) triggered dysfunctional thoughts, dysphoric mood, and an avoidance response. As will be shown in the next chapter, Dr. Kingdon's approach to Majir was geared toward modifying problems at two points in this diagram: 1) cognitive appraisal (self-condemning and paranoid thoughts); and 2) behaviors (acting like he is a loser who doesn't deserve to be in the company of others, inability to complete tasks, avoidance of social contacts). As shown in Figure 4–7, Dr. Kingdon simplified terms from the CBT model to help Majir understand the basics of their planned approach to his problems.

Mini-formulations can use other diagrams that may include basic schemas, coping strategies, or a variety of other basic CBT concepts or methods. However, in all cases it is best to keep the mini-formulation 1) simple, 2) practical, 3) easily understood, and 4) directed at meaningful change. We do not always write out mini-formulations in sessions, especially with patients who are difficult to engage or who may be quite fragile. But, efforts

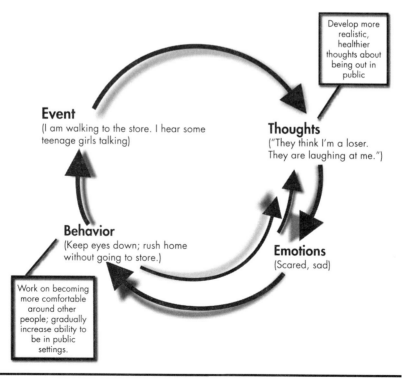

Figure 4–7. A mini-formulation: Majir's example.

are made to help all patients understand key concepts involved in the mini-formulation and to use this method to direct collaborative work. When possible, pen and paper or, even better, a whiteboard with some colored pens can be used in sessions so that patients and therapists can draw in the various elements of the mini-formulation.

Guided discovery is a fundamental process in developing mini-formulations. Patients are guided to explore their experiences to reach some new conclusions that will relieve symptoms and improve functioning. We usually start by asking the patient to tell us what she would really like to talk about (agenda setting). This may be a symptom like voice hearing or paranoia, but it could be a stressful event or a social problem. It is ideal if the patient is having the problem during the session (e.g., hallucinations, intense depressed mood, paranoia, grandiosity), because the symptoms are "fresh." When the problem is immediate, patients may be more likely to access intense, and especially salient, cognitions and emotions. If the symptom is not present during the interview, or if patients are having difficulty in remembering details of troubling situations or social difficulties, they can be asked to give an example of the problem that may have occurred during the previous week or to use imagery to recall automatic thoughts.

The following dialogue gives an example of the use of guided discovery in building a mini-formulation. The patient in this example, Terrance, has intense auditory hallucinations. The psychiatrist asks a series of questions that draw out the relationships between Terrance's thoughts and his behavior. They then begin to develop coping strategies, as shown below:

Psychiatrist: You want to feel less distressed by these nasty voices....How bad are they?
Terrance: Going nonstop, 24/7...giving me total hell.
Psychiatrist: How would you score them on a 0–10 point scale if 10 is the worst distress you can imagine?
Terrance: Ten, man...Ten!
Psychiatrist: Can you give me an example of what they might say?
Terrance: They say, "He is a waste...a total waste."
Psychiatrist: What goes through your mind at that point and how do you feel?
Terrance: I'm thinking, "How dare they—the scum..." I pace up and down and shout at them, "Shut up; leave me alone!" I'm furious with them.
Psychiatrist: What effect does this seem to have on the voices?
Terrance: They get worse for a while until I settle down.
Psychiatrist: So what might we do differently?
Terrance: Stay calm....Go for a walk....Put the TV on.
Psychiatrist: Sounds good...So we will put the TV on or go for a walk. Maybe we can also work on some calming thoughts, such as "It's only my illness acting up because of lack of sleep or stress" or "Lots of folks hear voices and live with it—so can I."

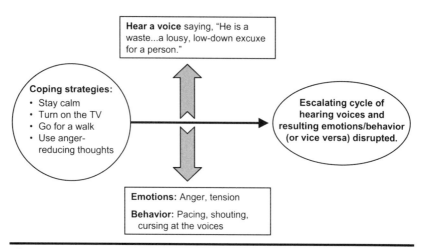

Figure 4–8. A mini-formulation: Terrance's example.

The mini-formulation developed with Terrance shows the disturbing emotional and behavioral effects of the voices. The potential coping strategies developed in the session are added to the diagram as a way of highlighting actions he can take to manage the problem. Thus, his mini-formulation includes the beginnings of a treatment plan (Figure 4–8).

After developing mini-formulations in treatment sessions, patients can be given a sheet of paper with the diagram on it to review for homework and to use for future reference. We often find that the simple explanations in mini-formulations have not been investigated by the patient previously and that efforts to develop these shorthand formulations can lead to highly significant treatment gains. Additional examples of mini-formulations can be found in Kingdon and Turkington (2002).

Summary

Key Points for Clinicians

- A full biopsychosocial formulation for CBT includes current symptoms, formative influences, stressors, biological factors, and patient strengths. The most important component is an understanding of the cognitive and behavioral elements of symptom development and maintenance.
- A timeline and Socratic questioning are useful tools for developing case conceptualizations.
- For many patients, the case formulation can be a very illuminating procedure. However, at times the process can be painful for patients

when they identify stresses, losses, and the impact of the illness on their lives.
- Mini-formulations are shorthand versions of more comprehensive case conceptualizations. These succinct explanations are used in sessions to help patients understand and use CBT methods to manage symptoms.
- CBT formulations are used to design the treatment plan.

Concepts and Skills for Patients to Learn

- Often symptoms can be better understood if stresses and vulnerabilities are recognized.
- It can be very helpful to work with a therapist on understanding how one's style of thinking, life history, physical health and biology, and social and cultural background can be involved in development of symptoms.
- In CBT, a brief written diagram (mini-formulation) is often used to sketch out coping strategies for common problems.
- It is extremely important to identify and draw on one's personal strengths. Everyone has strengths that can be used to fight illnesses and promote well-being.
- If it is stressful talking about any particular issue from the past, inform your therapist that this subject is upsetting. She should be able to help you cope with this stress.

References

Beck AT, Freeman A, Davis DD, et al: Cognitive Therapy of Personality Disorders, 2nd Edition. New York, Guilford, 2003

Clark DA, Beck AT, Alford BA: Scientific Foundations of Cognitive Theory and Therapy of Depression. New York, Wiley, 1999

Kingdon DG, Turkington D: A Case Study Guide to Cognitive Behavior Therapy of Psychosis. Chichester, England, Wiley, 2002

Read J, van Os J, Morrison AP, et al: Childhood trauma, psychosis and schizophrenia: a literature review with theoretical and clinical implications. Acta Psychiatr Scand 112:330–350, 2005

Wright JH, Basco MR, Thase ME: Learning Cognitive-Behavior Therapy: An Illustrated Guide. Washington, DC, American Psychiatric Publishing, 2006

5

Delusions

This chapter provides a description of the key elements involved in treating delusions with CBT. First we discuss how the general features of CBT can be employed to decrease delusional beliefs. We then explore how the classic definition of delusions may need revision if the clinician seeks to use cognitive-behavioral methods to induce change. The main emphasis of the chapter is on describing and illustrating specific CBT methods for modifying delusional beliefs in schizophrenia. Guidelines are also provided for dealing with resistant delusions and delusional beliefs in mood disorders.

Treating Delusions: Basic CBT Processes

The processes of engagement, assessment, formulation, normalizing, and educating described in earlier chapters are essential steps in therapeutic work with delusions:

- *Engagement* typically affects paranoia. When the therapist engages the patient effectively in CBT, trust begins to build, and the patient's paranoid beliefs about other individuals and the world in general are often undermined.
- *Assessment* takes patients through the development of their symptoms and life experiences and, in the process, stimulates a reexamination of assumptions and beliefs and a consideration of alternative explanations.

- *Formulation* is the process of making sense of predisposing, precipitating, perpetuating, and protective factors by examining thoughts, feelings, and behaviors within the social context. An effective formulation provides direction for specific interventions to modify delusions.
- *Normalization* destigmatizes psychotic illnesses, enhances the collaborative relationship, and promotes active coping.
- *Psychoeducation* helps patients understand their illnesses, accept treatment interventions, and learn effective tools to manage symptoms.

A good therapeutic relationship is necessary for CBT procedures to be utilized by the patient and for these methods to be effective. Initially, a working relationship may form the basis for assessment and formulation. But as the relationship strengthens over time, there can be greater amounts of disclosure, and sensitive areas can be more easily discussed. The process of examining beliefs and experiences in an accepting way, in itself, also builds the therapeutic relationship. Although beliefs may be resistant to change in the early phase of therapy, the process of engagement often is associated with the uncovering of important underlying issues or influences. Discussion and management of these concerns often results in significant behavioral change. Only later may the delusional beliefs fade in intensity or relevance.

When the clinician performs an assessment, it is very important to carefully examine historical details in the period leading up to the first episode. The circumstances surrounding onset of symptoms, including any possible stressful events, need to be outlined. Onset of the psychotic beliefs themselves should also be fully explored. The therapist attempts to uncover how thoughts were linked to specific triggers and how these came together to form strong, seemingly unshakable beliefs. Because most clinicians have not attempted to perform this sort of analysis before learning CBT methods for psychosis, the process of trying to understand and formulate associations between psychosocial influences and the development of psychotic symptoms may seem alien at first. It can be a big leap to switch from believing that psychotic symptoms have no specific meaning and can only be understood as faulty brain functioning to endorsing and effectively using a cognitive-behavioral-biological-social formulation that searches for stress-vulnerability explanations.

To some extent, work on developing CBT formulations requires that therapists believe that linkages among environmental events, patient vulnerabilities, and symptom expression exist and can be found. Our experience is that as therapists increasingly find such patterns in their clinical practices, such a belief becomes easier to hold. The triggers that are identified are not always major events. They can sometimes be reminders of past negative experiences or the final stage of an accumulation of minor, stressful events that have been sufficient to tip the person into a psychotic episode. The process of disease expression is then often amplified by negative experiences associated with becoming ill (e.g., hospital admission, family conflict, or discrimination in the workplace).

Normalizing and educating are other extremely important basic processes to use in CBT for delusions. If patients are heavily stigmatized and believe that they should be shunned by others, they may have difficulty engaging in good therapeutic relationships and accepting that CBT methods could help them make positive changes. On the other hand, patients who recognize that their problems are not vastly dissimilar from normal experiences, and who sense that their therapists view them as persons instead of illnesses, may be more likely to benefit from the CBT approach. Some of the useful normalizing and educating strategies for delusions include explaining that paranoia can occur when a person is under stress (e.g., if one walks into a room and it goes quiet, it is a perfectly natural, immediate, and common response to question whether one was being talked about). Suspiciousness or heightened vigilance is a normal adaptive response to feeling threatened in some way. It is then important to find out if the beliefs about being threatened are accurate or not. This might involve checking out whether a threat exists (e.g., to check if one was actually being spoken about by asking someone who was in the room at the time what the topic of conversation was before one arrived). As noted in Chapter 3 ("Normalizing and Educating"), readings and Web sites can also provide useful information to patients who experience delusions. See Appendix 2, "Cognitive-Behavior Therapy Resources," for additional reference.

Treatment of delusions in patients with schizophrenia usually requires a "go slow," gradual approach in which the therapist gears interventions to match the patient's degree of trust, level of thought disorder, and willingness to explore alternatives. Often, sessions are shorter than the traditional 45- to 50-minute sessions typically used with depressed or anxious outpatients. Feedback is given frequently, and therapists may often pause to check for understanding. Homework assignments are designed to be simple, practical, and achievable. These general procedures for treating patients with delusions are modeled throughout this chapter in video illustrations of Dr. Kingdon and Majir.

Before moving ahead to detail specific techniques for working with delusions, we need to consider just what is meant by the term *delusions* and to discuss indications for treating this symptom.

Defining Delusions

DSM-IV describes delusions as "erroneous beliefs that usually involve a misinterpretation of perceptions or experiences" (American Psychiatric Association 1994, p. 275). However this definition needs reconsideration:

1. Describing delusional beliefs as irrational or erroneous reflects an all-or-nothing approach. For many patients, understanding the origins of their beliefs leads to an appreciation of why they believe what they do. On occasion, beliefs initially described as delusional turn out to be true. More commonly, beliefs are not factually accurate but are based on actual circumstances. For example, John, age 61, was convinced that he was being persecuted by his employers because they were constantly moving him around his department and giving him menial tasks to do. He also began to believe that this persecution extended to his golf club and that he was being shunned by other club members because one of his employers was a member of the organizing committee there. His reaction was to repeatedly cross-question people at the club about his suspicions. Eventually, this behavior led to a request for him to leave, further reinforcing his belief that he was being persecuted. As these issues were discussed with John and his wife, it became clear that his employers had actually been using him at their convenience and without much appreciation. Unfortunately, his resentment and paranoia about the work situation spilled over to other environments and eventually became part of a system of paranoid beliefs.

2. Determining the influence of cultural background or "what everyone else believes" can be very difficult. Who decides if a belief is culturally appropriate or is a delusion? Family and friends may be able to help sort out the answer to this question. However, their beliefs about the patient may not be free of bias, especially when the patient has become alienated from them.

3. How does someone decide if a belief is not amenable to reason? Understanding beliefs can take time, and modification of beliefs may take much longer. The malleability of beliefs can be strongly dependent on factors such as the relationship with those trying to reason with the patient and the cogency of the arguments put forward. The idea that delusions are not amenable to reason is antithetical to the CBT approach and is not consistent with outcome research that shows reduced delusions in patients treated with CBT methods.

Our (the authors') alternative definition for a delusion might be "a strongly held belief that distresses the person or interferes with his functioning in a way that does not seem to be warranted by his circumstances." The strength of the belief is important, but interventions are appropriate only when the belief is distressing or disabling. Because culturally appropriate beliefs can be accompanied by symptomatic distress, a considered judgment is necessary to determine whether these beliefs are warranted by the circumstances. A conclusion that a strongly held belief is a delusion needs to be kept under review and revised if new evidence is accumulated to refute this conclusion.

If patients wish to discuss beliefs that interfere with functioning or are upsetting to them, CBT is usually indicated. However, when others (e.g., family, employers, schools, legal authorities) are concerned about these beliefs and are requesting intervention, decisions to treat can be more complex. In situations where the patient's delusional beliefs are interfering with others' functioning or distressing other people, or when there may be risk of danger to self or others, investigation of the delusions is usually warranted. Yet, balancing the needs of others with the right to eccentricity and individual freedoms can be a challenging task. Key factors to consider are listed in Table 5–1.

Measures for Delusions

A measure for rating the severity of delusions can allow tracking of change as it occurs and can be more sensitive than global estimations. A commonly used example is the Psychotic Symptom Rating Scales (PSYRATS; Haddock et al. 1999). The dimensions of delusions that are rated with this scale are very similar to the items in Table 5–1, but in this case the characteristic is given a specific rating, and a total score can be

Table 5–1. How do you decide if someone's belief is a delusion?

Strength	How strongly is the belief held?
Context	How unrelated is it to the person's situation and life circumstances?
Preoccupation	How much time does the person spend thinking about the experience?
Plausibility	How understandable is the belief?
Personalization	How much does the person relate an experience to himself?
Persistence	How long has the belief been present? Has it changed over time?

computed. The PSYRATS is provided in Appendix 1, "Worksheets and Checklists," for reference.

There are also valuable tools for assessing insight. For example, the Beck Cognitive Insight Scale (Beck et al. 2004) measures self-reflection and overconfidence in interpretations of experiences. The scale can be very useful in therapy with patients in identifying issues to discuss and monitoring change. Another instrument, the Scale for the Assessment of Insight (David et al. 1992) provides a useful and brief multidimensional evaluation.

In measuring insight, it is important to recognize that full acceptance and understanding of the illness, its symptoms, and treatment are ideal qualities but are not requirements for meaningful therapy with CBT. We frequently work with patients who do not believe that they are ill but are still willing to talk about their problems with us and often agree to take medication.

Discussing Delusions

During the process of establishing the therapeutic relationship, it is very likely that the person will speak about her delusional beliefs. As noted earlier in the section "Defining Delusions," it is often possible early in the assessment to trace the origins of these delusional beliefs. A picture can be constructed of the period leading up to the time when the person became convinced of the validity of the delusion. Sometimes a specific belief (e.g., being electrocuted by neighbors) can be traced back to relevant perceptions (e.g., tingling accompanying anxiety and hyperventilation) that have been misinterpreted (e.g., electricity running though the body). Circumstances may be described where it becomes apparent that the individual inappropriately took things personally, got things out of context, or jumped to unwarranted conclusions.

> ▶ **Video Illustration 5.** Tracing the Origins of
> Paranoia: Dr. Kingdon and Majir

After a few initial sessions with Majir in which a therapeutic relationship had gradually developed, Majir is asked whether he can talk about an earlier incident in his life that had considerable significance to him. When he was a teenager, he had a traumatic experience after drinking alcohol with two men that he had known as friends. Majir accompanied them back to their apartment and was asked to participate in an episode of sexual activity. In response, he left the apartment in a panic, never saw them again, and was never involved in any similar activities. However, Majir was now convinced that all the people around him, including strangers that he never had seen before, knew what had happened. In the video illustration, Dr. Kingdon uses sensitive guided discovery to draw out the beliefs associated with the aftermath of this incident and to explore Majir's reasoning behind these beliefs. This questioning process sets the stage for efforts to help Majir see that he may be personalizing or jumping to conclusions about the knowledge others have about him:

> Dr. Kingdon: This [incident] seemed to start these negative feelings toward other people. I can understand why you might have negative feelings toward those men but [why others]?
>
> Majir: When I ran out, there were a couple of guys standing there [outside the flat]....They knew what happened....So, I find it difficult to meet people. I think they know what happened.
>
> Dr. Kingdon: Can I ask about the two men [outside the flat]?...How did they know what happened if they were standing outside?
>
> Majir: I think...I was sweating...shaky...confused...in the middle of the night, so they must have known.
>
> Dr. Kingdon: What would they have known?...You were anxious and upset, but [how] would they know about this incident?
>
> Majir: Yes, I think they would know....That must be it....They knew what happened up in the flat.
>
> Dr. Kingdon: I wonder about that....It might be worth us exploring a bit further [later]....You also felt that others know because of these two men.
>
> Majir: I don't know....But when you talk to people, they know.

An advantage of CBT is that it can allow extensive exploration of the characteristics of delusions in a way that may be acceptable to the individual. In Video Illustration 5, Majir is very tentative at first in talking about the traumatic incident and how it has continued to affect his thinking. However, the collaborative and slowly paced style used by the therapist eventually pays dividends. Majir describes a set of illogical conclusions that appear to be amenable to change.

Another example of CBT methods for discussing delusions comes from work with patients who are deepening their problems by repeatedly haranguing others with their psychotic beliefs. In CBT, efforts can be made to develop alternative explanations that involve compromise. In this case, the therapist is giving the patient a tip that could help reduce strain in his close interpersonal relationships:

> We may not agree about your current beliefs, but telling your family, especially your son, that they are "the chosen ones" is just disturbing them and getting you admitted to the hospital. It might be more productive if you continue discussing these issues with us but not with them....After all, you've told them about your beliefs enough times. It's up to them now to make up their minds about what you've said. How do you think this kind of plan would work out?

Modifying Delusions

Examining the Evidence

The process of examining the evidence is the core of the CBT approach to modifying delusions. Often patients find it easier to begin with exploring the evidence *for* the delusion—why they believe it. Even when patients list key perceptions that seem to be very strong evidence (to them), the effort to identify evidence for a delusion almost always exposes areas of illogical thinking and uncertainty. Thus, listing evidence for delusions can provide the therapist with a trove of information that can be used to plan interventions.

Sometimes confirming evidence emerges (e.g., being taken into the hospital against one's will) that seems to validate the patient's belief that there is a conspiracy against him. Side effects of medication—such as interference in sexual function or gynecomastia from increase in prolactin levels—may lead to the belief that the person is changing gender. Or, sedation may promote thoughts that alien forces are interfering with his mind. When these types of arguments are made to support delusional beliefs, the therapist will need to use guided discovery and psychoeducation to help the patient understand the phenomena in a more rational way.

In developing evidence against a delusional belief, the therapist may need to be creative and persistent in asking Socratic questions and using other CBT procedures to encourage accurate reality testing. Often multiple sessions and a variety of homework exercises to collect evidence are needed. With particularly sensitive or fragile patients, the process of gathering evidence for and against a delusional belief may need to be woven into a very gentle questioning style instead of explicitly collecting and writing down evidence. Thus, the examining-the-evidence procedure may be more subtle and gradual than in patients with uncomplicated depression or anxiety.

> ▶ **Video Illustration 6.** Examining the Evidence for
> Paranoia: Dr. Kingdon and Majir

In this illustration, Dr. Kingdon helps Majir tell his story of a troubled attempt to visit a mall to buy a computer game. Majir experienced great difficulty when he began to believe that a group of teenagers knew all about him and were essentially able to read his mind. As a result, he returned home feeling very upset and without the game that he had intended to buy. This example shows how a cognitive-behavior therapist can elicit details about paranoid beliefs and can draw out evidence that can eventually be used to modify these beliefs:

Majir: As I was entering the mall, I heard this group of teenagers laughing loudly. And they suddenly stopped. One teenager looked at me. She knew everything about me. I started getting "vicious," having a go at me—"You're a failure, nothing is going to work...."

Dr. Kingdon: It does sound like a very distressing experience. Can I understand exactly what you experienced? You walked into the mall....Some teenagers were laughing and then stopped laughing. You believed they knew about what had happened previously.

Majir: I knew that....

Dr. Kingdon: Do the teenagers know you at all?

Majir: No, I don't think so.

Dr. Kingdon: So when they stopped laughing, you thought this was because of you. Was there any other possibility? (pause) Teenagers laughing and then they stopped laughing...any other possibilities for that happening?

Majir: I don't know....Maybe they finished talking and [were] going on their way....But I'm sure they stopped because of me...because of what they knew about me.

Dr. Kingdon: But if they didn't know you, how do you think they could have known something specific like that?

The discussion about Majir's distorted view of the specific situation and how others might know about him continues on Video Illustration 6, and a simple homework assignment is agreed upon. Although a full intervention for examining the evidence is not accomplished in this session, Dr. Kingdon and Majir have made a good start. Majir has talked about some of the experiences that make him think that others know what happened to him, has recognized that the teenagers do not really know him at all, and has begun to consider some alternative explanations (e.g., "Maybe they finished talking and were going on their way"). Obviously, a good deal of work still remains with examining the evidence and other CBT methods to help Majir modify his delusional beliefs.

Because examining the evidence is such an important technique for changing delusions, we provide another example here. In some respects, Rhonda, a 34-year-old patient with schizophrenia, was easier to treat than Majir. She was less depressed about her circumstances, was functioning better in managing everyday life as a mother of two young children, and was more verbal. Yet Rhonda had a rather fixed belief that required significant effort to change. She was certain that TV shows were sending her special messages and that the content of the show was written expressly for her. Like Majir, she thought that others knew all about her:

Rhonda: I'm convinced that this is happening. Yesterday, a woman on the Food Channel was cooking an Italian dish that she named for her husband. She was going on about their wonderful honeymoon in Italy. There was a definite message from the program about how my marriage is a disaster…how my husband just told me he would never travel anywhere with me again…that I will never be happy. Somehow they know exactly what is happening to me.

Therapist: How do you think they can know about the details of your life?

Rhonda: It's like they are filming right next door.

Therapist: Where do you think they actually film the show?

Rhonda: I guess in California or New York (patient lives in Louisville, Kentucky—a long distance from either city).

Therapist: And when do you think the show was filmed?

Rhonda: I don't know.

Therapist: Is there any way you could find out exactly where and when the show is filmed?

Rhonda: I suppose I could contact the Food Channel—call them or maybe get on the Internet.

Therapist: Could you actually do this?

Rhonda: I'm not sure.

Therapist: Do you know anyone you trust who could help you check with the Food Channel?

Rhonda: I guess I could ask my sister.

Therapist: Would you trust your sister to get accurate information?

Rhonda: Yes.

Therapist: OK. So would you be willing to ask your sister to help?

Rhonda: Yes, I could do that.

(The patient followed through with the assignment and came to the next session with the information that the shows are filmed in New York City and are taped several months in advance. The work on examining the evidence continued as follows.)

Therapist: So, you found out that the shows are taped in New York and that they are filmed way in advance of their being broadcast in Louisville.

Rhonda: That's right.

Therapist: Last week when we were checking your evidence for the idea that TV shows know all about you and are sending you special messages, you told me about the cooking show. Do you remember what you told me about the message you thought you received?

Rhonda: Yes. It was all about the host's perfect marriage and her honeymoon to Italy. They knew that my marriage is terrible and that my husband had just told me he would never go anywhere with me again.

Therapist: If the show is filmed in New York a couple months before it is broadcast, how could they possibly know what your husband had just told you? Could it be that you are really sensitive about the troubles in your marriage, and you got mixed up about what they were saying on the show?

Rhonda: You have a point there.

This chink in the armor of the patient's delusion was explored further, and the therapist and patient were eventually able to construct a fairly

---

Table 5–2. Examining the evidence for a delusion: Rhonda's example

---

Belief: TV shows are sending me messages. They know all about me.

Evidence for	Evidence against
Content of show often has same themes as problems in my life.	Filmed in other cities, often weeks or months before being shown.
Characters can be angry or can seem to tease me.	Why would writers of the show have any interest in my life here in Kentucky?
They are always going on about sex, and I don't get any.	My sister and mother tell me that there is no chance that the TV is sending me special messages.
	My illness makes me overly sensitive to things.
	I am paying too much attention to TV instead of other things in my life.

---

good case against the idea that TV shows know all about her and were sending her messages (Table 5–2).

The examining-the-evidence work with Rhonda was ultimately successful in helping her generate alternative explanations for her perceptions that TV shows knew all about her. She was able to recognize that the stress of problems in her marriage, coupled with her illness-related vulnerability to misperceive information, had fueled her delusion. Other patients with delusions may not be able to establish clear links with stressors, but yet are able to use examining the evidence as an effective tool. Thus, even if the formulation cannot identify detailed meanings for paranoid beliefs, such as were shown in the treatment of Majir and Rhonda, examining the evidence can still be a highly beneficial treatment intervention.

To practice examining the evidence for delusions, try the next learning exercise. It is designed to make you think of creative ways to help patients modify paranoid beliefs.

Learning Exercise 5–1. Examining the Evidence

1. Think of one of your patients who has a paranoid belief. Write down this belief on a piece of paper and then draw a two-column table as in Table 5–2 to record evidence for and against the belief.

2. In the "Evidence for" column, record the things you think your patient might say during the interview.

3. In the "Evidence against" column, record any items you believe that your patient might identify if she is simply asked to list this type of evidence. Assume that your patient will have significant problems working on this column.

4. Now, brainstorm some ideas for helping your patient overcome barriers to finding evidence against the belief. Write down at least two ideas for assisting your patient with this task, and then record any insights that you think the strategy might reveal. Are there customized homework assignments or other novel approaches that you think are worth a try?

Taking a Different Perspective

Another approach that can help patients examine their delusional beliefs is to ask them to put themselves in other peoples' positions, especially those whom they trust, or to consider their beliefs from a variety of other perspectives. For example, the following questions might be asked:

Why do you think that your husband (or mother) isn't convinced by this?

If you could put yourself in the position of your sister, what would you say about the belief that people on the TV shows know all about you?

If someone told you that they thought others could always read her mind, what would you think and how would you respond?

What do you think your pastor (priest, rabbi, etc.) would think about your belief that you are being poisoned by your family?

If you put yourself in the role of a scientist who was trying to find the truth about this situation, what questions would you ask? What information would you need to uncover?

Some patients may not be able to gain distance from their delusions by taking on a different perspective, but many patients may be prepared to consider alternative positions. The approach needs to be explorative and nonconfrontational, emphasizing collaboration with the patient as much as possible. Suggestions for alternative explanations are made only when the patient cannot think of useful ways to respond.

The ABC Technique

The ABC technique is derived from the basic CBT model described in Chapter 1 ("Introduction") and the mini-formulations described in Chapter 4 ("Case Formulation and Treatment Planning"). In this example (Table 5–3), Dr. Kingdon drew a diagram with Majir that summarized their work in understanding the relationship among the activating event, the consequence of the event, and the belief that mediated the consequence. This intervention is not shown in the video illustrations, but it occurred after they discussed the situation further. The ABC method can be a useful way of teaching patients about the impact of beliefs on behavior and can be used as a platform for implementing behavioral changes. In this case, Majir agreed to homework assignments to test the belief by gradual increases in trips to the mall and other public places.

Thought Records

Simplified thought records can sometimes be effective tools in modifying delusions. Patients need to be able to understand the basic principles of thought recording and to have a level of concentration that is compatible with doing this work. If they have difficulties in these areas, the therapist can assist them by doing at least part of the work in sessions. In treating patients with schizophrenia, it is usually best to pare down this activity to its bare bones. Thus, a classic five-column thought record (see Wright et al. 2006 for examples) rarely would be used. Instead, the therapist may suggest that the patient use a two- or three-column thought record. For example, the patient might be asked to record observations in the three columns (event, automatic thoughts, realistic thoughts) shown in Table 5–4.

Table 5–3. The ABC technique: Majir's trip to the mall

A	B	C
Activating event	**Belief**	**Consequence**
Teenage girls stop laughing as I enter the mall.	They know all about me and what happened when I met those men.	I return home immediately without buying the computer game.

Table 5–4. Susan's thought record

Event	Automatic thoughts	Realistic thoughts
Brother reaches for Kleenex and wipes nose.	I am in danger. He is sending me a sign to watch out. He would never hurt me. He is trying to protect me. He knows something he isn't telling me.	He has allergies and wipes his nose a lot. People would have to be absolutely still for me not to think they were sending signs—even then I might think that staying still was a sign. I'm just scared because bad things have happened to me. People have lots of other things to do besides worrying about sending signs to me. They have their own worries. It is unrealistic to think that I am getting signs all the time.

In this illustration, Susan, a 52-year-old woman with chronic paranoid schizophrenia, reported that she was very troubled because she thought that people were sending her "signs." She explained that in regular conversation, even with her family or her doctor, gestures such as reaching in a pocket for Kleenex, rubbing one's eyes, scratching one's head, or fidgeting in a chair were often interpreted as sending her a "sign" that she should look out because something bad might soon happen to her.

As part of a comprehensive strategy to reduce delusions, Susan worked with her therapist in treatment sessions to complete a thought record (Table 5–4). This work was accompanied by homework assignments to ask trusted people (i.e., brother, son, and therapist) about their gestures and whether they had any special meaning.

Schema Modification

With some delusional patients, underlying schemas about self-worth, acceptance, competence, lovability, and trust may emerge and undergird their maladaptive behaviors, and thus be useful targets for change (e.g., "I am a failure"; "I am worthless"; "I am stupid"; "I will always be alone"; "Nobody can be trusted"). However, there has been limited study of the effectiveness of direct work on schemas in facilitating change in psychosis. What does appear to effect change is modification of behavior. If there are positive behavior changes, there may be concomitant changes in beliefs about the self (e.g., by demonstration of mastery and receiving positive reinforcement from others).

In some cases, such as Majir, clear associations can be established with developmental problems or traumas. For other patients, the dysfunctional schemas can appear to be related largely to the impact of the severe mental illness. Living with a disorder such as schizophrenia or chronic depression can in itself promote negative self schemas because of stigma; actual personal failures (e.g., inability to sustain interpersonal relationships, school and work difficulties, declining social and cognitive skills); and other sequelae of the illness (e.g., victimization, repeated hospitalizations, interference with recreational and spiritual pursuits). When dysfunctional schemas are causing significant distress and are aggravating delusional thinking, the treatment plan may need to include methods to address these types of core beliefs.

Discussion of core beliefs must be sensitively handled. Therapists need to be aware that exposing beliefs such as "I am unlovable" can be highly emotionally arousing and could possibly lead to disengagement and an increase in symptoms. Where such core beliefs are detected, therapists may choose to focus on reducing the potential for overgeneralization (e.g., from being insufficiently loved by a parent to being unloved by all). For example, Paul had a seriously neglected childhood with little positive support from either parent. He had managed to find work and develop some relationships, but he still felt emotionally isolated. Eventually he began to believe that he was really a star football player waiting to be discovered and offered a multimillion dollar contract. This belief clearly related to his low self-esteem and underlying core beliefs. The approach to Paul's core beliefs was largely indirect. The therapist worked to develop a positive therapeutic relationship with Paul, discuss his delusional beliefs, and reinforce Paul's positive attributes. As a result, Paul's delusional beliefs became less prominent and his self-esteem began to improve.

CBT strategies for working with schemas about the self are detailed in Chapter 7 ("Depression"). These methods can be used, in modified form, for patients with schizophrenia, and in their classic form (as described in Chapter 7 and in Wright et al. 2006) for patients with mood disorders.

Resistant Delusions

When a patient's conviction in delusions is low to moderate, the reasoning approaches described so far may help shift them in a more rational direction. However, for many patients with strongly held delusions, this process may allow for greater understanding and better engagement but limited, direct observable effect on beliefs (e.g., as measured by a rating scale or as obvious to therapist, hospital staff, or family). Although aspiring therapists can become demoralized at this point, the improvement in understanding and engagement is a very important goal in its own right. Cognitive-behavior therapy is a process that is primarily aimed at improving patients' well-being. Cognitive change (e.g., reduced delusions, improved insight) may be part of this improvement in well-being but is not a sine qua non of treatment. Often the first sign of progress is that the patient's behavior begins to shift toward a more sociable and active lifestyle.

It is very important to recognize when an impasse has been reached in working on delusions and further efforts to directly question the validity of these beliefs are not likely to be of benefit. It is equally important not to prematurely close down such discussions. However, when a sense of going around in circles emerges, reasoning and cognitive restructuring may no longer help. At such points, a decision to *agree to differ* with the patient about her beliefs may be appropriate. If this process has been conducted collaboratively and with a genuine sense of trying to understand the beliefs, patients will often readily accept the therapist's position and allow movement onto other issues.

It is then time to stand back, review the formulation, and identify the remaining key issues and concerns. Having discussed delusional beliefs and their meaning with the patient, there may now be an opportunity to start to focus on significant stresses or other issues in her life. These concerns often have been evident from the original assessment (e.g., loneliness or poor self-esteem), and the delusions have acted in some respects as a diversion from them. With the patient now effectively engaged in a good therapeutic relationship, these issues can be tackled with CBT. An example of this work is illustrated in the treatment of James, a man with chronic delusions of religiosity:

> For many years, James believed that he literally was one of Jesus's disciples from the New Testament and spent his waking days preaching to others using idiosyncratic interpretations of the Bible. As a result, he was often getting into fights and had frequent hospital admissions. James had an aversion to using medication in between hospitalizations. Over the years, unsuccessful attempts had been made to engage him in CBT, until one day he approached his psychiatrist with a wad of papers and asked

him to read them out loud. This interchange occurred not in the psychiatrist's office but in the garden of the mental health unit where James was being treated. While attempting to conceal his own automatic thoughts of demoralized resignation, the psychiatrist sat down and began to read a series of quotations from the Bible, which did not appear connected to one another. As he progressed through the papers, however, sections emerged describing disturbing experiences that James had had in prison and traumatic abusive experiences in his childhood. Subsequently, it was possible to work with James on this previously undisclosed information and the effects these experiences had on him. These discussions were associated with James's emergence from a very isolated and lonely existence, his acceptance of medication, and reduced preaching.

When relevant material does not emerge spontaneously, as in the treatment of James, other routes can sometimes be used to identify it. *Inference chaining* is one approach to find out potential issues underpinning the delusional material. This process involves identifying a troubling belief and asking a series of questions to determine what the belief might imply or infer. In doing so, issues underlying delusional beliefs can often be reached and discussed. Examples are poor self-esteem or lack of respect, or sometimes more practical areas such as being isolated or having to struggle financially. For example, James was asked, "OK, I do have some problems with this [your belief that you are a disciple]....but if other people did accept what you are saying, what difference would that make to you?"

James replied that he would feel that others were listening to him and that he would be better regarded. It was then possible to discuss why he felt that others weren't listening to him: When did he first feel this way? How did he come to this conclusion? This type of questioning can open up areas of importance that might not be reachable with direct reality testing. Where beliefs have negative consequences, it might be worth asking what would distress the patient most about these ramifications: In what way does this belief cause you the most trouble? Is it important enough for you to devote your whole life to this particular cause, or do you deserve some life for yourself?

Therapeutic work on a resistant delusion is demonstrated in Video Illustration 7. The therapeutic relationship with Majir has improved as he and Dr. Kingdon have openly discussed the distressing incidents that Majir has experienced and the disturbing beliefs that he holds. Majir is becoming less preoccupied with these beliefs and is beginning to consider alternative strategies that might improve his quality of life.

▶ **Video Illustration 7.** Working With a Resistant Delusion: Dr. Kingdon and Majir

Dr. Kingdon: I can see why you believe what you believe—that people know what happened to you. I'm less convinced myself that that is occurring....It's very important though. What might you have liked out of your life if this was not happening?

Majir: Lot of stuff happening to normal people—having kids, a girlfriend, going on holiday.

Dr. Kingdon: It's really important to see if there are ways in which we can help you get these things, in time. Are there any positive things about yourself?

Majir: I'm good with kids...honest...can work the computer...reasonable intelligence...physically OK. If I'm to change my life...I may be able to speak to people.

Dr. Kingdon: Whatever is happening around you, you have the right to go out and live a life.

Majir's behavior and mood are strongly influenced by his belief that others know about him and particularly about the incident of which he is very ashamed. Direct discussion of this has been possible, and some doubt may have been sown about the validity of the belief. However, Dr. Kingdon recognizes that the delusion remains resistant to change. Because a detailed discussion of the belief and the reasoning behind it has occurred, it is now possible to work around the belief to encourage positive changes. Specifically, Majir is able to talk about things that he would have liked in his life. He can begin to consider the possibility that, despite his delusional beliefs, he does have significant strengths and that there may be alternative ways of achieving some of his life goals. The strategy used here by Dr. Kingdon is to focus on behavioral change while still acknowledging the importance of the delusional beliefs and the difficulties these may still cause.

Learning Exercise 5–2.   Modifying Delusions

1. Think of a patient with a specific delusional belief.

2. Think of precisely what the belief is and how it may have started.

3. Discuss and test the delusional belief, either using role-play with a colleague or by writing a brief script imagining your and the patient's responses.

4. Evaluate and discuss the effects of this process of reasoning.

5. Imagine that you are faced with a resistant delusion. Try to "agree to differ" and see if you can

develop other productive themes for therapeutic work. Think of questions you might ask, such as the following:

> "OK, I do have difficulty agreeing with you. But, if people did believe you, what would it mean to you? Why would it be important?"

> "Even though you are convinced it is true, is it possible to…(try going to the shops)? Does it have to stop you living your life?"

> "Is there any way of coping with these problems that might help (e.g., someone goes to the shop with you the first time)?"

6. Now, how about trying this approach with one of your patients?

Treating Delusions in Mood Disorders

In this chapter, the case illustrations and suggested methods for treating delusions described thus far have centered on treatment of patients with schizophrenia. However, the same basic CBT approach to delusions can also be used in treatment of mood disorders with psychotic features. In major depression, psychotic symptoms are quite common (Rush 2007). Typically, delusional symptoms in depression and mania are mood congruent. In depression, the delusional themes usually are concerned with failure, self-condemnation, somatic fears, or other negatively distorted beliefs (e.g., "Everyone knows that I am a failure, and they want me to make even a greater fool of myself"; "The police are after me because I have committed some terrible crime" [when no such "crime" has been committed and the patient cannot identify the crime]; "My insides are rotting out with cancer" [when a full medical evaluation has found no cancer or other significant physical illness to explain the symptoms]).

Often depressive delusions can be rather subtle and hard to spot. Thus, the clinician may not be fully aware that the patient has psychotic thinking. Negatively distorted thinking in depression follows a continuum from mild to severe, and defining the cutoff point between nonpsychotic thinking and delusional thinking can be difficult. For example, take the following negative cognitions: "I am a failure"; "I have messed up everything I ever touched"; "No one could possibly love me"; "I deserve to suffer"—when do these types of cognitions indicate that the line has been crossed from the typical, absolutistic thinking of a nonpsychotic patient to the more serious condition of psychotic depression?

Earlier in the chapter, we offered a definition for delusions ("a strongly held belief that distresses the person or interferes with his functioning in a way that does not seem to be warranted by his circumstances") that we believe is compatible with the CBT approach. In evaluating patients with mood disorders, the qualifiers from Table 5–1 (strength, context, preoccupation, plausibility, personalization, and persistence) may be useful in sorting out psychotic from nonpsychotic beliefs. For example, the belief may be clearly illogical (e.g., a depressed patient believes that the police are coming to get him when he has done nothing wrong; a manic patient believes that she has special powers to predict the stock market and then cashes in all her retirement savings to bet on a highly risky venture). Or the patient may not be able to accept any evidence against a strongly held negative belief (e.g., "I am totally to blame and deserve to be punished") when the evidence is very persuasive, at least to others (e.g., there were many contributors to a failed project at work, and the patient had only a small degree of responsibility for the negative outcome).

Even with using the qualifiers in Table 5–1 to evaluate possible delusional thinking, there can be many gray areas in which the therapist is not sure whether the cognitive distortions have reached the level of psychotic thinking. In these cases, it may be useful to consider the cognitive distortion a "quasi delusion" and to devote special effort to modifying the belief with CBT methods. Fully or partially developed psychotic thinking can be associated with dysfunctional behavior that perpetuates and/or aggravates the mood disorder.

Major Depression

Because patients with major depression with psychotic features typically have other severe symptoms (e.g., hopelessness, suicidality, marked anergia, agitation, poor concentration), work on delusions needs to be performed in concert with other procedures for depression described in Chapter 7 ("Depression"). If significant hopelessness and suicidality are present, efforts to modify delusions may assist in relieving these troubling symptoms. For example, patients' beliefs that they are experiencing personal financial ruin or are responsible for world disasters could increase suicidal thinking. Work with CBT could begin to sow doubt that these catastrophes have occurred—or, if actual negative events have occurred, to sow doubt that the patient was the sole cause of the calamity. In turn, standard CBT interventions for depression resulting in gains in energy and interest from behavioral interventions can have positive effects on the therapeutic relationship and make collaborative exploration of delusions more feasible.

Examining the evidence is one of the primary CBT procedures used for delusions in patients with depression, as it is in treatment of schizophrenia. Because depressed patients may have more acute delusions, the delusional beliefs may be more circumscribed and less intense, and reality testing may be more intact. Thus, methods for examining the evidence can usually be implemented more rapidly and thoroughly than in CBT for schizophrenia. Yet, the same basic rules apply. A solid therapeutic relationship must be established first, and then the therapist needs to pace interventions at a speed and intensity that matches the patient's level of symptoms and ability to participate in the reality-testing process.

Thought recording, schema modification, and asking the patient to take the perspective of a trusted other can also be applied in therapeutic work with psychotic depression. Of course, biological treatments such as combining antidepressants with antipsychotic medication or using ECT (either alone or with pharmacotherapy in some cases) are the mainstays of treatment of depression with psychotic features. CBT methods can provide a valuable adjunct to these treatments as demonstrated in the following case:

> Roberto was a 63-year-old man who had been admitted to the hospital after a suicide attempt by gunshot. Even though he had intended to die, the bullet had passed through his chest without hitting his heart or major blood vessels, and he had survived. After medical stabilization, he was transferred to the psychiatric unit for safety and for further therapy. During the psychiatric assessment, it was revealed that he had become depressed after losing a business—a small restaurant that had finally closed after he had fought a long battle against chain restaurants and other better-funded establishments. As Roberto had descended into depression, he had developed delusional and quasi-delusional thoughts, such as "They [family and friends] want me to die"; "John [a brother-in-law] and Marissa [sister] conspired to make this happen;" "It was because of my sin [had a short affair early in his married life] that God wants me to die and suffer forever."

In addition to the CBT methods for suicidality described in Chapter 7 ("Depression"), efforts were made to explore the beliefs that appeared to have possible delusional qualities and that had been driving Roberto to the point of self-destruction. It was possible that his family had turned against him or that his sister and brother-in-law were conspiring to do him harm, but it seemed unlikely that his perceptions were entirely accurate. One of the first steps was to ask questions that helped Roberto tell his story, using guided discovery to determine the strength of the delusions and to uncover possible leads for modifying them. At the same time, a detailed collateral history was taken from a variety of family members including his wife, a 35-year-old son, and a brother whom Roberto said he trusted. As expected, the family's version of events was much different than the picture painted by Roberto.

They described a situation in which the business had been declining for years, even though Roberto had worked valiantly to keep it going. There had been some strain with his sister and brother-in-law, who had been investors in the early days of the restaurant and had advised Roberto several years ago to sell it while he could still make a profit on the sale. However, they were not conspiring to harm him. In fact, they had offered to help him out by investing in a fast-food franchise that Roberto had talked about acquiring. There was good general support from the family and a sincere interest in helping him recover from depression. With this knowledge in hand, the therapist could proceed with using CBT methods to help Roberto develop more rational beliefs. One of the early interventions involved testing the belief "They want me to die":

Therapist: You told me that you believe your family wants you to die. What has made you think that they want you dead?

Roberto: I failed them. I lost everything. I deserve to die for what I did to them.

Therapist: I know that you have had a really tough time coping with closing your business—but it sounds like you are being very hard on yourself. I wonder if it is completely true that everyone in your family wants you to die for what happened. Is there anyone at all that might feel differently?

Roberto: I guess my son has stuck with me. He came to the hospital to see me today—but I was so ashamed to see him. How can I ever look anyone in the eye again?

Therapist: I'll try to help with your feelings of shame in just a bit, but let's just spend another few minutes checking to see if there are any other people who may still be on your side, even if times have also been hard for them.

(Roberto was then able to talk about his relationship with his wife and brother, and how they seemed mad at him because of the business failure but probably did not hate him so much that they wanted him to kill himself. Also, a pattern of isolation and lack of communication came to light.)

Roberto: I got so down about the way things turned out. I kept everything to myself and mostly stopped talking to them.

Therapist: Could it be that you were so down on yourself that you assumed everyone else felt exactly the same way?

Roberto: Maybe.

Therapist: So how could we find out the truth?

During the rest of this session, they planned how to arrange a family meeting with the people that he had trusted the most. Because Roberto was still not sure that he could talk openly about the problems or to ask questions that would draw out his family's true reactions, the therapist used role-play to prepare him for the meeting. After a successful family session, the therapist was able to use examining the evidence and other CBT methods to tackle Roberto's delusional beliefs about God wanting him to "die and suffer forever" and about a conspiracy between his sister and brother-in-law. One of the techniques used for the religious delusion was to "ask an expert." The therapist worked with Roberto to accept a visit from a hospital chaplain who was well versed in working with patients with severe depression and delusional beliefs of a religious nature.

The therapist's formulation in working with these distorted beliefs was that the conclusions about the conspiracy were quite delusional and would probably be the hardest to change. However, she was hopeful that early progress could be made with the belief about his family wanting him dead and that progress in this domain would make the later work more possible. As predicted, the conspiracy idea was more deeply held and was supported by some evidence that his sister and brother-in-law had often been critical of the way he ran the restaurant. Nevertheless, Roberto was able to modify this belief in a way that accurately accounted for the actual problems he was facing: "They know I messed up and are mad because they lost money, but they didn't plot to make me fail."

As the therapy progressed, much of the effort was directed at Roberto's very low self-esteem and intense guilt. Schemas related to competence and acceptance were identified and modified where possible, and behavioral assignments were used to help him regain functionality. Methods for working with schemas related to self-esteem are discussed in Chapter 7 ("Depression").

Mania

As noted in Chapter 8 ("Mania"), CBT for bipolar disorder is primarily directed at relapse prevention, and therapy interventions may work best when performed as preventive measures between episodes of severe symptoms such as florid mania with pronounced grandiose delusions. However, efforts to help manic patients test mildly to moderately delusional beliefs may be worthwhile in some cases, especially when the delusions are leading to disinhibited, risky, or damaging behavior (e.g., arguments with employers, family, or others because of grandiose beliefs). For example, Colin claimed, incorrectly, to be the chief psychiatrist of the hospital. Therefore, he concluded that he should be prescribing medication to all the other patients and, naturally, did not require it himself. An explanation was provided that as for all doctors joining the staff, he would need to produce his professional documentation and references and apply for a vacant post before being allowed to prescribe. The discussion did not abolish the belief, which receded as his mania came under control—but it did reduce his attempts to treat the remainder of the ward population.

CBT methods for working with grandiosity or paranoia in mania need to account for the pressured thinking and distractibility that are so common in this state. Thus, therapists often use structuring and focusing procedures to help patients settle down so they can consider alternatives to delusional beliefs. CBT interventions for grandiose beliefs are detailed and illustrated in Chapter 8 ("Mania").

Summary

Key Points for Clinicians

- The CBT approach for delusions starts with the development of a sound therapeutic relationship, a detailed assessment, and a comprehensive formulation. These steps provide an essential platform for implementation of specific techniques.
- Discussing the circumstances leading up to delusion formation can provide valuable clues for understanding and treating delusional beliefs.
- Weighing the evidence for and then against a strongly held belief is one of the most useful CBT methods for modifying delusions.
- Standard CBT methods, such as thought recording, can be modified for work with delusions.
- In situations where change in the belief is not occurring, a strategy of "agreeing to differ" can be employed. Then the focus can be transitioned to other areas highlighted by the formulation (e.g., other symptoms, social issues, behavioral goals).
- Although resistant beliefs may be slow to change, the behavioral patterns associated with the delusion can start to shift. For example, there may be decreased preoccupation with the belief and increased socialization.

Concepts and Skills for Patients to Learn

- A large number of people experience suspicious thoughts, paranoia, and delusional thinking.
- If strongly held beliefs are causing distress, it can help to trace them back to their possible origins.

- One of the best ways to sort out strongly held beliefs is to weigh the evidence for and against the beliefs.
- Another good method of checking out beliefs is to ask someone you trust. This can be a family member, a friend, or a therapist.
- One of the most important goals of CBT is to help people develop an accurate and realistic view of problems. When people see things accurately, they can usually find good ways to cope.

References

American Psychiatric Association: Diagnostic and Statistical Manual of Mental Disorders, 4th Edition. Washington, DC, American Psychiatric Association, 1994

Beck AT, Baruch E, Balter JM, et al: A new instrument for measuring insight: the Beck Cognitive Insight Scale. Schizophr Res 68:319–329, 2004

David A, Buchanan A, Reed A, et al: The assessment of insight in psychosis. Br J Psychiatry 161:599–602, 1992

Haddock G, McCarron J, Tarrier N, et al: Scales to measure dimensions of hallucinations and delusions: the psychotic symptom rating scales (PSYRATS). Psychol Med 29:879–889, 1999

Rush AJ: The varied clinical presentations of major depressive disorder. J Clin Psychiatry 68 (suppl 8):4–10, 2007

Wright JH, Basco MR, Thase ME: Learning Cognitive-Behavior Therapy: An Illustrated Guide. Washington, DC, American Psychiatric Publishing, 2006

6

Hallucinations

Hallucinations are some of the most troubling symptoms of severe mental illness. Although it was thought at one time that hallucinations were largely resistant to psychotherapeutic interventions, specific CBT interventions have been developed to help patients reduce their distress and build coping skills for managing these symptoms. This chapter outlines practical CBT methods for understanding and managing hallucinatory experiences.

Impact of Hallucinations

Hallucinations are of course most common in schizophrenia. They are typically derogatory and critical but can be positive or friendly in some instances. Command hallucinations are particularly important because of their link to an increased risk of violence to others or to self when these hallucinations are acted on. A hallucination is described phenomenologically as being "a perception which occurs in the absence of an appropriate sensory stimulus but which has all of the characteristics of a real perception" (Sims 2003).

Certain types of hallucinations are commonly observed in the illness of schizophrenia. These include the following:

1. Voices that address the patient in the third person, for example, "He is useless" or "She will never find a job."
2. Voices that deliver a running commentary on the patient, for example,

"Look, she is going up the stairs....perhaps she should stop and rest now."

3. Voices that speak the patient's own personal thoughts out loud.

Hallucinations are less common in affective disorder but do occur in psychotic depression. Here the content is typically in keeping with the patient's severely depressed state. Thus, voices are often nihilistic, for example, "He should commit suicide now" or "He is penniless and bad through and through." Hallucinations can occur in mania but are fleeting and very rarely dominate the clinical presentation. In many patients with schizophrenia, auditory hallucinations and delusions often occur together. Patients with these conditions may also experience visual hallucinations, for example, "seeing blood running down the walls," or olfactory hallucinations, such as "smelling the horrible stench of decay." Gustatory hallucinations, such as "tasting the poison in the food" also occur, but are much less common, as are somatic hallucinations such as "feeling shocks going through the whole body" or "feelings of sexual interference."

Some of the problems that are frequently associated with hallucinations include perplexity, demoralization, exhaustion, anger, anxiety, shame, and sadness. Often patients with hallucinations decide to hide away from social interaction and normal day-to-day duties and activities. Such patients rarely utilize effective coping strategies for these symptoms.

Video Illustration 4 (first discussed in Chapter 3, "Normalizing and Educating") demonstrates the impact of command hallucinations on Brenda, a patient with schizophrenia. Brenda stops seeing her granddaughter Maria after starting to hear voices that tell her to "Hurt Maria." Brenda exhibits the anxiety and shame that patients typically experience in the face of such commands.

Interestingly, many patients hear positive voices, which can be benign or even encouraging. Patients rarely request help with these types of voices; however, it is usually the case that when negative voices start to improve, positive voices also diminish.

Learning Exercise 6–1.   The Impact of Voices

This exercise needs to be done with the help of two colleagues.

1. Sit facing one of your colleagues who will be attempting to have a discussion with you. Another colleague stands to the side and speaks directly into your ear telling you that you are a complete loser, a bum, and so forth.

2. Experience how difficult it is to think clearly, communicate, and function socially when auditory hallucinations are prominent.

3. Now give your colleagues a chance to be the voice hearer.

The CBT Approach to the Hallucinating Patient

Engaging the Patient

Before a psychotic patient can begin to build her understanding and use of CBT techniques, a period of engaging, socializing, and gaining of trust is needed with the therapist (see Chapter 2, "Engaging and Assessing"). Why would a frightened psychotic patient disclose painful personal information to someone she hardly knows? Engaging and assessing proceed together and will take more than one discussion with a hallucinating patient. It is particularly important that patients be allowed to tell their own story of how the voices began. They should then describe in some detail how the voices interfere with their activities.

The CBT approach to hallucinations is based on an empathic, open questioning approach with psychiatrist and patient exploring the voice hearing experience together like two scientists testing hypotheses. This *collaborative empiricism* approach avoids confrontation or collusion, which would both be distinctly unhelpful.

Evaluating Hallucinations

The main purpose of evaluating the nature of hallucinations is to assist patients in obtaining a more objective perspective on this phenomenon. Socratic questions are used to help patients better understand hallucinations and to move toward rational explanations for these symptoms. Instruments such as the Psychotic Symptom Rating Scales (Haddock et al. 1999; see Appendix 1, "Worksheets and Checklists," for the scale) can also be used to evaluate the impact of the hallucinatory experiences. Rating hallucinations on a specific scale can help patients realize that their voices must be similar in form and content to those experienced by other people. Additional benefits of using a rating scale are 1) obtaining extensive information on the dimensions of hallucinations to plan interventions; 2) demonstrating to patients that the intensity of hallucinations can vary depending on stress levels, coping skills applied, and other influences; and 3) having a useful measure of progress.

Table 6–1 contains examples of questions therapists can ask to help patients characterize auditory hallucinations, pin down the geographical location of voices, and begin to question their validity. Patients often aren't quite sure where the voices are coming from. They also may suspect that other people, including the therapist, can hear their voices, at least some of the time. When they come to this conclusion, they may experience intense anxiety and shame—especially if the voices are derogatory, critical, demeaning, insulting, or frankly sexual in nature. Thus, therapists need to be very sensitive to patients' reactions as they ask the types of questions in Table 6–1. If the voice hearer has a successful experience in discussing hallucinations at this point, then further engagement can be expected.

A homework assignment for patients that might flow from work on characterizing auditory hallucinations follows:

1. Ask a family member or close friend about the voices. When you are hearing voices and are in the same room with this person, does he hear the voices?
2. Try to identify exactly where the voices are coming from. Write down your observations on a piece of paper.
3. Make an audio recording of the voices using a tape recorder or other audio-recording device.

Normalizing Hallucinations

Patients will often not be aware that voice hearing is an extremely common experience. Thus, it can be very helpful to explain that voice hearing is a frequent occurrence in the general population. In Video Illustration 4, Brenda was told, "You are not alone"; "Lots of people hear voices"; "The figure is in the order of 2%–3%"; "One person in each high school class is or has been a voice hearer." In normalizing hallucinations, the attitude of the clinician should remain comfortable and genuine, making clear points and designing easy homework experiments. These experiments might include reading a pamphlet about the causes of voice hearing (e.g., sleep deprivation, sensory impairment, or triggering of voices with background noise). Table 6–2 outlines various causes for hearing voices in the general population. Patients can put a checkmark beside the points in the handout that might be pertinent to their own situation and try to apply this information to their own life.

If the patient asks the therapist for an opinion on any of these matters, the clinician should give a response that is as true and honest as possible. One example might be if the patient has underlined in the pamphlet that voice hearing is common. The patient might ask the therapist, "Have you

Table 6–1.   Key questions to evaluate auditory hallucinations

Is the voice male or female?

Do you recognize the voice?

How forceful or loud is the voice?

Is it a voice of a clever person?

Is the voice stronger or weaker than you?

Where does the voice appear to be coming from?

Can you point to the general area in the room?

Shall we go to that point in the room and have a search?

If it is coming from there, will the voice get louder as we get nearer?

Can you do anything to make the voice louder? How can we explain this?

Have you told anyone else about the voice?

What did that person say about the voice? Could they hear it?

Do you think I would be able to hear the voice?

Shall we turn on the tape recorder and see if we can hear the voices when we play it back?

ever heard a voice?" The clinician might honestly answer that he has not heard voices as such but has occasionally woken from a deep sleep, believing that the phone was ringing or that somebody had called his name when this had not happened. This phenomenon can be described as a very common form of hallucination—the hypnagogic hallucination.

The Patient's Explanation for Hallucinations

When the patient does have an explanation for his hallucinations, then this explanation should be explored first. If the patient's view is not openly discussed, further progress is likely to be derailed. Table 6–3 shows how patients can appear to draw explanations from current world events or from the popular press. These explanations are often culturally and personally syntonic but at variance with a medical model of illness. A collaborative and empirical approach should be used to evaluate dysfunctional explanations. After examining the evidence to support or refute the belief, guided discovery can be used to help patients move toward more rational alternatives for explaining their symptoms. Such explanations and action plans can reveal key elements of the patient's

---

Table 6–2.   Causes of voice hearing in the "normal" population

---

Bereavement: Has there been a death in the family? Have you been able to grieve? (Many people hallucinate the presence, touch, smell, or voice of the deceased.)

Sleep deprivation: Were you, or are you, lacking sleep? The severity of voices is very closely related to the severity of sleep disturbance.

Sensory deprivation: Are you sitting all day for long periods of time in a darkened room?

Noise: Is there persistent traffic or machinery noise? Perhaps double glazing for a window or switching off a fan can help.

History of trauma: Have you been the victim of sexual or physical assault? Researchers (Read et al. 2005) have shown that trauma is linked to voice hearing.

Hostage situations/solitary confinement: Hostages and prisoners kept in solitary confinement often end up hallucinating.

Depression: Have you been seriously depressed?

Illegal drug use: LSD, cocaine, "mushrooms," and amphetamine can all cause hallucinations. Were you, or are you, using any of these drugs?

Temporal lobe epilepsy: Certain forms of brain injuries or seizures can cause hallucinations. Do you have seizures or any other neurological problems?

---

thinking that help explain adherence problems, provide valuable insights on risk assessment, and suggest possible targets for interventions.

Introducing the Basic CBT Model

The early sessions when patients are being engaged in therapy provide an excellent opportunity to show openness and respect for their explanations of their hallucinations while introducing the basic CBT model as a method for understanding and coping with symptoms. We often begin with a "decentering" approach, in which examples are provided of how the CBT model can explain emotional and behavioral reactions in everyday life. Common situations that many people experience (e.g., anger at other drivers or anxiety when speaking in public) can be used to show how environmental events can trigger cognitions, emotional responses, and behavior. Patients can then be asked what they might be thinking in these situations and what emotions they might be feeling. They also can be prompted to generate some other ways of thinking in these situations

Table 6–3. Patients' explanations and their behavioral plans for hallucinations

Patients' explanations	Patients' behavioral plans
"It is the voice of a ghost."	Have an exorcism.
"It is the voice of the police from the phone lines."	Destroy the phone lines.
"It is the voice of the Communists."	Buy weapons for defense.
"It is the voice of a five-star general."	Practice marching; buy army clothes.

(rational responses). The therapist might even disclose some personal problem that he has tackled with CBT. The best examples are usually of mild phobias or of stress management.

Another useful strategy can be to illustrate the CBT model using an anonymous example of another patient's voice hearing. Using a white board or a piece of paper, the therapist diagrams the relationships between triggering events (if present), hallucinations, automatic thoughts about the voices, emotions, and behavior, as in the mini-formulations described in Chapter 4 ("Case Formulation and Treatment Planning"). The key message to convey in providing an anonymous example is that the automatic thoughts (e.g., dysfunctional meanings attached to voices), emotions (e.g., fear, anger, sadness) and behaviors (e.g., avoidance, hiding away, yelling at voices, abusing drugs or alcohol) associated with hallucinations can be problematic—instead of helping to cope with the problem, they can make it worse. After discussing the maladaptive responses of this hypothetical patient, the therapist can explain how CBT might be directed at making positive changes.

Generating a Problem List and Targets for Treatment

Effective interventions with a hallucinating patient often include the development of a problem list. The question needs to be asked, "Is the voice itself the problem, or is anxiety or some other problem linked to the experience?" The patient might want to work directly on the voices or might have some other difficulty to discuss (e.g., finances, housing, interpersonal conflict). Once a problem list is decided on, clinician and patient can set specific targets—for example, to understand more about the voices or to reduce anxiety. If the target is a reduction in the distress linked to the voice-hearing experience, then a measuring system can be introduced. One example might be as follows: "You currently score yourself as a 9 on a 10-point distress scale. Would you know what it would feel like if you could reduce your distress to a 4 on this scale? OK. So, let's score the distress at the end of each day and see if our CBT techniques can help us reach this goal."

Specific CBT Techniques for Hallucinations

Developing Rational Explanations

Once a collaborative empirical relationship has been established and patients have begun to show an interest in understanding more about their voices, they usually become more agreeable to the use of specific CBT techniques. One of the most valuable interventions is to help patients develop more adaptive explanations for their hallucinations. Techniques such as Socratic questions, examining the evidence, and checking out beliefs with homework assignments are usually used in the process of modifying explanations. Often these methods can be very helpful in generating alternative ideas. However, there often can be a lack of real-world knowledge (e.g., How many exorcisms were actually done in the state last year and who did them? Can phone lines transmit sound without the receiver being lifted? Is there a local Communist party and how active are they? Can we speak to them?). Thus, the therapist may need to be creative in helping the patient find data to check out dysfunctional beliefs.

Illustrations of modifications of maladaptive explanations are shown in Table 6–4.

Video Illustrations 8 and 9 show CBT interventions geared toward helping a patient with hallucinations develop an adaptive explanation for

Table 6–4. Modified explanations for hallucinations

Dysfunctional explanations	Functional explanations
"It is a bug in my ear/brain planted by the CIA/police."	"It is my schizophrenia acting up."
"It is radio waves from terrorists."	"It is due to stress."
"It is an evil spirit talking to me."	"Maybe my medications need to be adjusted."
"Aliens are communicating with me."	"Maybe the problem is that I am not getting enough sleep."
"It's all caused by witchcraft."	"These voices are a special gift."

the phenomenon. Unfortunately, Brenda had a very dysfunctional explanation for her voices. She had come to believe that it was the devil that was speaking to her and was terrified as a result.

> ▶ **Video Illustration 8.** Explaining Hallucinations: Dr. Turkington and Brenda

> ▶ **Video Illustration 9.** Coping With Hallucinations: Dr. Turkington and Brenda

In the beginning of Video Illustration 8, Brenda tells Dr. Turkington that she is 100% certain that it is the devil who is telling her to harm her granddaughter, Maria. The therapist's first attempt to shake this belief is to ask her about the pamphlet that she read about hallucinations. Did Brenda learn anything in the pamphlet that gave her ideas for other possibilities? Although she mentions sleep problems, it is obvious that the reading assignment didn't have a significant impact on the strength of her belief. When Brenda is unable on her own to generate any other alternative explanations, Dr. Turkington proposes an interesting idea:

> Dr. Turkington: Is there any place where we could find out what the devil has actually said to people in the past?
> Brenda: (Ponders for a moment then responds with a question of her own.) The Bible?

Because Brenda is a church attendee who regularly reads the Bible, the therapist then suggests a homework assignment in which Brenda will do research on what the devil actually says in the Bible and use a double-column method to compare these statements with the character of the voices she is hearing. In order to improve the chances of success, Dr. Turkington helps Brenda explore places she could get help in doing the assignment. She notes her pastor would be an excellent resource. They then agree that Dr. Turkington will call the pastor to explain the project, and Brenda will complete the assignment before the next session. This example demonstrates how a therapist may need to devise a unique plan for each patient to help break through firmly held beliefs about hallucinations.

In the next session (Video Illustration 9), there is evidence that Dr. Turkington's strategy is working:

> Brenda: The pastor said the Bible said that Satan was deceptive—he asks questions and kind of twists things around a little bit....He was a trickster. He never said really bad things to people—he would try to sugarcoat it...so he could win people over.

Dr Turkington: (Comments that the voices she hears are just nasty and that they give her commands to do things.) So what's your conclusion? Are these from the same person?

Brenda: No, maybe it's not the devil, but I still don't know what it is.

(Dr. Turkington asks Brenda to try again to think of an alternative explanation.)

Brenda: Maybe I'm getting sick like the last time.

Dr. Turkington: So, it could be some type of illness in which voices are one of the symptoms. That's not necessarily bad news, Brenda.... Because we know that stress makes certain illnesses worse, and there are certain things you can do to get on top of an illness, aren't there? What kind of things did you do last time to get on top of it?

This illustration shows how reworking a patient's explanation for hallucinations can be a springboard to developing effective coping strategies. After Brenda and Dr. Turkington set a target of learning skills that can reduce her anxiety from a rating of 10 (on a 10-point scale) down to 5, a voice diary is suggested as a good way to monitor hallucinations and to check out the usefulness of ways of coping.

Voice Diaries

Much like thought records are used in treatment of depression and anxiety (see Wright et al. 2006 for examples), voice diaries can be customized to fit the stage of treatment and the cognitive capacity of the patient. Brenda appeared to be grasping the concepts well and was motivated to work on her hallucinations, so a four-column diary was suggested. The elements were 1) what the voices say; 2) emotions associated with voices; 3) coping strategies that were tried; and 4) outcome (changes, if any, in anxiety or other emotions). In this case, the voice diary was used to try to build coping skills.

Other forms of voice diaries can be used early in therapy when patients are just beginning to learn about voices and how they may be influenced by stressors or other environmental events. An example of this type of voice diary—a simple three-column diary—is provided in Table 6–5.

These diaries can show patterns of voice hearing linked to specific triggers and a clear fluctuation in the severity of the experience. Triggers can be extremely variable from patient to patient. Some individuals are more likely to hallucinate when among a group of people, whereas others are more likely to hallucinate when they are on their own. Some patients hallucinate at particular times of day. Others may not have distinct patterns of reactions to environmental influences but have rather autonomous hallucinations.

Table 6–5. A three-column voice diary

What was I doing at that time?	How strong was the voice?[a]	How did I feel at the time?
Boiling the kettle	4	Bored
At the mall	9	Very nervous and ashamed
Walking the dog	2	Relaxed
Arguing with parents	9	Panicky and ashamed
Listening to the radio	2	Interested

[a]Rated on a 0–10 scale, with 10 being the strongest.

The review of a voice diary can be an important phase in beginning to see links between triggers, when present, and the variations in voice hearing intensity. It also may be possible to identify specific emotions linked to the voice hearing and to recognize patterns that can lead to recommendations for coping strategies. In the example in Table 6–5, anxiety and shame are strongly linked with being in enclosed places with other people (e.g., at the mall; arguing with parents). This patient believed that other people could hear the same voices that he heard and might act on them to harm him. A technique that might be used here is a homework assignment to attempt to audiorecord the voices.

Building Coping Strategies

Coping-strategy enhancement is one of the most valuable CBT methods for helping people control hallucinations. In Video Illustration 9, Brenda relates that loud music aggravates her voices, but soft music eases the hallucinations. Therefore, she and Dr. Turkington work out a plan to increase the time that she listens to soft jazz (Brenda's choice to dampen the voices) and to hum a song that pleases and comforts her ("Amazing Grace"). When Dr. Turkington asks Brenda if she can think of any other possible coping methods, she brings up a helpful message from her pastor and says that she will remember what he said: "I am a child of God; I do not need to be afraid of the devil." The latter coping strategy is a good example of the unique methods that patients can sometimes generate. We try to encourage patients to come up with any idea that might help control voices, and are often pleasantly surprised by their creative responses.

In building coping strategies, we explain that everyone is different and that what works for one person may not work for another. Thus, it is a good idea to keep trying methods until the most effective ones are identified. As noted in Table 6–6, a large number of possibilities can be considered. Coping strategies can be grouped into three general categories:

1. Distraction
2. Focusing
3. Schematic and metacognitive (developing an overarching attitude about one's self and the hallucinations that promotes acceptance and healthy adjustment)

Coping strategies are chosen collaboratively and are often demonstrated and practiced during the session, especially if the patient does not clearly understand how to use the skill. The rationale for using the method should also be explained, and the results of attempts to use coping methods should be monitored. An example of a monitoring method is an extended voice diary. Brenda used a four-column thought diary for this purpose. An example of a five-column diary is provided in Table 6–7. If after a week or two, the coping strategy is not working, then another should be chosen. If patients have trouble identifying strategies, a list of possibilities can be provided (Appendix 1, "Worksheets and Checklists," contains a list of 60 potential coping strategies for hallucinations; see also Kingdon and Turkington 2005). In this way, patients can systematically work their way through a variety of strategies and decide which ones provide the most help. As this effort progresses, patients often learn more about their voices and become more confident in controlling them.

Table 6–6.   Coping strategies for hallucinations

Distraction	Focusing	Schematic/metacognitive
Listen to music	Subvocalization	Schema modification
Practice a hobby	Rational responding	Acceptance
Play a computer game	Giving the voices time to talk later	
Exercise	Dismissing the voices	
Pray	Positive imagery	
Use a mantra	Mindfulness	
Sing a song		

Table 6–7. A five-column voice diary

Activity	Voice intensity[a]	Emotion	Coping strategy	Voice result[a]
Sitting smoking	6	Angry	Whistle a tune	8
Father called	9	Angry	Do some painting	3
Having lunch	4	Relaxed	Whistle a tune	4

[a]Rated on a 0–10 scale, with 10 being the strongest.

Distraction

We typically begin our work in building coping strategies with distraction techniques because these are easier for patients to understand and implement. For example, Brenda chose to listen to soft jazz and to hum the tune "Amazing Grace." The patient who completed the voice diary in Table 6–7 had suggested two possible distracting activities, but only one seemed to work. His first choice of a coping strategy, whistling a tune, did not appear to be helpful. However, he discovered that distraction by doing some painting seemed better for him. After patients build their confidence with distraction, they can move on to learning more complex techniques.

Focusing Approaches

If subvocalization is chosen as a coping strategy, it should be explained that whispering internally at a subvocal level can help some people reduce the activity in the voice-generating area of the brain (Fannon et al. 2000). A specific plan for using the subvocalization technique needs to be chosen, demonstrated, and rehearsed. Examples of subvocalization activities could be a song, poem, or a rhyme.

As some patients become more engaged in tackling their voices, they may begin to question their voices and produce rational responses. It is often a good plan to write down what the voices say on a piece of paper or a whiteboard and then to check them for truthfulness. Initially, therapists can guide patients into thinking about whether the voices "have got it right." The therapist becomes a joint listener: "Let's tune into the voices and see what they have to say for themselves today." As the voice content is written down, therapist and patient can look for cognitive distortions and produce rational responses (Table 6–8). If progress is made, the re-

Table 6–8. Responding rationally to voices

Examples of voice	Rational response
"He is a waste of space."	"I'm a person, a human being with rights."
"She has no friends."	"OK, so I don't have many friends, but I have my brother and the two people at the center."
"He is gay."	"My sexuality is my own business."
"She is trash."	"Not true. I've only had a couple of boyfriends."
"Die, you should die now."	"I don't want to die. I have plenty of reasons to live."

sults should be recorded on a card or an audiotape to help the patient re-member and use the information.

As patients begin to assert themselves and refute their voices, they need to be warned that hallucinations can become a bit nastier or louder for a while before they start to come under control. We sometimes tell our patients, "The voices might get louder temporarily, but that is a sign that you have got them on the run!" Obviously, there is some concern that patients could be ostracized for seeming to speak back to nobody. This problem can be dealt with by using a cell phone. The patient is instructed to speak into her cell phone (not switched on) whenever responding to the voices and to always speak in a reasoned and calm tone. Other focusing techniques, such as assertively dismissing the voices or allowing them to have their say at a later time, can also work for some people.

Positive imagery is another technique that can be used to cope with hallucinations. For example, we have a patient who uses imagery to reduce the intensity of a voice that tells him to poison his parents. He imagines the voice going into a closet, being covered with a blanket, and then having the door closed on it. Each step in this progression is associated with a lessening of the volume and intensity of the voice. By the time the imagery is complete, the voice is just a whisper or can't be heard at all. Other imagery possibilities include the use of pleasing or calming scenes (e.g., spending imaginal time on a beach or walking in a meadow on a fine spring day) to focus attention away from hallucinations.

Mindfulness, a technique described in more detail in Chapter 7 ("Depression"), may be used effectively by some patients to focus their attention away from hallucinations. We do not recommend that patients with psychosis use the meditation techniques that are involved in full implementation of mindfulness (Kabat-Zinn 1990). However, a mindful approach to appreciating everyday things (e.g., savoring the flavors and textures of food, paying increased attention to objects and scenes in nature, listening carefully to music) can be a valuable focusing method for patients who have sufficient concentration to use this approach.

Schematic and Metacognitive Approaches

Patients often believe what their voices say about them because they have negative core schemas about themselves. Typical core beliefs in schizophrenia may include "I am worthless"; "I am useless"; "I am evil"; "I am damaged"; "I am different." These types of beliefs tend to mediate the low self-esteem so commonly seen in schizophrenia. Negative beliefs about the self can be elicited with guided discovery and also detected by using measures such as the Schema Inventory provided in Appendix 1 ("Worksheets and Checklists") or the Brief Core Schema Scales (BCSS; Fowler et al. 2006).

Maladaptive schemas can be challenged in CBT, and if they can be modified there can be a change in attitude toward critical and unpleasant hallucinations. For example, if a patient had the belief "I am useless," the therapist might comment, "Calling yourself completely useless is a very absolute statement, could we check it out to see if it is entirely true?" Techniques such as examining the evidence or the cognitive continuum (detailed in Chapter 7, "Depression") could then be used to find areas in which the patient has made some contributions and to put the self-condemning belief into a more rational perspective. Even a small shift in a core negative schema can be very worthwhile. Methods for working with core beliefs related to self-esteem are discussed at more length in Chapter 7.

The term *metacognitive* is used here to refer to shifts in attitudes about the self and the illness that involve acceptance of the condition. There is no specific CBT method that, in itself, is directed at acceptance of illness. However, the engaging, normalizing, and educating procedures described previously, in addition to the cognitive restructuring techniques detailed throughout the book, can promote increased levels of acceptance. For a significant number of patients with hallucinations, pharmacotherapy plus CBT will not eliminate this symptom. In this case, the goals of treatment are to accept that hallucinations may be ongoing and to learn how best to live with this malady. CBT strategies for enhancing acceptance are discussed further in Chapter 13, "Maintaining Treatment Gains."

Graded Exposure

Some auditory hallucinations have the characteristics of flashbacks or obsessional thoughts. Often this type of mental imagery can be linked to avoidance of situations that seem to stimulate the hallucinations. At times, Brenda's voices were telling her to injure her baby granddaughter Maria. These command hallucinations of an obsessional quality were quite out of character with Brenda's nature. She had never harmed anyone and had no intent or desire to hurt the baby. In fact, she was a very religious person with strong positive values who sincerely liked to help others.

Command hallucinations, such as the ones reported by Brenda, can be addressed with techniques of graded exposure and response prevention—but only after adequate coping strategies have been established. Graded exposure can be practiced in therapy sessions using imagery. At a later session not shown in the video illustrations, Brenda was instructed as follows:

> Imagine you are walking into your son's house and you are starting to feel nervous....What would the voices be saying? Imagine hearing these voices now, and describe how you feel....Now in your imagination, let's stay in the room with the voices instead of running home. Let's see what happens.

She was then asked to practice letting the voice be there and "do its worst" while using some of her coping strategies. As the imaginal exposure proceeded, Brenda noticed that her anxiety levels started to fall.

When Brenda became more confident, she agreed to spend 10 minutes in the room with Maria, but only if other people were present. The command hallucinations settled, and gradually she spent more time holding and nurturing the baby. Obviously, the issue of risk is crucial here in designing interventions such as these. A detailed assessment of risk and thorough preparation are essential before these kinds of homework assignments are implemented.

Coping Cards

In order to help reinforce the use of strategies learned in sessions, the key elements of the plan to manage hallucinations can be recorded on a coping card. We highly recommend use of this method because patients may not carry the insights from therapy appointments into the real world unless efforts are made to encourage learning and repeated skill rehearsal. An example of a coping card developed by Brenda is displayed in Table 6–9. This coping card captures the methods articulated in Video Illustrations 8 and 9 and in a few subsequent sessions.

To gain skills in using CBT for hallucinations, try the following learning exercise.

Table 6–9. Brenda's coping card

Listen to soft music, especially jazz.

Hum "Amazing Grace."

Remind myself that "I am a child of God; I do not need to be afraid of the devil."

Remember that it is my illness that causes the voice, not the devil.

Take it a step at a time in getting back to being comfortable around Maria.

Respond to the voice by saying "I would never hurt anyone, I am a good grandmother."

Realize there is no risk that I would hurt Maria, because I have no reason to follow the voice.

Take the medication for voices every day as scheduled.

Learning Exercise 6–2.   Coping With Hallucinations

1. Ask one of your colleagues to role-play a patient with auditory hallucinations.

2. Ask a series of questions to determine what things appear to make this patient's voices both better and worse.

3. Now try to build up the patient's coping strategies by listing at least three additional methods that can be tried for homework.

4. List all of the adaptive strategies on a coping card.

5. Use the same procedures with your patients who experience hallucinations.

Summary

Key Points for Clinicians

- The CBT approach to hallucinations starts with a detailed evaluation of the dimensions (e.g., severity, location, malleability) of these symptoms.

- As in treatment of other symptoms of severe mental illness, normalization is an important early step in CBT for hallucinations.
- After exploring the patient's explanations for hallucinations, the basic CBT model can be introduced and illustrated.
- Maladaptive explanations for hallucinations can be modified with a variety of CBT techniques, including Socratic questioning, examining the evidence, and homework assignments to test the validity of beliefs.
- Voice diaries can help patients understand hallucinations better and gauge the success of coping strategies.
- Building coping strategies is a centerpiece in the CBT approach to hallucinations. Therapists can help patients identify and strengthen coping strategies in three main categories: distraction, focusing, and schematic/metacognitive.
- Graded exposure—a core behavioral strategy from CBT—can assist hallucinating patients in reversing patterns of avoidance and improve social functioning.
- Coping cards are useful in reinforcing CBT methods for managing hallucinations.

Concepts and Skills for Patients to Learn

- A realistic explanation for hallucinations usually helps people cope better with this problem.
- It can be very useful to work with a therapist, or perhaps a trusted family member or friend, to help check out the validity of hallucinations. An example of a good question to ask is "Can anyone else hear the voices?"
- Coping strategies for hallucinations can be very helpful in reducing distress. Experiment with different coping strategies until the most effective ones are identified and learned.
- Despite the best treatment with medication and CBT, some people will continue to have residual hallucinations. When this happens, one may need to accept the facts of the illness and then try to maximize the use of coping strategies.

References

Fannon D, Chitnis X, Doku V, et al: Features of structural brain abnormality detected in first episode psychosis. Am J Psychiatry 157:1829–1834, 2000

Fowler D, Freeman D, Smith B, et al: The Brief Core Schema Scales (BCSS): psychometric properties and associations with paranoia and grandiosity in nonclinical and clinical samples. Psychol Med 36:749–759, 2006

Haddock G, McCarron J, Tarrier N, et al: Scales to measure dimensions of hallucinations and delusions: The psychotic symptom rating scales (PSYRATS). Psychol Med 29:879–889, 1999

Kabat-Zinn J: Full Catastrophe Living: Using the Wisdom of Your Body to Fight Stress, Pain, and Illness. New York, Hyperion, 1990

Kingdon DG, Turkington D: Cognitive Therapy of Schizophrenia. New York, Guilford, 2005

Read J, van Os J, Morrison AP, et al: Childhood trauma, psychosis and schizophrenia: a literature review with theoretical and clinical implications. Acta Psychiatr Scand 112:330–350, 2005

Sims A: Symptoms in the Mind: An Introduction to Descriptive Psychopathology, 3rd Edition. London, Saunders, 2003

Wright JH, Basco MR, Thase ME: Learning Cognitive-Behavior Therapy: An Illustrated Guide. Washington, DC, American Psychiatric Publishing, 2006

7

Depression

This chapter focuses primarily on severe and treatment-resistant depression. However, the methods described here can be applied in CBT with other severe mental illnesses. For example, suicidality in patients with schizophrenia or bipolar disorder can be addressed with the same type of antisuicide plan used in persons with major depression. Also, methods for increasing pleasure and involvement in activities can be modified for use in patients with psychosis who have apathy, social withdrawal, or secondary depression. Thus, this chapter is designed to help clinicians treat patients who have a broad range of depressive symptoms and a variety of diagnoses.

We discuss CBT interventions for three main clusters of problems in severe or treatment-resistant depression: hopelessness and suicidality, low energy and anhedonia, and low self-esteem.

Two principal forms of CBT are used for chronic depression: 1) standard "Beckian" methods as modified by Fava and coworkers (1996, 1997, 1998, 2002) and others (Luty et al. 2007; Wright 2003); and 2) McCullough's Cognitive Behavioral Analysis System of Psychotherapy (CBASP; Keller et al. 2000; McCullough 2000). McCullough's method focuses more on interpersonal and transference-related therapy processes than standard CBT and is not used as widely as Beck's classic techniques. The standard form of Beck's CBT has been shown to be effective for severe depression (DeRubeis et al. 1999; Luty et al. 2007) and in one recent study was found to be more effective than interpersonal therapy in patients with more severe symptoms (Luty et al. 2007). We describe how to implement standard CBT in this chapter. Interpersonal aspects of CBT for depression and other severe mental disorders are explored in Chapter 9 ("Interpersonal Problems").

Hopelessness and Suicidality

Hopelessness

Hopeless thinking is one of the most ominous symptoms of severe depression. A number of studies have found that hopelessness is strongly associated with suicide risk (A.T. Beck et al. 1975, 1985; Fawcett et al. 1987). For example, an investigation by A.T. Beck et al. (1975) discovered that the overall level of depressive symptoms, as measured by the Beck Depression Inventory (A.T. Beck et al. 1961), was less predictive of suicide risk than scores on the Beck Hopelessness Scale (BHS; A.T. Beck et al. 1974). Another study found that elevated BHS values on discharge from a psychiatric hospital were the strongest predictor of risk for future suicide (A.T. Beck et al. 1985).

The tie between hopelessness and suicidality is understandable. If one has given up all hope and can see nothing in the future except pain and despair, suicide may seem like a reasonable choice. On the other hand, if the patient believes that recovery is possible or likely, has genuine reasons to live, and can see possible solutions for problems, he may be able to tolerate extreme levels of depression without seriously considering self-harm. An especially appealing feature of CBT for depression is that it has been shown to reduce hopelessness and the risk of subsequent suicide attempts (Brown et al. 2005; Rush et al. 1982). In one influential study, Brown and associates (2005) found that patients who had attempted suicide and were treated with CBT had substantially fewer subsequent suicide attempts than those who received standard care.

The rationale for vigorously addressing hopelessness goes beyond the reduction of suicide risk. Patients with significant hopelessness may be reticent to fully engage in treatment because they believe that there is little or no chance that it will work (Wright 2003). They may become mired in patterns of low activity, social withdrawal, and procrastination because they think, "What's the use?" And their pessimism is likely to be contributing to self-defeating behavior and deepening their low self-esteem. Thus, the dampening effect of hopelessness may need to be countered before significant therapeutic gains can be realized.

Table 7–1 lists some of the key CBT methods for building hope. These methods can be used to stimulate a more optimistic viewpoint and to reduce suicidal thinking, if present. We will more specifically detail CBT

Table 7–1. CBT methods for building hope

Use the therapeutic relationship to instill hope.

Educate about reasons for an optimistic outcome.

Structure treatment.

Set realistic goals.

Suggest behavioral assignments that demonstrate ability to change.

Challenge hopeless cognitions.

Identify strengths and positive core beliefs.

Use cognitive methods to develop a more optimistic thinking style.

Directly address suicidal thinking.

strategies for developing antisuicide plans later in this chapter. Here we describe and illustrate general CBT methods for treating hopelessness.

In many ways, Table 7–1 reads as if it were a list of CBT methods used for any problem or condition—form a good relationship; educate; structure; set goals; use behavioral methods; and so on. These commonly used procedures are listed here because basic CBT methods, in themselves, serve to reduce hopelessness. Think for a moment how you might feel if you were demoralized, hopeless, and had run out of ideas on how to solve your problems. If you went to a therapist who was kind, empathic, understanding, and reasonably optimistic—who additionally offered a structured, clearly understandable, and sensible path to recovery—it is likely that you would begin to be more optimistic yourself. If instead you happened to see a therapist who seemed aloof and disengaged and presented a rather aimless or clouded picture of the therapeutic process, you might actually feel worse.

In our work with persons with significant hopelessness, we make a special effort from the first session onward to generate realistic optimism by trying to establish the best possible therapeutic relationship and to model a balanced but hopeful outlook. Because depressed persons are so good at viewing themselves and the world through a negative lens, it is easy to get caught up in their hopelessness. Conversely, therapists can fail to perceive the seriousness of problems, have difficulties expressing accurate empathy, and exude an overly cheery or optimistic tone. To some extent, the therapist's own worldview may pervade and influence, either directly or indirectly, the process of conveying (or failing to convey) a sense of hope.

The next time you work with a patient with significant hopelessness, you might ask yourself some of these questions: Am I fully appreciating the depth of the patient's symptoms and problems? Am I expressing an appropriate level of empathy while still conveying realistic hope for change? Could my own degree of pessimism/optimism be having a deleterious effect on the patient's ability to develop genuine hope? Am I modeling too little hope, or am I expecting too much positive gain from the therapy?

In concert with efforts to maximize the hope-engendering aspects of the therapeutic relationship, cognitive-behavior therapists can use the educating, structuring, and goal-setting features of CBT to help patients begin to see possibilities for improvement. Dr. Wright demonstrates these methods in Video Illustration 3 (first shown in Chapter 2, "Engaging and Assessing") when he explains to Mary, a middle-aged depressed woman, how CBT is different from other therapies, points out how her depressive perspective interferes with developing hope for the future, structures and paces the session to keep Mary focused on reaching more positive outcomes, and collaboratively develops some initial goals for treatment. At the beginning of this first session, Mary reports that she sees herself as a "hopeless case," but by the end of the session she is able to identify two goals for treatment (i.e., to start "getting out of the house" and to "do something about my marriage") and to have at least some sense that she might be able to reach them. Although her mood is still quite depressed, she appears to be less despairing and more willing to engage in treatment. Mary is so deeply and chronically depressed that it would be unlikely that she would be able to build a great deal of hope in only one session. Nevertheless, the process of developing more optimistic expectations was under way.

Behavioral assignments can be very powerful ways of generating hope, especially if they reactivate patients and demonstrate to them that change is possible. Sometimes these assignments can provide a large boost in hope, even if the behavioral intervention is relatively simple. An example from our practices includes a 40-year-old man with severe depression who believed that he wasn't "fit to be around people" because he was a total failure who had "nothing to offer." He had refused multiple invitations from old friends to sit in on their weekly "jam session" where they played rock music. He had played guitar in a band when he was younger. After agreeing to a behavioral plan of accepting their invitation and spending at least 1 hour at the jam session, he had a very positive experience that gave him considerable hope that he could begin to turn his life around.

Because hopeless cognitions can have such intensely negative consequences, their validity should be challenged with all of the skill and creativity that the therapist can muster. If the therapist does not aim toward modifying these cognitions, a tacit validation of the beliefs may occur, and the therapy process may be undermined. Any of the basic cognitive restructuring methods (e.g., Socratic questioning, examining the evidence, finding rational alternatives, spotting cognitive errors, thought recording, and others) can be used to revise hopeless cognitions. These basic procedures are explained in core texts such as *Learning Cognitive-Behavior Therapy: An Illustrated Guide* (Wright et al. 2006) and will not be detailed here.

Video Illustration 3 demonstrates several examples of cognitive restructuring methods for hopelessness. After Mary exudes pessimism in reporting that her previous psychiatrist had essentially given up on her, psychotherapy hadn't helped in the past, and virtually all medications had been tried without any lasting benefit, Dr. Wright asks a Socratic question: "You don't seem to have much hope, yet you came to this session....There must be something in you that thinks there might be a chance for success." In asking this question, he is trying to draw out some positive reasons for her engaging in treatment. Having Mary try to uncover these reasons may be more effective than simply telling her why treatment could be beneficial.

Dr. Wright also does some early cognitive restructuring in the first session by asking Mary to review times in the past when she was functioning better and to start to identify several of her strengths. Although still in the opening phase of therapy, work has begun on developing a more optimistic thinking style. Mary did not express significant suicidal ideation in the first interview, but later in treatment an argument with her husband stimulated suicidal thoughts that were addressed with a CBT intervention.

Suicidality

CBT strategies can be used to develop effective plans to reduce the risk of suicide (Brown et al. 2005). Many of the items in an antisuicide plan can be drawn directly from work on hopelessness, but other interventions can add power to the plan (Table 7–2). For example, agreement to specify a person(s) to contact if suicidal thoughts emerge can provide a needed margin of safety. Also, if possible triggers for symptom worsening and increased suicidality can be identified, plans can be made in advance for how to best cope with these stressors. CBT rehearsal can be used to recognize maladaptive automatic thoughts and behavior in projected stressful situations and to practice more adaptive responses. These positive strategies can be recorded on a coping card that can become part of the antisuicide plan. A variety of other customized interventions can be developed if needed.

Table 7–2.   Key features of effective antisuicide plans

Identify specific reasons to live.

Collaboratively agree to safety precautions.

  Commit to contact/call a specific person(s) (list contact information).

  Commit to contact therapist or get other help (list contact information).

  Block or reduce access to guns or other dangers (e.g., have a family member lock up all medications and supply only one day's dose at a time).

Identify adaptive cognitions and behaviors that may help patient fight despair, anxiety, or other symptoms.

Develop coping strategies for possible triggers for increased suicidal thinking.

Write out plan and review it frequently.

Therapists and patients should use their creativity to generate antisuicide plans that are—

1.   Meaningful (the plan is highly significant to the patient)
2.   Specific (detailed enough to give clear specifications and instructions)
3.   Committed (patients have a genuine commitment to the key features of their plan)
4.   Collaborative (patients are fully involved in generating the plan)

CBT methods for suicidality are shown in Video Illustration 10, the third CBT session with Mary. The video illustration depicts a portion of a session in which Mary begins to build an antisuicide plan. Because only brief vignettes are included in this book, a full assessment of suicide risk is not displayed on the video. However, Dr. Wright completed an extensive risk assessment before the interview concluded and was prepared to implement precautions, including hospitalization, as needed. Fortunately, Mary was able to respond positively to efforts to generate hope and decrease suicidality.

▶ **Video Illustration 10.**   An Antisuicide Plan: Dr. Wright and Mary

List of Reasons to Live

Dr. Wright's strategy for helping Mary overcome her suicidal thinking began with generating a list of reasons to live—one of the especially useful elements of effective antisuicide plans. Even with patients who have had a recent suicide attempt or who are seriously considering suicide, judicious and well-phrased questions about positive reasons to live can yield considerable benefits. These types of questions often serve as a "wake-up call" by alerting patients to very meaningful aspects of their lives that have been temporarily obscured by the monolithic, hopeless outlook of depression.

Mary had noted that an argument with her husband had been laced with critical remarks ("You're not pulling your weight"; "You can't do anything"; "You aren't any fun anymore") that had driven her deeper into depression and to the potentially dangerous thought "My husband and kids would be better off with me dead." Instead of challenging this cognitive distortion immediately, Dr. Wright first asked Mary to reflect on her previous suicide attempt that occurred over 20 years ago. He remembered that Mary had rallied after that attempt, had coped with a divorce, and had been able to work steadily to support her young daughter—so there must have been reasons to live at that time. Could any of these reasons help Mary see that there was hope for improving the current situation? Mary responded to Dr. Wright's question by noting that after the previous suicide attempt by an overdose, she called the ambulance immediately because she suddenly realized that she didn't want to hurt her daughter.

When Mary was asked about current reasons to live, she replied, "My kids—my boys are still at home." If she had not identified her children as a current reason to live and had gone on to talk about how her children would easily get over her death, there would have been greater concern about suicide risk. However, the emotional attachment to her children and the great significance she attributed to their relationship became evident as the interview proceeded.

In developing a list of reasons to live, it is important to identify as many elements as possible from varied domains of the patient's life. Also, it can be very helpful to ask questions that give specific details about the reason to live. These details build the case for living instead of dying. Thus, in the video illustration, many questions are asked to assist Mary in identifying multiple reasons to live and to expand Mary's view of herself as a mother. At first, Mary only reports that she is needed by her children because she helps them with homework and she does the chores. But, with additional questions, she is able to recognize that there is a deep bond of love with her children and that she is extremely important to them.

Mary's entire list of reasons to live is shown in Table 7–3. It includes details on living for her children, the positive features and potentials of her marriage, the possibility of developing a closer relationship with her father, and a personal goal for the future. The last item on the list did not come easily to Mary. In fact, a "hint" was needed that she was ignoring personal goals. Often patients with severe depression have difficulty thinking of any reasons to live except for their family or to adhere to spiritual beliefs that prohibit self-harm. Because Mary's self-esteem was so low, she didn't give any consideration to things that she might like to live for in her own personal life. After the hint was given, Mary was able to note that she wanted to finish school to become a licensed practical nurse.

In addition to helping counteract suicidal thinking, the list of reasons to live can give the therapist and patient direction for further CBT interventions. Mary's list of reasons to live included several good possibilities. For example, her relationship with her husband could become an agenda item for future sessions, behavioral assignments could be developed to capitalize on her father's renewed interest in the family, and CBT methods could be employed to build self-esteem and help Mary return to school. Some of these interventions are detailed later in the chapter.

A Multifaceted Antisuicide Plan

At the end of Video Illustration 10, Dr. Wright asks Mary if she is ready to work on a plan to reduce her risk for suicide. The remainder of the ses-

---

Table 7–3.   Mary's list of reasons to live

My children
  I don't want to hurt them.
  I am very important to them.
  I love them deeply.

My husband
  I really care about him.
  He hasn't left; he is sticking by me.

My father is back in my life.
  He wants to do things with the kids and me.
  This is a good opportunity for me.

I would like to go back to school to become a nurse.
  I want to be a nurse and help people.
  I need to work and to make money.

---

sion (not shown in the video) was then devoted to a full assessment of suicide risk and the development of a multifaceted antisuicide plan, including safety precautions, positive cognitions and behaviors to fight despair, and plans to cope with potential triggers that could produce suicidal thoughts. A multifaceted antisuicide plan is detailed below.

Develop Safety Precautions.   Although it is impossible to "suicide proof" a home, or even a hospital, reasonable precautions will give the patient at least some protection in case suicidal thoughts return or become stronger. If the patient can genuinely commit to interventions such as contacting a family member or clinician, or removing especially dangerous methods such as guns or large amounts of potentially lethal medication, the antisuicide plan will gain significant specificity and strength. Mary's antisuicide plan included an agreement to call her sister for help if she had increased suicidal thinking, to contact the clinician on 24-hour duty in Dr. Wright's practice, and to have only a 2-week supply (14 pills) of her citalopram (20 mg) at any time. She was taking no other medications.

Identify Adaptive Cognitions and Behaviors.   Adaptive cognitions and behaviors may help patients fight despair, anxiety, or other symptoms. A variety of CBT methods can be used to develop healthy cognitions and behaviors that reduce suicidality. For example, a patient might be taught to identify habitual patterns of automatic thoughts or core beliefs and to list more rational thoughts for the antisuicide plan (e.g., "I will spot beliefs such as 'I can never do anything right' or 'I'm not lovable' and replace them with more reasonable beliefs, such as 'I do many things right, but I need to keep learning how to do better'; 'I've had trouble with some relationships, but I am still capable of love'"). Another strategy could be for patients to remind themselves of positive beliefs or behaviors that become submerged when depressive thinking is at its peak. Mary used this technique in her antisuicide plan when she wrote: "Think of the things that I have done well—raised my children, coped with a divorce, ran a day care operation, helped lots of families and children."

Another example of a cognitive intervention that became part of an effective antisuicide plan comes from the treatment of Larry, a patient with depression and ulcerative colitis who had just attempted suicide. This 53-year-old man had taken a very large overdose with a clear intent to die. He had concluded that he couldn't live with ulcerative colitis because he had no energy, had no interest in life, and couldn't face a continued existence of pain and disability. When seen for the first time in the intensive care unit, he was disappointed that the suicide attempt had not worked.

Over the course of two additional daily visits, his psychiatrist found that Larry had been focusing so much on his medical condition that virtually all other aspects of his life had been abandoned or ignored. She asked Larry to complete a pie graph to depict how much of his life had been occupied by his bowel problems in the few weeks preceding his suicide attempt (Figure 7–1). Then she asked him to draw a graph to indicate his future plans. If he were thinking in a healthy direction, how much time would he like to devote to the physical illness compared to other aspects of his life?

The CBT strategy that was used here is often termed *reattribution*. This method involves identifying an attribution (assignment of meaning or significance about a problem or stressor) that is distorted or inaccurate and then helping the patient develop a more reasonable way of viewing the situation. Larry had been making global and absolute attributions about the significance of the ulcerative colitis, and these misattributions were fueling his suicidal thoughts.

The reattribution technique worked rapidly to help reduce hopelessness and suicidal thinking. Among other items in his antisuicide plan, Larry noted that "I will only allow myself to devote 20% or less of my time and energy to colitis—I will build up the other parts of my life that make it worth living." He was discharged from the hospital after a 5-day stay and then received a course of outpatient CBT. Larry had a full remission from depression and learned to cope effectively with the symptoms of ulcerative colitis. Suicidal thinking did not return.

Behavioral methods can also be very useful components of antisuicide plans. Although simple behavioral assignments can seem somewhat superficial at first glance, patients who are experiencing deep despair, intense anxiety, sleeplessness, or other troubling symptoms need relief. If behavioral interventions can lessen these symptoms, then they are well worth including in the plan. The activity should be something that the patient can realistically perform and is likely to be helpful. Examples of simple behavioral plans include 1) devoting at least an hour a day to pleasurable activities (e.g., reading, cooking a new recipe, talking on the phone with a friend); 2) following sleep hygiene recommendations; and 3) listening to a relaxation tape.

Mary was having trouble fighting low energy and anhedonia, but she was able to list two activities as part of her antisuicide plan. She noted that having her sister visit, even if they only watched a TV program together, helped relieve her despair. She felt connected to someone who accepted her for who she was and would support her "no matter what." Another positive activity was "spend time with kids—help them do homework, read with them, play a game." Later in the chapter, we give more detail on using behavioral methods and explain how these techniques were used to help Mary relieve depressive symptoms.

A. How much my life is occupied by colitis now.

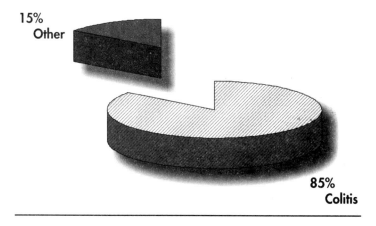

15%
Other

85%
Colitis

B. How much I plan my life to be occupied by colitis in the future.

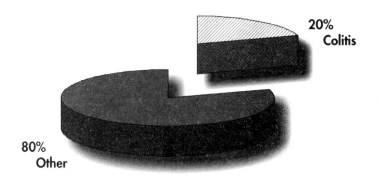

20%
Colitis

80%
Other

Figure 7–1. Reattribution: Larry's example.

Develop Coping Strategies for Possible Triggers of Hopelessness or Increased Suicidal Thinking. Planning ahead for ways to cope with potential stressors may be particularly important for long-term success. If patients can identify possible future problems or events that could stimulate suicidal thinking, then CBT strategies can be developed for effectively managing these situations. Examples of possible triggers are getting fired or laid off from a job, finding out that your wife is actually having an affair that she denied previously, financial reversals, diagnosis of a severe medical illness, and return of depression that appeared to be under control. Sometimes cognitive-behavior therapists use a "worst-case scenario" technique in which the patient is asked to imagine that a feared outcome actually occurs. By bringing these fears out into the open, therapists can help patients build strategies for coping in advance. Thus, patients are prepared to manage events that previously may have set off a downward spiral into suicidality.

To help strengthen Mary's antisuicide plan, Dr. Wright asked her to imagine a bad argument with her husband that might make her suicidal thoughts return. He then asked her to identify the negative automatic thoughts, emotions, and behavioral responses that would occur in this situation. Mary noted that she might think, "I'm worthless"; "I'm never good enough"; "What's the use?" and that she would feel very depressed and angry. Her likely behavioral response would be to shout a few critical remarks and then to isolate herself and brood over the argument. After Dr. Wright and Mary used examining the evidence and other CBT methods to develop more rational thinking, they role-played more adaptive and assertive behavioral responses. These strategies were recorded on a coping card that Mary kept in her pocketbook.

Write Out the Plan and Review It Frequently.   Writing out the key elements of the plan can help patients remember strategies developed in sessions and promote use of CBT antisuicide methods. We typically recommend that patients carry the plan with them and review it on a regular basis. In work with inpatients who have attempted suicide or have been admitted because of severe suicidal risk, we often begin a CBT intervention on the first day with a list of reasons to live and post this in their room where they will see it frequently. They are asked to add items to the list for homework and to discuss the list with nurses and others who may be able to help. By the time of discharge, the list of reasons to live is gradually expanded to a fully developed, written antisuicide plan. Mary's antisuicide plan is shown in Table 7–4.

An Antisuicide Plan for a Patient With Schizophrenia

To illustrate how an intervention similar to the one used with Mary could be adapted for other conditions, we will briefly describe an antisuicide plan for a patient with psychosis. Antonio was a 38-year-old man who had been diagnosed with schizophrenia at age 17. Since that time, he had struggled with thoughts of uselessness and defeat. He had married once in his early 20s, but the relationship fell apart quickly after he was hospitalized with severe paranoia. Attempts to work had been similarly unsuccessful. Although he had completed high school, the best job he ever held was as a fast-food worker for a few weeks. Currently, he was living alone and was receiving a monthly disability payment. His positive symptoms of psychosis

---

Table 7–4.   Mary's antisuicide plan

Remind self of "My Reasons to Live": children, husband and hope for improved marriage, father is back in my life, return to school for nursing degree.

Contact others if suicidal thinking gets stronger: sister's number [list] and 24-hour emergency number [list].

Keep only a 2-week supply of antidepressant.

Think of the things that I have done well: raised my children, coped with a divorce, ran a day care operation, helped lots of families and children.

Do positive things that improve my mood: ask sister to visit, spend time with kids.

Use coping card for dealing with possible future arguments with husband. Spot automatic thoughts and try to avoid excessive self-criticism.

---

had been under fairly good control with antipsychotic medication that he took regularly, but he had noticed the return of voices in the last 3–4 weeks.

Antonio had just been admitted to the hospital because he was having increasing thoughts of self-harm, including stepping in front of a car or bus. The only stressors that he could identify were an upcoming high school reunion, which he had decided not to attend, and the news that his only sibling, a 32-year-old sister, had just become pregnant for the first time. The thought of attending the reunion filled him with dread because he was so ashamed of the way his life had turned out. Although Antonio said he was happy for his sister, he admitted that this event highlighted his failure to have his own family or to have any other successes.

The initial interview after hospitalization also revealed that Antonio had started to hear voices telling him that he was a loser and that he should jump in front of a car. He was quite hopeless and at first could see no reason to fight against the voices that were calling for his death. The psychiatrist revised Antonio's antipsychotic medication regimen, and CBT was used to build hope and lower the risk for suicide.

The intervention with Antonio did not start directly with generating a list of reasons to live. He was so defeated and beaten down that the therapeutic work began with simple behavioral activation—finding a few things that he could do on the inpatient unit that gave him a bit of respite from his condemning voices and despair. A daily activity schedule was implemented, and it was found that he got some relief from participating in board games and being able to use an exercise bike on the unit. He also reported enjoying sessions with his psychiatrist and a nurse—both of whom had experience in CBT.

After achieving at least a small benefit from behavioral activation and building the therapeutic relationship, the psychiatrist gently started to question Antonio about reasons to live:

> Psychiatrist: I know that you said that you feel like you are totally alone and that it wouldn't make any difference to anyone if you committed suicide. But, just for a moment let's see if there is any other way to look at the situation. Could it be that you have been so discouraged and depressed that you haven't been able to recognize the importance of some of your relationships?
>
> Antonio: I still have my parents.
>
> Psychiatrist: And how would your suicide affect them?
>
> Antonio: It would probably kill my mother. She has been sick anyway—she has a heart problem.
>
> Psychiatrist: So if we started a list of reasons to fight the voices and keep living, what do you think about writing down something about your parents?
>
> Antonio: Yes, I don't want to cause them any pain.

After starting the list of reasons to live, the psychiatrist explored some other possibilities:

> Psychiatrist: What do you do besides sitting alone in your apartment?
>
> Antonio: I go to the program at the community center 3 or 4 days a week.
>
> Psychiatrist: And what do you do there?
>
> Antonio: I answer the phones, make copies, and help out around the office. (Mood appears to lift slightly.)
>
> Psychiatrist: You look a bit happier. Do you enjoy the work at the center?
>
> Antonio: Sure. I feel like I'm sort of needed. I do something useful for a change. And, I have some friends there.
>
> Psychiatrist: (Hands list of reasons to live to Antonio). Can you think of anything to say about your work at the center that you could add to the list?
>
> Antonio: Yes, It's good for me to go to the center. I actually am needed. People notice when I don't attend.

Over a period of about 10 days, the psychiatrist, the nursing staff, and the group CBT therapist worked together with Antonio on developing an antisuicide plan that used some of the standard items in Table 7–1, but also included customized interventions targeted at his psychotic symptoms and his social isolation (Table 7–5). For example, they developed several useful coping strategies for reducing the intensity and believability of his voices. Also, the antisuicide plan was communicated to the staff at his day program who agreed to help Antonio follow the plan.

Table 7–5. Antonio's antisuicide plan

Think of my positive reasons to live.
  My parents
  I am needed at the community center, and I enjoy working there.
  I am basically a good person who deserves to live, just like anyone else. It isn't my fault that I hear voices. Lots of people hear voices.
  I can learn to enjoy things more and make new friends.

Use coping skills for voices.
  Listen to soft music. Use earphones.
  Learn to shift my attention to other things like reading, paying attention to my meals, painting, walking.
  Remind myself that I do not have to pay attention to the voices or do what they say.
  Take medication every day at the same time, when I am brushing my teeth before going to bed.

Spend less time alone.
  Attend community center five times a week.
  Accept the invitation of a friend at the center to have dinner together.
  See parents at least two times a week.
  Resume attending free concerts. Go with other people if possible.

If thoughts of suicide get stronger and I need help—
  Call my therapist's emergency number [list].
  Call my parents.

If you have not developed CBT antisuicide plans for your own patients, such as the ones shown in this chapter for Mary and Antonio, or if you do not use these plans routinely in clinical practice with patients at risk for suicide, take some time now to do the next learning exercise.

Learning Exercise 7–1. Developing an Antisuicide Plan

1. Think of one of your patients who has expressed significant suicidal thoughts.

2. Imagine your asking this person for a list of reasons to live. Write down some responses that might be likely.

3. Now, write down at least two ideas you have for adding additional items or more detail to the list. How could you help the patient build an effective case against suicide?

4. Next write out a full antisuicide plan, including a list of reasons to live, safety precautions, and at least two other cognitive or behavioral interventions to build hope or reduce suicide risk.

Low Energy and Lack of Interest

Reduced energy levels and anhedonia are very common symptoms in both acute and chronic forms of depression. Fava and coworkers (1996, 1997, 1998, 2002), who have completed a number of studies of CBT for treatment-resistant depression, recommend a vigorous effort to improve energy and stimulate interest. Their research has shown a solid effect for CBT in treating resistant or residual depression.

Most of the work in treating low energy and lack of interest utilizes standard CBT methods, especially behavioral techniques such as activity scheduling and graded task assignments. However, Fava's group has suggested that a focus on promoting the patient's positive attributes and potentials can add an important dimension to the therapy process. Table 7–6 lists some of the most useful CBT methods for building energy and interest.

Behavioral Interventions

In many respects, the behavioral methods used for treating low energy and interest involve "trench work." These techniques aren't fancy or particularly stimulating for therapists. They can be repetitive and may lack interest to clinicians who have done them many times over with a myriad of patients. However, the core behavioral methods of CBT for depression can pay great dividends in treating patients with severe or treatment-resistant depression (Dimidjian et al. 2006). In this section, we describe how basic behavioral methods can be directed at reversing the difficult-to-treat problems of poor energy and anhedonia and completing effortful tasks.

Behavioral Activation

The term *behavioral activation* is sometimes used to describe any effort to increase the patient's level of activity. However, we use this term in a narrower manner to refer to simple behavioral plans—collaborative agree-

Table 7–6. CBT strategies to improve energy and interest

Use basic behavioral methods.

　Behavioral activation

　Activity scheduling

　Graded task assignments

Pitch interventions at appropriate level for patient.

Be a good coach—persistent, collaborative, creative.

Use cognitive methods to enhance behavioral initiatives.

Capitalize on patient's strengths; build sense of well-being.

Use mindfulness techniques.

Focus on rhythms of daily life—sleep-wake cycle and meals.

ments to engage in one or a limited number of activities that the patient believes would make him or her feel better (Wright et al. 2006). A few examples of behavioral activation (e.g., "ask sister to visit, spend time with kids") were given earlier in the chapter when we discussed treatment of hopelessness and development of antisuicide plans. Often behavioral activation is used early in treatment before more detailed behavioral interventions can be organized or attempted. Behavioral activation can give the patient a sense of accomplishment and positive movement, which then has a ripple effect on other therapy initiatives.

In performing behavioral activation or any other behavioral technique, it is important to fully collaborate with the patient in choosing appropriate targets for change and to select targets that are reachable, yet meaningful. For some patients with pronounced depression, the assignments may need to be rudimentary at first (e.g., walk around the block at least once this week, eat at least three meals at home this week instead of eating all meals at the fast-food restaurant; look at one of the magazines that is in the pile at home). In preparing for such assignments, it can be useful to normalize the struggle to pull out of depression and to educate the patient with statements such as "It can help to do anything to get moving again, even if you start with a small step"; "It can be very difficult to fight the low energy of depression"; "Can you just give it a try, and if it doesn't work out, we'll come up with another plan the next time we talk?"

Depending on the level of depression and the patient's capacities and previous experiences, behavioral activation can sometimes achieve more rapid results. For example, Beth, a 72-year-old woman with moderate, chronic depression, noted that she had stopped almost all of the pleasurable activities that she had engaged in before her husband's death 2 years ago. Among other activities, she had played bingo with her female friends, had gone to church regularly, had enjoyed cooking classes, had traveled widely with her husband, and had volunteered to record books for visually handicapped persons. During the first CBT session, Beth reported that her grief had been so intense that she couldn't "enjoy anything" and had been living out her days in "miserable loneliness." A behavioral activation assignment to resume attending her bingo games and church led very quickly to increased socialization and reduced depression.

When patients with severe or treatment-resistant depression come to therapy they often have good ideas about what they need to do to get going again, but they haven't been able to make changes on their own. So, how does a meeting with a cognitive-behavior therapist help break the gridlock in the patient's life? The decision to meet with a therapist often indicates that patients have the motivation to change; and if they form an effective bond with the clinician, it may take just a nudge from the therapist to begin a process of reengagement in activities. Also, therapists can provide support and effective coaching on how to overcome barriers to change.

Using a problem-solving approach, therapists can identify possible obstacles to completing a behavioral assignment and then develop strategies to overcome these difficulties. In treatment of Beth, the therapist asked if there might be anything that could get in the way of her attending church again. Beth admitted that she would be embarrassed to see the pastor because she hadn't been to church for several years, and that the fear of embarrassment could make her stay at home. The therapist then helped her reframe the experience by realizing that the pastor would be likely to be happy about her return because of his concern for her and because he probably wanted as many people as possible to attend his services. They also developed a short list of positive reasons to resume going to church (e.g., "I will be around lots of people"; "I like to hear the choir music"; "I've missed paying attention to my spiritual side"; "I could get involved in volunteer activities there").

Activity Scheduling

Many patients with difficult-to-treat depression can benefit from activity scheduling—a more organized and methodical reactivation technique used frequently in CBT (Wright et al. 2006). We will not give a detailed explanation of this method here because it is covered in basic texts (A.T. Beck et al. 1979; Wright et al. 2006). *Learning Cognitive-Behavior Therapy: An Illustrated Guide* (Wright et al. 2006) gives a full description of this technique and also includes a video illustration. A weekly activity schedule is included in Appendix 1 ("Worksheets and Checklists") and can be downloaded from the American Psychiatric Publishing Web site (www.appi.org/pdf/62321).

Activity scheduling involves asking the patient to record activities for a week, a day, or a portion of a day and then to rate the activities for mastery (sense of achievement) and pleasure on scales of 0–10 or 0–5 points. The ratings often display modulations in mastery or pleasure, which can be used to demonstrate to patients that they are able to perform tasks and experience enjoyment. In addition, the activity schedule may indicate 1) types of activities that could be increased to help reverse anhedonia; and 2) activities that could be decreased, or managed in a more adaptive manner, because they are associated with symptom worsening.

Because patients with resistant depression are often stuck in maladaptive behavioral patterns, it can be helpful to use brainstorming to generate interesting or previously unconsidered ideas for change. Also, therapists can ask patients to reflect on activities that were important before their depression clouded daily life or to imagine that the depression is gone and they can engage in any activity they desire. These brainstorming and imagery methods can help patients generate good options for modifying their activities to fight low energy and anhedonia.

When deep or chronic depression is present, the therapist may need to be persistent and not give up easily when patients seem to resist changing their behavioral patterns. Good coaching techniques are often required. If the therapist can remain supportive while still encouraging change, and be creative in suggesting options for finding new or stimulating activities, it is often possible to effectively treat anhedonia in patients with long-standing symptoms.

The next video illustration shows Dr. Wright helping Mary use activity scheduling to break out of the rut of spending most of her time at home in front of the TV. Mary rated the amount of pleasure she had watching TV as only a 2 on a 10-point scale. Yet she was doing very little else with her time and was berating herself for being so unproductive. After explaining the activity scale and mastery and pleasure ratings, Dr. Wright introduces the brainstorming technique. This strategy proves successful in helping Mary generate some excellent ideas for change. As more ideas come forth, Mary's mood lightens and she seems more optimistic. The vignette ends with Mary agreeing to accept an invitation to go fishing with her father and her sons—an activity that seems likely to boost interest and open doors to additional opportunities for change.

▶ **Video Illustration 11.** Behavioral Intervention for Anhedonia: Dr. Wright and Mary

Graded Task Assignments

When patients appear to be stuck in depression and are overwhelmed by problems that seem insurmountable, a step-by-step approach can often help them achieve success. For example, Rick, a 48-year-old salesman, had fallen behind on meeting his sales goals after struggling with depression that had lasted over a year. He had valiantly tried to keep up with work, but now he was thinking that he would be defeated by the depression, would fall further behind, and would certainly lose his job. In the last month, he had made no sales calls and was spending his time at home worrying how he would ever pay his bills. He reported very low interest and energy.

One of the strategies used with Rick was to help him break down the task of getting back to making sales calls into a series of gradual steps that could build confidence and help him reach his goal. The first step was to sort through his e-mail and voice mail to discard any junk mail and to place contacts from prospective customers into a separate file. He had been ignoring his e-mail and voice mail for over 2 weeks. Next he prioritized the list of potential customers by ranking them in categories: 1) people I know well—old customers who would be easy to call; 2) possible leads, but contacts whom I don't know well; 3) people I don't know at all—probably very "tough sells." Then he further broke down the first category into contacts that would be likely to place an order and those who would be less likely to buy his product. Then he agreed to a first step of making three calls a day to "easy sells" in category 1. Further graded task assignments were developed to assist Rick in getting back into as productive a mode as possible.

The method of graded task assignment is a very common-sense approach that is used routinely in managing daily life by most people. Yet when depression becomes severe or long-lasting, patients may forget how to use this method or seem paralyzed by inaction. Their efficiency plummets, and problems with low energy and task completion escalate. Coaching on the graded task method needs to be done judiciously so that patients do not feel demeaned or put down by suggestions that they use these simple methods to help organize their efforts. Therapists can make comments such as "When you are feeling well, I'm sure that you can do these things naturally; however, depression gets in the way of thinking clearly to organize plans to solve problems. Can I suggest some methods that can help you get back on track?" Readers who are interested in learning more about graded task assignments and wish to view a video illustration can consult Wright et al. (2006).

Cognitive Methods for Improving Energy and Interest

Cognitive methods can be interwoven with behavioral techniques in an overall CBT strategy for treating low interest and anhedonia. Often behavioral initiatives will uncover maladaptive cognitions that are fueling the problem. In the example of a graded task assignment given above, Rick had a number of self-defeating automatic thoughts as he began to organize a plan to get back to work. These thoughts (e.g., "It's too much for me"; "I can't handle it"; "I'll never get back to normal"; "I can't face my boss") were loaded with cognitive errors such as absolutistic thinking, catastrophizing, and magnifying. He was also ignoring the evidence that he still had many job skills and that he had some excellent contacts for potential sales. Thus, the treatment plan included work on revising maladaptive automatic thoughts and helping Rick develop a realistic assessment of the path ahead. He had challenges to face, but he had significant assets to bring to the task.

Another common example of a behavioral assignment that can trigger negative automatic thoughts is activity scheduling. Persons with deep depression can report that they have little or no interest in activities or tasks and are so fatigued that they can't accomplish anything. Yet when an activity schedule is completed, it is discovered that they have at least some capacity to enjoy themselves and be productive. After documenting these findings on the activity schedule, the therapist can use this evidence to test the validity of the absolutistic statements about interest and energy.

Maladaptive schemas can also play a role in anhedonia or low productivity. For example, in Video Illustration 3, Dr. Wright demonstrated a CBT initiative to directly challenge a very destructive belief ("I'm a hopeless case") that Mary had developed after a series of unsuccessful treatments. He asked Socratic questions that helped Mary revise this belief and then devote energy to using CBT to overcome her depression. As she changed this belief, she became more animated and started to show more interest in activities.

Although any of the basic cognitive interventions (e.g., Socratic questioning, modifying automatic thoughts, thought records, examining the evidence, reattribution, revising schemas) can be used to stimulate improvement in energy and interest, Fava and coworkers (1996, 1997, 1998, 2002) have recommended that an emphasis be placed on promoting potential strengths. They make a special attempt to help patients develop cognitions and behaviors that enhance a sense of well-being. Thus, the therapist using Fava's modifications may spend less time identifying negative automatic thoughts and schemas and more time working to reinforce and build positive or adaptive thoughts and beliefs. Also, behavioral strategies may lean toward recognizing and facilitating the growth of constructive and affirmative behaviors.

Mindfulness

Mindfulness is being used increasingly in CBT for depression and may have a useful role to play in patients with anhedonia. Studies of mindfulness approaches have typically focused on use of these methods to prevent relapse in patients who have responded to other treatments and are not currently depressed (Ma and Teasdale 2004; Teasdale et al. 2000). The reason that mindfulness-based approaches are not recommended as the primary treatment for acute or chronic depression is that a full mindfulness intervention involves training in meditation—an activity that may be difficult for persons with significant depression.

One of the precepts of mindfulness is that many people become preoccupied with unproductive worries and become stuck in rigid and maladaptive behavioral patterns because they are not mindful or aware of the everyday sensations that they experience as human beings. People can conduct their lives as if they are robots that place one foot in front of the other in a mechanical and disconnected march through life. Instead, the mindful approach encourages an exploration of senses and perceptions, especially for everyday activities that often are overlooked. For example, people can learn to truly experience and savor the food that they eat, allow themselves to fully appreciate all the stimuli in nature, or open their minds to the words they read in books or to the sounds they hear in music.

Extensive treatment with mindfulness approaches involves training in meditation and development of a metacognitive perspective (i.e., negative thoughts come to be viewed as mental events instead of a perception of the whole self) (Segal et al. 2002), but we have found that the general concept of mindfulness (without formal training in meditation) can help some persons with resistant depression build their level of interest for both the routine and the special things in their lives. Good books about mindfulness to recommend to patients are *Full Catastrophe Living: Using the Wisdom of Your Body to Fight Stress, Pain, and Illness* (Kabat-Zinn 1990) and *The Mindful Way Through Depression: Freeing Yourself From Chronic Unhappiness* (Williams et al. 2007).

Regulating the Sleep-Wake Cycle and Other Daily Rhythms

Insomnia, one of the trademark symptoms of depression, can be part of a vicious cycle that accompanies low energy and interest. People who have very poor sleep are likely to be exhausted and depleted during their waking hours and may not want to participate in enjoyable, diverting, or productive activities. In turn, those who spend their days in boredom, inactivity, or repetitive cycles of unproductive worry may have difficulty falling asleep at night. CBT has much to offer in treating insomnia and thus helping with low energy and other symptoms of depression. Studies of CBT for insomnia have found that CBT may be more effective than benzodiazepines or similar medications (Edinger et al. 2007; Sivertsen et al. 2006). CBT methods for insomnia are described in Chapter 8, "Mania."

The major regulator of circadian rhythms is the sleep-wake cycle, but other daily activities such as meal times, work and recreational schedules, and periods of exercise can either stabilize or dysregulate the "biological clock." Recent research has suggested that regularizing the sleep-wake cycle and other daily rhythms can be helpful in the treatment of bipolar disorder (Frank 2007; Frank et al. 2005). Interpersonal and social rhythms therapy as developed by Frank (2005) seeks to stabilize daily rhythms and thus correct irregularities in the circadian secretion of cortisol, thyroid hormone, growth hormone, and other hormones; and perhaps promote normal functioning of neurotransmitter and second messenger systems in the brain. Although social rhythms therapy is not typically a part of CBT for depression, we think it is reasonable to advise regularity of the daily schedule as part of an overall plan to restore normal sleep patterns and energy.

> **Learning Exercise 7–2.** Using CBT for Low Energy and Anhedonia
>
> 1. Think of a depressed patient you are seeing, or have seen, who has difficult-to-treat low energy and anhedonia.
>
> 2. Write out a treatment plan for using CBT for these symptoms.
>
> 3. List at least three ideas for breaking the pattern of low energy and anhedonia. Detail these interventions with specific examples.
>
> 4. Be creative in thinking of possible ways to stimulate energy and interest.

Treating Low Energy and Anhedonia in Schizophrenia

The behavioral and cognitive methods for treatment of unipolar and bipolar depression described in this chapter can be modified for use in patients with schizophrenia and other psychoses. In general, the goals and pace of interventions are reduced to be consistent with the patient's ability to engage in treatment and to work toward change. As noted in Chapter 11 ("Negative Symptoms"), patients with significant negative symptoms, such as severe apathy or social withdrawal, may require slow, very gradual efforts to help them engage in activities or to participate in rehabilitation efforts. Also, patients who have marked disorganization of thinking may not be good candidates for using CBT methods for low energy and interest. Some of the patient characteristics or symptoms that may suggest that classic CBT methods, such as behavioral activation, activity scheduling, and graded task assignments, may be useful are listed in Table 7–7.

Earlier in this chapter, we discussed how behavioral activation and activity scheduling were used to help Antonio, the man with schizophrenia who was quite depressed and hearing voices telling him to kill himself. In Chapter 11 ("Negative Symptoms"), additional examples are provided of behavioral methods for psychotic patients who are experiencing negative symptoms, social withdrawal, and anhedonia.

Low Self-Esteem

Patients with chronic and treatment-resistant depression often have low self-esteem that can be quite entrenched and difficult to treat (Wright 2003). They may describe years of disappointments and perceived failures that appear to prove the case that they are doomed to a lifetime of rejection, loneliness, and lack of achievement or love. In this section, we describe strategies for building self-esteem and self-efficacy in chronic depression (Table 7–8). These techniques may also be useful in patients with bipolar disorder who primarily have recurrent depressive episodes, in bipolar patients who have low self-esteem despite periods of mania, and in modified form for patients with schizophrenia.

Identifying Cognitions and Behaviors That Control Self-Esteem

One of the most important steps in tackling chronic self-esteem difficulties is to identify the key cognitions and behavioral strategies that define the patient's self-concept (A.T. Beck et al. 2003). Because schemas are the enduring, deeply held beliefs that regulate self-concept (Clark et al. 1999), they are often a primary target of CBT for long-standing self-esteem problems. We emphasize CBT methods for core beliefs and associated behavior patterns here, but also recommend that standard CBT interventions for identifying and modifying automatic thoughts be used in treating low self-

Table 7–7. Treating low energy and interest in schizophrenia

When may CBT interventions be most useful?

A good working relationship has been established.

Severity of thought disorder is low to moderate.

Effort can be sustained for at least short periods of time.

Patient appears to have some interest in feeling better and working toward change.

There is at least some support from family, friends, or persons in a therapy group.

esteem. Techniques for working with automatic thoughts are described elsewhere in this book and in standard texts (A.T. Beck et al. 1979; Wright et al. 2006).

Because chronic depression is often associated with problems that have actually occurred or are occurring (e.g., hypercritical parents, difficulties with acceptance by family or peers, traumatic events, school underachievement, job underperformance or loss, marital distress or divorce, and social skills deficits), it is important for the clinician to recognize and validate these real-life influences. Yet, persons with chronic depression often have developed a cognitive and behavioral style that serves as a "self-fulfilling prophecy." If someone believes "I've been so damaged that no one could ever love me" or "I'm a failure," he may act in a manner consistent with the belief (e.g., avoidance of relationships or of commitment to relationships; not recognizing or rejecting valuable opportunities for education, work advancement, or personal growth).

Sometimes core beliefs that influence self-esteem are readily apparent, but often underlying schemas can be submerged or obscured. Thus, a special effort may be required to uncover them and begin the process of change. The most commonly used technique for identifying schemas

Table 7–8. CBT principles for treating chronic low self-esteem

Identify self-defeating automatic thoughts and schemas.

Identify behavioral patterns associated with maladaptive beliefs.

Use cognitive strategies to modify automatic thoughts and schemas.

Work on behavioral change.

Practice, practice, practice.

is the collaborative questioning style of CBT (Wright et al. 2006). Therapists ask good questions that help patients tell their story and verbalize important cognitive and behavioral themes. This type of questioning is modeled in a number of the video illustrations, including the videos of Dr. Wright and Mary and of Dr. Kingdon and Majir.

Psychoeducation also can play an important part in identifying schemas. Patients usually are not fully aware that negatively biased schemas can be based on misinterpretations of the meanings of events or communications from others. Instead, patients may regard these beliefs as established facts that are not open to question. Lack of knowledge about schemas also frequently extends to limited awareness of the positive coping value of adaptive schemas and the importance of recognizing, promoting, and more fully developing these beliefs. Therapists can briefly explain these concepts, give illustrations from the patient's life, suggest readings, and provide other learning experiences.

The basic goal of the educational process is to show patients that schemas form the basis of their self-esteem and that people can build a healthy self-concept by 1) revising inaccurate and self-limiting core beliefs, 2) cultivating self-affirming schemas, and 3) practicing more effective behaviors that are consistent with adaptive beliefs.

Another method for helping patients recognize their core beliefs is to spot recurring patterns of automatic thoughts—the more superficial level of cognitions that are typically driven by underlying schemas (A.T. Beck et al. 1979; Clark et al. 1999; Wright et al. 2006). For example, automatic thoughts with themes of unacceptance or unlovability (e.g., "I don't measure up to her expectations"; "Nothing I do ever pleases her"; "She is bound to leave me") could be associated with core beliefs such as "No matter what I do, I won't be accepted" or "I will always be rejected."

One of the most useful methods of identifying schemas in persons with chronic low self-esteem is to infer their presence by spotting repetitive, problematic behavioral patterns. Then a hypothesis is formed about a possible underlying schema, and collaborative questioning is used to determine if the hypothesized core belief is actually present. Some examples of chronic behavioral patterns that might predict the presence of self-defeating schemas are perfectionism ("I'm never good enough"); going overboard to please others ("No one could accept me for the way I am"); and lack of effort in school or work ("I'm stupid").

The method of uncovering schemas by first characterizing habitual behavioral patterns can also be used when psychotic symptoms are present. Examples include these possible behavior-schema links: shame and social isolation ("I'm so different from others that I should stay away from people"; "I'm not fit to be with others"); avoidance of church or other spiritual activities that were once important to the patient ("Because the devil talks to me, I'm evil"); and self-effacing behavior, such as always glancing away from others or trying to remain "invisible" ("I'm worthless"; "I don't count").

Cognitive Methods for Building Self-Esteem

The classic methods of CBT for depression described by Aaron Beck and colleagues (A. T. Beck et al. 1979; J. Beck 1995; Wright et al. 2006) provide highly useful tools for building self-esteem in chronic depression. Some of the most frequently used cognitive techniques for low self-esteem are Socratic questioning, thought change records, examining the evidence for schemas, listing advantages and disadvantages for schemas, using a cognitive continuum, reattribution, generating alternative schemas, and rehearsing modified schemas (J. Beck 1995; Wright et al. 2006). In all of these procedures, a well-being emphasis, as recommended by Fava and coworkers (Fava 1999; Fava and Ruini 2003; Fava et al. 1996, 1997, 1998, 2004) may be particularly useful for residual or treatment-resistant depression.

Video Illustration 12 gives an example of cognitive interventions for low self-esteem. Mary, a woman with chronic depression, has revealed a core belief ("I'll never succeed") and other related beliefs ("I really haven't ever done anything"; "I'm never good enough") that are centered on the theme of personal competence. Mary tells Dr. Wright that she received constant criticism from her mother and "never did what my mother wanted me to do." Her father was always working and was "never at home" so she did not have role models for people who were successful. Nor did she seem to receive much support for using her strengths to achieve success. Later, a failed marriage, financial problems, and recurrent depression added credence to the belief that she would never succeed. Yet, Mary had significant strengths that she was largely ignoring, and she had experienced successes that were either minimized or forgotten.

> ▶ **Video Illustration 12.** Building Self-Esteem:
> Dr. Wright and Mary

When the therapist first introduced examining the evidence in this video illustration, Mary had trouble finding any clear evidence against her maladaptive belief "I'll never succeed." She noted one positive element from her past ("I did work for a while at UPS") but then quickly discounted this fact ("But then I had to quit"; "I didn't finish school"; "I haven't been doing anything since then"). Slipping almost immediately back into a very self-condemning cognitive style is a common problem in patients with chronic low self-esteem. They seem to be masters at minimizing strengths or positive contributions and maximizing perceived weaknesses or negative outcomes.

In this video illustration, the therapist did several things to try to help Mary develop a more balanced view of herself. First, he explained the concept of schemas as beliefs that "have been stamped into your mind" and can "drag you down and keep you from reaching your potential." In framing schemas in this manner, he was explaining that core beliefs are changeable and that such changes could free Mary from the negative messages of the past and open doors to positive growth.

After this brief psychoeducational intervention, Mary begins to present some evidence against her pejorative core beliefs about success and competence (e.g., "I feel good about my daughter"; "She's finishing up technical school"; "I'm proud of her; she is pretty successful"). However, she still has difficulty seeing through the negative filter of chronic depression to identify more examples of possible successes or achievements. The video illustration shows Dr. Wright subtly prompting Mary with ideas for places to look for evidence against her negative beliefs (i.e., her work operating a day care program, her strengths in fighting adversity, her marriage). Although it is best if patients can do the majority of the work themselves in recognizing counterbalancing experiences or attributes, patients with deeply held negative beliefs and very resistant low self-esteem may need help in this process.

After Mary is able to recognize several good lines of evidence against her dysfunctional belief (Table 7–9 contains the entire exercise for examining the evidence that Mary did in session and completed for homework), Dr. Wright begins an intervention to modify the schema. He asks her, "If you carry around with you this belief 'I'll never succeed' or 'I'm not a success,' how does this affect things that might happen from here on out? How does this influence your effort, whatever you might do in your life...from this day forward?" Mary's answer is predictable: "I just don't do anything, I don't try to do anything." The link between the negative core belief and the self-defeating behavioral pattern is now clear to both patient and therapist, and the need for change is boldly evident. A somewhat dramatic or expressive way of making key points to the patient, as exemplified in this interchange, may be needed to break through the rigid thinking style of patients with chronic low self-esteem.

The remainder of Video Illustration 12 shows efforts to develop a modified schema and to start planning targets for behavioral change. Mary relates that she wants to revise the schema to "I would like to succeed....I would like to help others." This modification still does not reflect

Table 7–9. Examining the evidence for Mary's schema "I'll never succeed"

Evidence for	Evidence against
I don't do anything.	My daughter is a success; I'm proud of her.
I didn't finish nursing school.	I did a good job in day care; the parents were grateful.
I quit my job.	I have fought financial problems and depression.
I haven't returned to school.	I've been with my husband for 16 years; maybe the marriage is a success.
	I really enjoy being with my kids, and I'm a good parent.
	I want to return to school to become a practical nurse.
	I really like to help people, and I think I can do this.

a balanced, or particularly positive, self-concept—but now there is potential for moving away from her rigidly held, absolutistic beliefs about personal failure and the futility of trying to achieve success.

The video shows only a small sample of therapeutic interventions to build self-esteem. Typically this type of work takes considerable time and effort, especially if there have been many real-life traumas or failures and there have been many months or years of acting in ways that are consistent with core beliefs about low self-esteem. Dr. Wright's plans to help Mary build self-esteem included some of these items:

1. Set reachable short- and long-term goals for increasing mastery of meaningful and productive pursuits (i.e., move from "I do nothing" to "I do lots of things well, have many interests, and am achieving success").
2. Engage in step-wise behavioral plans to act on revised schemas about self-efficacy.
3. Consider use of a cognitive continuum to help her view herself more accurately (i.e., use a 0–100 point scale with total success at one pole and total failure at other pole; have her give ratings for how she sees herself now and how she would like to see herself in the future).

4. Continue to work on revising schemas related to self-esteem.
5. Identify positive attributes that can serve as building blocks for personal growth and increased well-being.
6. Implement behavioral assignments to increase use of positive attributes.

Behavioral Change— A Necessary Step in Building Self-Esteem

To build self-esteem, patients need to take action to change the way they have been behaving. Even if Mary is able to develop further schema revisions, such as "I have had some successes in my life and want to have more," a continued pattern of inactivity and lack of any significant movement toward meeting goals would probably lead to a reinforcement of her old beliefs and stalling of any progress toward improved self-esteem.

Some of the major behavioral methods to put revised schemas into action have been described earlier in the section "Low Energy and Lack of Interest." Behavioral activation, activity scheduling, and graded task assignments can be adapted nicely for self-esteem–related interventions. For example, Mary could use activity scheduling to reduce the time she spends "doing nothing" and increase time spent in productive activities, such as doing things with her children or investigating options for returning to school. Graded task assignments could be used to break a big challenge (e.g., returning to school, getting a job) into manageable pieces.

Because patients with chronic depression may be confronting difficult problems and may have actual skills deficits (e.g., finding a job, being assertive in personal communications, negotiating a divorce), coaching or CBT rehearsal may be needed to give behavioral plans a better opportunity for success. As noted earlier in the chapter, rehearsal techniques involve practicing adaptive ways of thinking and behaving in advance of a projected stressful situation. Another valuable method for enhancing behavioral change is to use coping cards that list specific self-affirming actions.

A likely scenario in Mary's subsequent treatment would be the development of positive coping strategies for applying for licensed practical nurse training and participating in an admission interview. Her behavior in this interview could be rehearsed in a therapy session, and a coping card could be developed (Table 7–10).

Practice, Practice, Practice

Repeated rehearsal and real-world experiences in behavioral change are often integral parts of achieving enduring improvements in self-esteem.

Table 7–10. Mary's coping card: an interview for nursing school

---

Remind myself that I did well in school last time, and only had to drop out because I had small children and couldn't afford the tuition.

Remind myself that I have lots of life experience and have been successful at running a day care program.

Keep my "head up" during the interview and speak clearly.

Effectively communicate my desire to help others.

Thus, we recommend that therapists frequently use homework assignments to put revised schemas into practice. If patients have difficulty with assignments, then the experiences can be used to identify barriers to change or to spot skill deficits that may require more coaching and rehearsal. A few examples of homework assignments to put modified schemas to work are 1) a woman with perfectionistic schemas and low self-esteem who had been spending large amounts of time cooking family dinners agrees that "spending only 30 minutes preparing dinner is acceptable" and agrees to the assignment "I will make dinner in less than 30 minutes at least half of the times I cook"; 2) a man who has believed "I am unlovable" and has been avoiding situations where he might meet women states, "I will do research on clubs such as a bicycling group where I could meet appropriate women....I will join one of these clubs and work on building up my conversational skills"; and 3) a man who has been struggling with schemas about failure participates in a homework assignment to "accept an invitation to a neighborhood dinner party and prepare in advance by making a list of topics that show some of my interests and strengths."

Learning Exercise 7–3. Modifying Schemas to Improve Self-Esteem

1. Think of a patient that you are seeing, or have seen, who has entrenched low self-esteem.

2. List at least two core beliefs and associated behavioral patterns that appear to be involved with the self-esteem problem.

3. Write down a strategy for reversing low self-esteem by modifying core beliefs and behaviors. Give specific examples of the content of the patient's thinking and the methods you plan to use.

4. Describe at least two homework assignments to put a modified schema into action.

5. Identify a barrier that you might encounter in implementing strategies for low self-esteem and write a plan for overcoming this barrier.

Building Self-Esteem in Schizophrenia

Patients with schizophrenia also can have low self-esteem as a result of traumas, stigma, relationship difficulties, secondary depression, and other problems common to this disorder. The type of detailed schema work described for treatment of chronic depression is rarely possible in patients with schizophrenia. Yet attention to core beliefs or delusional cognitions that influence self-esteem can be beneficial in some cases. Also, behavioral interventions that stimulate meaningful interests and activities can help enhance self-esteem. Dr. Kingdon's treatment of Majir (Video Illustrations 1, 5, 6, and 7) demonstrates a gentle, "go slow" approach to helping a man with paranoia and very low self-esteem. Majir sees himself as being rather incapable (only babysits for sister's children and can't accomplish going to the mall to buy a computer game), and he believes that others know about past traumatic experiences. Whenever he goes out in public, he feels estranged and singled out for ridicule. In this treatment situation, gradual empirical testing of the paranoid beliefs and development of alternative explanations help reduce Majir's self-condemnation. Also, Dr. Kingdon suggests unpressured behavioral assignments ("perhaps you could try again to buy that computer game") to help increase self-esteem and self-efficacy.

Other strategies for building self-esteem in patients with schizophrenia can be to 1) destigmatize the illness, thereby reducing sense of alienation or shame; 2) work on building coping skills for hallucinations, thus improving one's sense of control; 3) engage in rehabilitation efforts to enhance communication, recreation, and job skills; 4) encourage use of sense of humor; and 5) help patient find activities that he or she values and finds satisfying. These types of interventions can be implemented in either individual or group settings. For patients who are able to participate in group therapy, the setting may offer useful opportunities for receiving and giving support, being accepted and valued by others, and seeing models for use of effective coping strategies.

Summary

Key Points for Clinicians

- CBT methods have been shown to be effective for reducing hopelessness and suicidality.
- Development of a specific antisuicide plan is a powerful method of using CBT to reduce suicide risk.
- Although behavioral interventions for low energy and interest can seem like "trench work" to clinicians, these procedures can be very valuable to patients.
- CBT methods for regulating the sleep-wake cycle can have positive effects on energy, interest, and other symptoms of depression.
- In treatment of chronic low self-esteem, it is important to repeatedly practice modifications in schemas and associated behavioral patterns.
- Patients with schizophrenia can benefit from CBT methods to improve self-esteem.

Concepts and Skills for Patients to Learn

- Hopelessness is a symptom of depression. It can be effectively treated with CBT.
- To build hope, it is important to recognize and build strengths that may have been hidden by depression.
- If suicidal thoughts are present, it is important to work with a therapist on a safety plan.
- A vital step in fighting depression is to find things that can stimulate your interest and get you back into a good mood. A therapist can help you develop a plan to become more active.
- Getting a good night's sleep and keeping a regular schedule can help relieve symptoms of depression. CBT can help people improve sleep and better organize their lives.
- CBT can improve self-esteem and build people's abilities to accomplish goals.

References

Beck AT, Ward CH, Mendelson M, et al: An inventory of measuring depression. Arch Gen Psychiatry 4:53–63, 1961

Beck AT, Weissman A, Lester D, et al: Measurement of pessimism: the hopelessness scale. J Clin Psychol 42:861–865, 1974

Beck AT, Kovacs M, Weissman A: Hopelessness and suicidal behavior—an overview. JAMA 234:1146–1149, 1975

Beck AT, Rush AJ, Shaw BF, et al: Cognitive Therapy of Depression. New York, Guilford, 1979

Beck AT, Steer RA, Kovacs M, et al: Hopelessness and eventual suicide: a 10-year prospective study of patients hospitalized with suicidal ideation. Am J Psychiatry 142:559–562, 1985

Beck AT, Freeman A, Davis DD, et al: Cognitive Therapy of Personality Disorders, 2nd Edition. New York, Guilford, 2003

Beck JS: Cognitive Therapy: Basics and Beyond. New York, Guilford, 1995

Brown GK, Ten Have T, Henriques GR, et al: Cognitive therapy for the prevention of suicide attempts: a randomized controlled trial. JAMA 294:563–570, 2005

Clark DA, Beck AT, Alford BA: Scientific Foundations of Cognitive Theory and Therapy of Depression. New York, Wiley, 1999

DeRubeis RJ, Gelfand LA, Tang TZ, et al: Medication versus cognitive behavior therapy for severely depressed outpatients: mega-analysis of four randomized comparisons. Am J Psychiatry 156:1007–1013, 1999

Dimidjian S, Hollon SD, Dobson KS, et al: Randomized trial of behavioral activation, cognitive therapy, and antidepressant medication in the acute treatment of adults with major depression. J Consult Clin Psychol 74:658–670, 2006

Edinger JD, Wohlgemuth WK, Radtke RA, et al: Dose-response effects of cognitive-behavioral insomnia therapy: a randomized clinical trial. Sleep 30:203–212, 2007

Fava GA: Well-being therapy: conceptual and technical issues. Psychother Psychosom 68:171–179, 1999

Fava GA, Ruini C: Development and characteristics of a well-being enhancing psychotherapeutic strategy: well-being therapy. J Behav Ther Exp Psychiatry 34:45–63, 2003

Fava GA, Grandi S, Zielezny M, et al: Four-year outcome for cognitive behavioral treatment of residual symptoms in major depression. Am J Psychiatry 153:945–947, 1996

Fava GA, Savron G, Grandi S, et al: Cognitive-behavioral management of drug-resistant major depressive disorder. J Clin Psychiatry 58:278–282, 1997

Fava GA, Rafanelli C, Grandi S, et al: Prevention of recurrent depression with cognitive behavioral therapy. Arch Gen Psychiatry 55:816–820, 1998

Fava GA, Ruini C, Rafanelli C, et al: Cognitive behavior approach to loss of clinical effect during long-term antidepressant treatment: a pilot study. Am J Psychiatry 159:2094–2095, 2002

Fava GA, Ruini C, Rafanelli C, et al: Six-year outcome of cognitive behavior therapy for prevention of recurrent depression. Am J Psychiatry 161:1872–1876, 2004

Fawcett J, Scheftner W, Clark D, et al: Clinical predictors of suicide in patients with major affective disorders: a controlled prospective study. Am J Psychiatry 144:35–40, 1987

Frank E: Treating Bipolar Disorder: A Clinician's Guide to Interpersonal and Social Rhythm Therapy. New York, Guilford, 2005

Frank E: Interpersonal and social rhythm therapy: a means of improving depression and preventing relapse in bipolar disorder. J Clin Psychol 63:463–473, 2007

Frank E, Kupfer DJ, Thase ME, et al: Two-year outcomes for interpersonal and social rhythm therapy in individuals with bipolar I disorder. Arch Gen Psychiatry 62:996–1004, 2005

Kabat-Zinn J: Full Catastrophe Living: Using the Wisdom of Your Body to Fight Stress, Pain, and Illness. New York, Hyperion, 1990

Keller MB, McCullough JP, Klein DN, et al: A comparison of nefazodone, the cognitive behavioral-analysis system of psychotherapy, and their combination for the treatment of chronic depression. N Engl J Med 342:1462–1470, 2000

Luty SE, Carter JD, McKensie JM, et al: Randomised controlled trial of interpersonal psychotherapy and cognitive-behavioral therapy for depression. Br J Psychiatry 190:496–502, 2007

Ma SH, Teasdale JD: Mindfulness-based cognitive therapy for depression: replication and exploration of differential relapse prevention effects. J Consult Clin Psychol 72:31–40, 2004

McCullough JP Jr: Treatment for Chronic Depression: Cognitive Behavioral Analysis System of Psychotherapy. New York, Guilford, 2000

Rush AJ, Beck AT, Kovacs M, et al: Comparison of the effects of cognitive therapy and pharmacotherapy on hopelessness and self-concept. Am J Psychiatry 139:862–866, 1982

Segal Z, Williams JMG, Teasdale JD: Mindfulness-Based Cognitive Therapy for Depression: A New Approach to Preventing Relapse. New York, Guilford, 2002

Sivertsen B, Omvik S, Pallesen S, et al: Cognitive behavioral therapy vs zopiclone for treatment of chronic primary insomnia in older adults: a randomized controlled trial. JAMA 295:2851–2858, 2006

Teasdale JD, Segal ZV, Williams JM, et al: Prevention of relapse/recurrence in major depression by mindfulness-based cognitive therapy. J Consult Clin Psychol 68:615–623, 2000

Williams M, Teasdale J, Segal Z, et al: The Mindful Way Through Depression: Freeing Yourself From Chronic Unhappiness. New York, Guilford, 2007

Wright JH: Cognitive-behavior therapy for chronic depression. Psychiatr Ann 33:777–784, 2003

Wright JH, Basco MR, Thase ME: Learning Cognitive-Behavior Therapy: An Illustrated Guide. Washington, DC, American Psychiatric Publishing, 2006

8

Mania

It may go without saying, but the peak of a manic episode when thoughts are racing, sleep loss is causing fatigue, mood is irritable, and agitation is high may not be the best time to teach CBT skills. Interventions can have greater impact and information is more likely to be retained if conveyed when the person is much less symptomatic. As manic symptoms emerge, the patient can call on previously acquired skills to help manage them. As symptoms worsen, clinician guidance is usually needed to help the patient slow down, focus on one symptom at a time, and utilize structured interventions.

The primary emphasis of CBT for mania is on prevention of recurrences through recognition of symptoms as they begin to develop and quick intervention to slow or stop their progress. To accomplish these goals, the patient must be able to recognize mania as it approaches and be motivated to stop its progression. Mania can evolve rapidly and may not be obvious to the person until symptoms begin to impair functioning. By that time, mania may be too severe to control without aggressive changes in the pharmacological regimen. Those who have had pleasant experiences with mania, or who have been in a depressive episode for some time and welcome the perceived improvement, may not be highly motivated to avert a full manic episode. In these cases, skills training may not be useful until the individual has had an opportunity to consider the pros and cons of controlling mania and has concluded that it is worth her time and effort. Standard CBT methods can be used for comparing the advantages and disadvantages of controlling mania or of allowing the symptoms to evolve (see Basco and Rush 2005). Patients who have had euphoric manic episodes and have suffered few negative consequences from them may not be ready to learn strategies for prevention. They look forward to what they perceive as the freedom that comes with euphoria, the boost in self-esteem, and the ability to overcome inertia, especially after experiencing a lengthy period of depression. These same individuals may be highly motivated to avoid future depressive episodes, however. Therefore, the rationale for learning to prevent or control manic episodes should be framed as an overall strategy for managing the illness and reducing the recurrence of mood swings.

Mania Prevention Plan

The cognitive-behavioral approach to management of mania is based on the treatment approach of Basco and Rush (2005). The plan includes five components: 1) lifestyle management, 2) symptom recognition, 3) preparation for recurrence, 4) symptom control, and 5) postepisode analysis. Targets of intervention for each component include medication adherence, sleep hygiene, overstimulation, cognitive distortions, and escalation of emotions. The plan is to equip patients with the skills to lessen the likelihood of mania and to manage the symptoms once they begin to evolve. Each manic episode provides an opportunity to learn more about the factors that trigger recurrence and escalate symptoms, as well as the strategies that prove most helpful in their control. Over time and recurrences, the clinician, the patient, and his family members and friends can strengthen their mania prevention skills.

Not all patients realize that mania can recur and therefore, introduction of a mania prevention plan may be unsettling. Thus, clinicians should take time to educate patients about the recurrent nature of mania and the other features of bipolar illnesses. Table 8–1 provides a mania prevention plan.

Lessen the Risk of Mania with Lifestyle Management

Manage Medications

The most common precipitant of manic episodes is discontinuation of mood stabilizing medications (Keck et al. 1996). Some people become disorganized in their thoughts and actions as mania develops, the consequence of which is forgetting to take their medication. In this situation, the mania starts first and the adherence problems are a result. For other people, there is a decision to use less medication and this reduction lifts the barrier to relapse that treatment had previously provided. Chapter 12

Table 8–1. Mania prevention plan

1. Lessen the risk of mania with lifestyle management.
2. Learn to recognize the emergence of symptoms.
3. Plan ahead for future recurrences.
4. Take action to control symptoms.
5. Learn from the experience.

("Promoting Adherence") is dedicated to the problem of medication non-adherence across disorders. It provides information relevant to the control of mania and a case illustration in which Angela, who questions the validity of her diagnosis of bipolar disorder, discusses the obstacles she encounters when attempting to be consistent with her medication treatment.

Manage Sleep

A decreased need for sleep is a common symptom of mania. Some find it difficult to fall asleep because racing thoughts keep the mind alert. Others enjoy the night and do not want to give in to sleep. They feel their best at the end of the day and enjoy nighttime activities such as watching TV, sex, surfing the Internet, and socializing. During a manic episode, those who are able to fall asleep at their normally scheduled bedtime might find themselves waking earlier than normal and unable to go back to sleep. Rather than toss and turn in a futile attempt to return to sleep, they wake and begin their day. Whichever the case, sleep loss has been found to precipitate and escalate mania—and must therefore be avoided when possible.

The behaviors that enhance sleep are listed in Table 8–2. Briefly, they include 1) preventive strategies, such as reduction in stimulant use near bedtime; and 2) stimulus control, in which the bed is associated with sleep rather than activities not conducive to sleep, such as eating, watching TV, or paying bills. Physical comfort is encouraged in nightwear and bedding, and a calm atmosphere should be created—all of which increase the likelihood of relaxing enough to fall asleep. Perhaps more importantly, regularity in sleep schedule, including the avoidance of daytime napping, can help to prevent sleep loss. The reader is directed to Basco and Rush (2005) for a more complete description of strategies for enhancing sleep in bipolar disorder.

Table 8–2.   Managing sleep and activity to prevent mania

Discontinue activity at least 1 hour before bedtime.

Choose sleep over extending nighttime activity.

Mentally disengage from activities or interactions before bedtime.

Resist the urge to multitask. Do one thing at a time.

Finish one activity before starting another.

Prioritize tasks.

Plan activities to keep expectations and demands at a reasonable level.

For people who experience episodic mania, overstimulation can contribute to sleep loss, particularly sleep onset. Environmental stimulation such as noise or bright lights and consumable stimulants such as caffeine may be relatively easy to control. However, people do not always associate these sources of stimulation with insomnia, so education about stimulants may be useful. When Angela wakens during the night and can't easily go back to sleep, she makes herself a cup of coffee, sits in her favorite chair, and picks up a book. Her favorites are crime stories. She fancies herself an amateur criminologist and enjoys the challenge of figuring out who committed the crime before the author gives it away. The caffeine in her coffee coupled with a cliffhanger worsens Angela's ability to fall back to sleep. She believed, however, that drinking something warm and getting her mind off of her worries by reading a book was a good way to ease herself back into sleep. This is a common scenario. The therapist can troubleshoot sleeping practices with patients by inquiring about what they do when they cannot sleep. In addition to preventive strategies, suggest new strategies that reduce mental and physical stimulation when the patient awakens during the night.

Another simple preventive intervention is to plan ahead for schedule changes that might interfere with sleep. That would include travel, especially travel that includes time zone changes and changes in work schedules. Prescription of sleep agents in anticipation of insomnia can be part of the preventive plan. Patients often find it helpful to think through their schedule changes, especially for their regimen of psychiatric and other medications. Medications taken at bedtime that can cause sleepiness may be impractical if patients have to work or otherwise function at the time that would usually be their bedtime. Adjustments to the regimen should be planned together, otherwise patients will alter their regimens on their own to avoid the side effect of sleepiness when it is inconvenient.

Cognitive and affective interventions can also be part of a sleep management plan. For example, cognitive interventions for reducing worry before going to sleep can help, especially when coupled with problem solving. Patients can be encouraged to create plans for addressing difficulties before they go to sleep so that rumination at bedtime becomes unnecessary. Making relaxation exercises or meditation at night a routine practice can also help set the stage for a good night's sleep. These activities help ease the transition between daily activity and sleep.

For those who work or attend school during the day, the evening—including bedtime—is often the time for addressing life issues, problems, worries, and conflicts. Angela jokingly claimed that she and her boyfriend always fight at night because they don't have time to fight during the day. When she is more vulnerable to mania such as when her sleep has been disrupted by travel or she has forgotten to take her medication for several days, those arguments can keep her awake at night long after the conflict has ended and her boyfriend has gone home. For these circumstances, learning to manage stress and conflict also facilitate sleep.

Manage Stress

Psychiatric symptoms are often sensitive to stress, escalating when tension, worry, or pressures increase. Actively managing stress on a regular basis reduces the risk of symptom exacerbations. The standard cognitive and behavioral interventions aimed at reducing emotions such as anxiety or depression can help to reduce stress when applied to the negative thinking, poor coping behaviors, and emotions stimulated by psychosocial stressors and life events. Active rather than passive coping strategies should be developed and strengthened so that an accumulation of stress can be minimized. Unfortunately, the lives of people with chronic mental illnesses are often filled with difficulties. Work disruptions due to symptoms lead to financial problems. Lack of resources is often at the root of homelessness, the inability to secure treatment, and the disruption of family life. Avoidance of stress may be impossible, but psychotherapy can be helpful in providing a forum for patients with chronic mental illnesses to work through difficulties on a regular basis. Problem-solving skills can be taught, but many patients need the ongoing support of a therapist to use those skills. Depending on the patient's life circumstances, it can be helpful to schedule psychotherapy sessions on a bi-weekly or monthly basis for the purpose of stress management even after symptoms stabilize.

Conflict with others is another common source of stress. Arguments at night have been a problem for Angela because they keep her from sleeping. Even when conflict occurs early in the day, the resulting emotions can persist as people continue to think about what happened, what was said, what should have been said, and any consequences they anticipate. If the conflict has been resolved but the person continues to review the incident in her mind, thought stopping procedures can be useful (Backhaus et al. 2001; Peden et al. 2005). If worry persists, decatastrophizing methods can be used to reduce distortions and focus the patient on ways to prevent catastrophic outcomes and how to cope if the feared outcomes occur. If what remains from the conflict is regret for things said or not said, assertiveness training may help prepare the patient for a follow-up conversation to resolve what remains of the original argument. Role-playing in session is particularly useful in these circumstances if the therapist plays the role of the listener while the patient practices communicating concerns in an assertive manner. Therapists are cautioned not to instruct patients on what to say to others, but to help the patient put feelings into her own words.

It is a common mistake in CBT for newly trained therapists to bypass Socratic questioning in these circumstances. It is important to remember that in CBT the process of teaching an intervention is as important as resolving the problem under discussion. Although patients might ask therapists for advice on what to say in a particular circumstance, these quick answers should be avoided. Instead, patients should be asked what they would like to communicate if they could. These words are then rehearsed in session. Troubleshooting should occur to help the patient anticipate a negative reaction by the listener so that a proper response can be planned. This is a lengthy process, and therapists can become impatient and just tell patients what to say, especially when running out of time in session. Teaching someone to be assertive is important enough to do a thorough job, so it is better to postpone such skill training for another session than to rush through it and revert to giving advice.

Manage Activity

It is difficult to know whether increased activity is being caused by the emergence of hypomania or mania or if the activity itself is overstimulating the patient and precipitating the episode via sleep loss. As hypomania begins, the increased energy, motivation, and capacity for pleasure increases the desire for social, work, recreational, and family activities. This is a welcomed change from the lethargy of depression. Therapists should recognize these positive aspects of hypomania and may not want to discourage patients' efforts to overcome prior procrastination and stagnation. The trick is to find a level of activity that is satisfying and productive, but not overstimulating. This balance is not always easy to achieve. See Table 8–2 for strategies patients can use to manage activity and sleep.

To determine the optimal level of activity, it is useful to monitor symptoms of hypomania. Signs that activity should be reduced include sleep disruption and increased racing thoughts. Table 8–3 lists some common symptoms that activity may be exacerbating hypomanic or manic symptoms.

Manage Symptom Triggers

Some people have predictable episodes of mania. There may be seasonal changes; spring to early summer is often a time of increased mania (D'Mello et al. 1995; Goodwin and Jamison 1990; Hallam et al. 2006; Kerr-Corrêa et al. 1998; Volpe and Del Porto 2006). However, each person may have a unique time period associated with mania, such as light-exposure changes, idiosyncratic biological rhythms, or activity changes, such as increased work hours or increased travel. The advantage of a predictable pattern of mania onset is that preventive measures can be taken, including both pharmacological interventions and behavior management. For example, Angela's periods of mania generally occurred in March. For her, preventive measures can be started in February. These might include being more diligent with medication adherence or increasing the dose of antimanic medications. A more concerted effort can also be made to follow the lifestyle management strategies described previously, as in the following case of Mark:

> Mark takes an annual trip with his family to Las Vegas. It is a chance for him to get together with his siblings and parents, who otherwise see each other infrequently. A week in Las Vegas usually means late nights, overstimulation with noise and lights, increased alcohol intake, and gambling. All of these factors usually result in Mark's interrupted sleep and less consistent use of medication, the latter of which Mark justifies because he

---

Table 8–3. Signs that activity may be overstimulating

Unable to turn off thoughts about activities at bedtime

Stress or pressure to complete tasks increases.

Several tasks are started but not completed.

Feelings of agitation, irritation, or anxiety during activities

Feeling driven to complete tasks

Enjoyment of activities is lessened.

---

knows he is going to drink excessively. These annual trips usually lead to the emergence of hypomanic symptoms and, on occasion, have precipitated a full manic episode.

Although it would not be reasonable to ask Mark to abstain from this annual family event, it would be helpful for him to look at the trip more objectively. If Mark has not associated his actions in Las Vegas with the onset of manic symptoms, some education on these matters is indicated. If he is fully aware, he might benefit from weighing the pros and cons of his behaviors in Las Vegas and to consider some risk management strategies. These might include finding ways to enjoy his family while being more consistent with his self-care behaviors. The therapist's role in this situation is to facilitate Mark's consideration of setting limits on himself rather than to instruct Mark to set limits. The motivation to prevent mania must come from him. Below is an example of how Mark and his therapist worked through this issue:

> Therapist: So Mark, it sounds like you have a great time when you visit with your family in Las Vegas.
> Mark: Oh, yeah.
> Therapist: It also sounds like you are aware of how it can lead to you getting manic.
> Mark: Yeah, I get it. But I don't always have a problem. Last year was fine. I had a great time, other than losing a little too much at the slots. I felt a little stirred up, but not in a bad way. It took a while to settle down once I got back, but I didn't miss work or anything.
> Therapist: How worried are you that something could go wrong this time?
> Mark: Not very worried.
> Therapist: What makes you so confident? Is it because the last trip went well?
> Mark: Yeah, I guess. I try not to worry about it.
> Therapist: Would it be worth our time today to come up with a plan to avoid problems like getting manic?
> Mark: We can do that.
> Therapist: OK. Maybe you could start by telling me what you already know about getting manic after your trips to Las Vegas.
> Mark: I usually start off OK. When my big brother comes into town, it usually starts to get a little hairy.
> Therapist: What do you mean?
> Mark: He is a party animal. When he is on vacation, he goes all out. We spend the day out at the lake fishing and drinking beer. When we come back into town, we have a late dinner and hit the casinos. He isn't married, so he doesn't have a wife that controls the money. He makes enough to play

> hard. I don't gamble as much, but I try to stay up with him because he's fun to watch. He drinks like a fish too. I can't match him on that, but after being out a few hours we can put away quite a bit. The problem for me is that when we go back to the room, he crashes and sleeps until early afternoon. I can't do that. I try to sleep, but I have trouble turning off my brain, and when I finally get to sleep, I'm up when the sun comes up. A few days of that and I start to get high.
>
> Therapist: High?
>
> Mark: Manic.
>
> Therapist: How long does it take to get back to normal?
>
> Mark: It probably takes me a couple weeks or so to get my head right and to be able to sleep normal again.
>
> Therapist: Do you want to do anything differently this time to avoid getting high like that?
>
> Mark: I probably should. Two years ago I nearly ended up in the hospital.
>
> Therapist: You know yourself pretty well. What do you think you need to do?

This conversation led to Mark creating a plan for being consistent with medication and going to bed at an earlier hour than his brother. He liked being up with his brother, but too much of a fun time had consequences for him. The compromise was to have fun with his family, but to try to keep his sleep and medication as consistent as possible. He also found that if he took a break from the noise and activity in the casinos by spending some time alone in his room, he was less exhausted and edgy by the end of the day. By staying relatively neutral and allowing Mark to make the decision to take precautions, Mark and his therapist were able to work out a plan collaboratively.

Taking the position of lecturing patients about the evils of alcohol, gambling, and staying out late would have had less impact overall, and adherence with the instruction to set limits probably would have been very limited. Empowering patients to choose to take preventive actions increases the likelihood that they will take responsibility for their self-care while maintaining and even strengthening the therapeutic alliance.

Manage Substances

The lifetime prevalence of substance abuse in people with a history of mania is approximately 60%–70% (Brady et al. 1991; Strakowski et al. 1992; Weissman and Johnson 1991). They use substances such as alcohol to control symptoms of agitation or insomnia, to slow racing thoughts, or to dull the senses when irritability is more than can be tolerated. Most clinicians feel strongly that substance use should be avoided by these patients.

However, many patients do not want to give up drinking or recreational drug use. They believe that it is their right, and many believe that it helps to control symptoms. Substance use at the level of abuse or dependence, however, requires treatment. It is beyond the scope of this book to discuss interventions for substance abuse. The reader is referred to the work of Weiss and coworkers for detailed information on treatment of comorbid substance abuse and bipolar disorder (Weiss 2004; Weiss et al. 2007). Also, references for CBT methods for substance abuse are supplied in Chapter 1 ("Introduction"), and readings on substance abuse are listed in Appendix 2, "Cognitive-Behavior Therapy Resources" (see "Recommended Readings").

Learn to Recognize the Emergence of Symptoms

The second component of the mania prevention plan is to teach patients how to recognize the onset of mania. Subtle changes that are precursors to the symptoms that constitute the diagnostic criteria for mania should be the monitored targets. Because individual patients often have different hallmark signs or symptoms of mania, a customized monitoring plan is more useful and more personally relevant than standardized mania rating scales.

Symptom Recognition

Development of a plan begins with getting to know the patient. When taking a history of the presenting illness, listen for circumstances surrounding the onset of mania to try to determine which kind of changes occurred first. For example, some people will experience sleep loss as their first sign of mania, for others it will be an increased sex drive. Table 8–4 shows a list of typical mild, moderate, and severe symptoms of mania.

This table can be used as a worksheet (see Basco 2006) to familiarize patients with the early signs of mania. Review the list of symptoms in session and allow the patient to take a copy of the list home to share with family and friends. Ask the patient to mark the symptoms he has experienced during manic episodes. Get sufficient elaboration so that both you and the patient have a clear idea of how each symptom might manifest itself early in a manic episode. Family members and friends are generally good observers and may be able to recognize the subtle changes in behavior, emotions, and thought processes that signal the onset of mania. Conjoint sessions with close family members or friends might expedite this process.

Keep in mind that the more easily identified indicators of the onset of mania might not be the common symptoms listed in Table 8–4. What

Table 8–4. Mild, moderate, and severe symptoms of mania

Mild	Moderate	Severe
Everything seems like a hassle; impatience or anxiety	More easily angered	Irritability
Happier than usual; positive outlook	Increased laughter and joking	Euphoric mood; on top of the world
More talkative; better sense of humor	In the mood to socialize and talk with others	Pressured or rapid speech
More thoughts; mentally sharp, quick; lose focus	Disorganized thinking; poor concentration	Racing thoughts
More self-confident than usual; less pessimistic	Feeling smart; not afraid to try; overly optimistic	Grandiosity—delusions of grandeur
Creative ideas, new interests; change sounds good	Plan to make changes; disorganized in actions; drinking or smoking more	Disorganized activity; starting more things than finishing them
Fidgety; nervous behaviors like nail biting	Restless; prefer movement over sedentary activities	Psychomotor agitation; cannot sit still
Not as effective at work; having trouble keeping mind on tasks	Not completing tasks; late for work; annoying others	Cannot complete usual work or home activities
Uncomfortable with other people	Suspicious	Paranoia
More sexually interested	Sexual dreams; seeking out or noticing sexual stimulation	Increased sex drive; seek out sexual activity; more promiscuous
Notice sounds and annoying people; lose train of thought	Noises seem louder, colors seem brighter, mind wanders easily; need quieter environment to focus thoughts	Distractibility—have to work hard to focus thoughts or cannot focus thoughts at all

Source. Reprinted from Basco MR: *The Bipolar Workbook: Tools for Controlling Your Mood Swings.* New York, Guilford Press, 2006, p. 60. Used with permission.

Table 8–5.   Additional changes that occur during manic episodes

Category	Increases in	Decreases in
Preferences	Visiting with friends; listening to music	Solitude; quiet; darker environment
Habits	Rising earlier; drinking coffee	Overeating; working crossword puzzles
Routines	Bathing right after waking; cooking	Watching TV in the middle of the day
Interests	Hobbies; making crafts; learning something new	Watching violent or sad movies; playing computer solitaire
Motivations	Desiring change; pleasing others	Saving money; going to bed early

patients may notice instead of symptoms are changes in preferences, habits, routines, interests, and motivations. Table 8–5 provides an example of common changes that can occur in the course of a manic episode.

Symptom Monitoring

Once key presenting symptoms have been identified, a monitoring system can be designed to assess their presence and severity. The symptom summary worksheet (Basco 2006) presented in Figure 8–1 can be used to help patients and therapists gain a better understanding of the fluctuation of symptoms between depression and mania and how these differ from an asymptomatic or normal state. The worksheet includes three columns for contrasting subjective experiences and symptoms in mania and depression with usual or normal functioning. Completing this form is highly educational for the patient who has not previously considered how factors such as mood, sleep, appetite, and cognitive processing can differ in these three states. Understanding these variations will allow the patient to distinguish between symptoms and normal experiences, thereby alerting them to the possible recurrence of depression and mania. Completion of the worksheet can be initiated in session and completed as homework. Copies of the completed form should be provided for the patient, therapist, psychiatrist, and any significant family members who might be in a position to help identify symptomatic relapses in the patient.

Mood graphs (see Basco 2006 or Basco and Rush 2005) are commonly used tools for symptom monitoring and are widely available. These tools can be customized to measure symptoms other than mood. For example,

Category	When manic	When depressed	When feeling OK
Mood			
Attitude toward self; self-confidence			
Outlook on the future; thoughts about suicide			
Usual activities			
Social activity			
Ability to function			
Sleep habits			
Appetite/eating habits			
Concentration and decision-making ability			
Energy level			
Creativity			
Speech patterns			

Figure 8–1. Symptom summary worksheet.

Source. Adapted from Basco MR: *The Bipolar Workbook: Tools for Controlling Your Mood Swings.* New York, Guilford Press, 2006, p. 63. Used with permission.

energy level, ability to concentrate, speed of thought, or quality of sleep can be rated daily in the same format as mood. When initiating CBT, it is helpful if patients keep mood or symptom graphs daily. These will allow the therapist to better understand the degree of fluctuation the person experiences on a day-to-day basis. Once this is established, symptom monitoring can be tailored to the needs of the patient. For example, if the patient has predictable times when mania is likely to occur, symptoms should be monitored closely in the month before the usual time of onset. This monitoring will allow the patient and the therapist to observe the onset of mania. Another critical time to monitor symptoms is when medication changes occur. Rather than relying on patients' retrospective self-reports of symptom changes, a daily mood or symptom graph is somewhat more reliable. Figure 8–2 provides an example of mood graph.

Recognizing Manic Episodes

If patients detect the onset of mania or hypomania, they should be told to alert their health care providers. Even if well instructed in symptom detection, patients will not always feel confident in their abilities to correctly identify the onset of mania. In fact, the most that some patients may be able to do is know when they are not doing well and need assistance. This puts the burden on the health care provider to figure out what is happening from the patient's report. If you are familiar with a patient's symptoms of mania, they can be reviewed by phone or during a session. In addition to inquiring about common symptoms of mania, a mixed state should be considered if the patient reports dysphoria along with typical manic symptoms. If the patient is unable to describe symptoms well, it may be necessary to "read between the lines" of his story. Inquire about changes in medication regimen, missed doses, and changes in routine and behavior that might be consistent with the onset of mania. If the patient focuses on psychosocial stressors ask about the degree of distress experienced and any sleep disruption from worry. Also inquire about health problems that might keep the patient up at night and any somatic treatments that might interfere with the patient's psychiatric medications. If the onset of mania seems likely, it is time to take action.

Plan Ahead for Future Recurrences

Avoid Exacerbating Stimuli

People who have experienced mania in the past are usually fairly aware of what can escalate an episode once it begins. Table 8–6 is a list of typical examples of the activities, events, and experiences that can escalate

Date:							
Check (✓) the box to rate mood	Sun	Mon	Tues	Wed	Thur	Fri	Sat
Manic +5 Psychotic							
+4 Manic, poor judgment, impaired functioning							
+3 Hypomanic, elevated mood, judgment OK							
+2 Hyper, busy, restless, more energy							
+1 Happy, up							
0 Normal							
−1 Low, down, blue							
−2 Sad, tearful, negative thoughts, withdrawn							
−3 Depressed; decreased activity							
−4 Immobilized, hopeless							
−5 Suicidal Depressed							

Figure 8–2.   Mood graph.

Source.   Adapted from Basco MR: *The Bipolar Workbook: Tools for Controlling Your Mood Swings.* New York, Guilford Press, 2006, p. 73. Used with permission.

Table 8–6. Activities, events, and experiences that can escalate mania

---

Not taking medication

Drinking too much alcohol or using stimulant drugs

Thrill seeking

Risk taking

Arguments with people

Staying up all night

Loud music

Travel

Family gatherings

Upsetting movies that stimulate rumination

Trying to do too much

Pursuing a new romantic relationship

Changing jobs

Moving to a new city or new apartment

---

mania. The goal of mania prevention is to avoid these situations when the person feels vulnerable to the onset of mania. It should be emphasized that the goal is not to avoid these things altogether, but to limit them when they will cause an exacerbation of manic symptoms. In other words, when it seems that mania may be starting, try not to make matters worse. A mania prevention plan should include a list of things to avoid written in the patient's handwriting. The use of index cards can be helpful for this exercise. When mania begins and the therapist refers the patient to that list, it will be more compelling if the patient is reminded that these were her own instructions for controlling symptoms.

If it is difficult to resist temptations such as drinking, risk taking, or arguments once manic symptoms begin, it is best to avoid places and people associated with these temptations until the patient feels more self-control. Therefore, the patient's prevention plan should include avoidance of situations where symptoms can create new problems, which in turn escalate symptoms. For example, it may be too difficult for the person to sit still in church when agitated. Attempting to do so could escalate agitation rather than reduce it as intended. If the patient is irritable, it may be best to avoid people that tend to be annoying or seem to create conflict. Angela, for example, avoids calling her mother when she is agitated because she inevitably overreacts to her mother's words at those times. The argument increases her agitation. To avoid becoming embroiled in an overstimulating debate, patients should probably avoid conversations in which it would be best to keep their opinions to themselves. Discussion of these risky situations should result in a written plan for situations to avoid when mania begins.

Plan for Temptations

If the patient has had prior experience with mania, she probably knows the temptations that are hard to resist. For example, Joanna is very lonely and somewhat shy. When she is becoming manic, she loses her inhibitions and seeks out romantic companions. At the time, the attention she receives for dressing and acting in a seductive manner feels good. She only has regrets after the fact when she realizes that she has put herself at risk by having unsafe sex or by opening her heart to someone who will not stay with her as her illness worsens. Although she hates the pain that goes with heartbreak, the desire to be loved coupled with the freedom to express her sexuality when she is manic leaves her uncertain about giving up the freedom of mania next time her symptoms return. She knows this is her weakness, and she cannot promise that she won't allow herself to become manic again.

Using the advantages and disadvantages comparison exercise from standard CBT (see Wright et al. 2006), Joanna can more closely examine her choices. If she can work on ways to maximize the advantages of being disinhibited and minimize the risks of getting hurt in the process, she might be willing to set a limit on her mania. Gaining comfort in social situations, improving her relationship skills, and seeking out a romantic partner could become therapy goals that are pursued after containment of the episode.

Most patients who have experienced mania in the past will be able to identify their weaknesses during a manic episode. These weaknesses might be similar to Joanna's or might include overspending, driving too fast, using substances of abuse, or changing jobs or places of residence. If they decide to control these urges, a plan can be made to lessen the risk, delay decisions, or otherwise use stimulus control strategies. *Stimulus control* is placing constraints on actions and limiting access to environmental circumstances that lead to the unwanted behavior. For example, if overspending is an issue, the person may decide not to shop or to leave money or credit cards at home so that they can't be used in times of weakness. If change is suddenly desired, a plan can be made to delay the decision and get the opinion of two trusted people before any change is made. If the patient knows that alcohol is hard to resist during manic periods, the person may decide beforehand to drink only water or soda in social situations until the manic symptoms pass. The point is that decisions can be made to address the patient's weaknesses. However, there is no guarantee that when in a tempting situation during a manic episode, the patient will make the healthier decision. If the temptations are overwhelming, the patient may give in and hope for the best. If no negative consequences occur, this experience will increase the likelihood that risks will be taken during the next manic episode. If negative consequences are experienced, this information will likely inform the prevention plan for the next manic episode; see the section later in this chapter, "Learn From the Experience," for additional discussion.

Discuss Treatment Adherence

The best time to discuss medication adherence is long before it is a problem. Given that skipping doses or discontinuing medication is a common precipitant of mania (Keck et al. 1996), it will be necessary to inquire about adherence when symptoms worsen. Prior discussion of treatment adherence sets the stage for these future conversations and lessens the chance that the patient will feel attacked or offended when questioned about missing doses of medication.

Chapter 12 ("Promoting Adherence") will provide a more thorough discussion of treatment adherence, but for the purpose of developing a mania prevention plan, it should be discussed with the patient how missing doses might impact the illness. Not all patients understand the need for consistency in pharmacotherapy or the consequences of missing or lowering doses. This type of education should occur early in therapy. Discussion of adherence can be made easier by inquiring about it regularly. In this way, it becomes a normal topic of conversation and therefore easier to talk about when the onset of mania is suspected. Therapists should empathize with the difficulty of taking medication everyday and normalize adherence problems by sharing with patients how others often struggle with the same challenges. Also, positive reinforcement should be provided when adherence is stable.

Stabilize Sleep

Any mania prevention plan should include regulation of sleep. This would include reducing daytime napping, which tends to be a normal response to nighttime insomnia. It is easy for patients to become phase shifted as they stay awake later and later at night and awaken later in the day. To remedy the problem, it is easier to eliminate napping and rise earlier than it is to force sleep onset earlier in the evening.

Help patients to anticipate any negative reactions they might have to the suggestion that they go to bed earlier at night. A useful strategy is to assist the patient in preparing a counterresponse and writing this down on an index card. On one side of the card have the patient write the objection to an earlier bedtime and on the back write out the rational response. For example, the objection might read, "I feel my best at night. I don't want to go to bed early and lose that feeling." The counterresponse might be, "Too many nights without enough sleep will make me manic. It's not worth it." With this preparation, the therapist is removed from the role of encouraging a manic person to get some sleep. Instead, reading the rational response encourages the patient to carry out his own plan.

Encourage Patients to Call for Help

Clinicians can play helpful roles in reducing manic symptoms if the patient feels comfortable in asking for help. Two obstacles for patients in engaging care providers are that patients 1) may not know when to ask for help and 2) may not know what doctors and other therapists can do. Many people have survived manic episodes without assistance or did not activate their support system when it was available. Assuming that patients are motivated to avoid a full episode of mania, some discussion is necessary of how to use care providers in this process. A good way to clarify roles and possible responses is to develop the mania prevention plan and then ask patients how you and/or other clinicians can be helpful when symptoms begin to emerge.

One useful intervention is to provide patients with feedback on their symptoms when they do not appear to be aware of them. Rapid speech, tangential thinking, psychomotor agitation, and elevated mood may be apparent to the therapist who sees the patient infrequently, but less obvious to the patient who acclimates to subtle changes over time. Early in treatment, therapists should offer to give feedback to patients when they see symptoms appearing. The feedback should be presented in the form of hypotheses to allow the patient to consider the possibility that symptoms are present rather than given as statements of fact. For example, "You seem different to me today. Are you feeling any differently than usual?" or "You seem to be talking more rapidly than usual. Do you hear it or is it just me?" If the patient is willing to consider these changes as symptoms, the therapist can follow with "Should we be concerned that you are getting manic?" Showing concern will prevent the patient's perception of being condemned or labeled in a negative way.

Another way to encourage patients to call for help before they become fully manic is to offer to help them figure out if mania is returning. Some patients will be fearful of becoming manic and will call when symptoms are at a minimal level or will misinterpret normal joy or excitement as symptoms. Praise should be given for self-awareness and for calling for help before problems developed. This interaction allows the therapist an opportunity to reinforce prevention. If it is unclear whether or not mania is returning, it can be helpful to suggest symptom or mood monitoring, reinforce healthy lifestyle management, and schedule a follow-up visit within a week to assess any symptom exacerbations.

Take Action to Control Symptoms

The fourth component in the mania prevention plan is activated when manic symptoms are present. In general, the goal is for the patient to use the lifestyle management strategies previously described. In other words, to reduce overstimulation, take medication consistently, add other optional medication if necessary, avoid substances of abuse, and get adequate sleep. In addition, once symptoms are recognized, the patient should alert his psychiatrist to discuss the need for additional antimanic medications and/or sleep agents, because merely resuming the usual regimen, if doses have been missed, may be insufficient to contain symptoms. If the therapist is not the treating psychiatrist, it may take some coaxing to get the patient to call his doctor, as many patients are initially reluctant. If the patient approves, the therapist can call the doctor during the therapy session with the patient present. This method is more easily accomplished if the therapist and the psychiatrist have previously discussed the care of the patient and both have a copy of the patient's list of common symptoms of mania.

Specific interventions for helping patients contain the symptoms of mania will be described. These interventions target three general areas: behavioral symptoms, cognitive changes, and mood swings.

Behavioral Interventions

The first behavioral assessment to consider when mania is suspected is to check on medication adherence and substance abuse. If the preparatory work has been done on treatment adherence as described above, this discussion should be fairly straightforward. If medications have not been taken, they need to be resumed. If substances are being abused, they should be discontinued. If the patient is not convinced that he is manic or that changes in medication or substance use are necessary, you may need to use cognitive interventions to work through this difference of opinion before you can use more behavioral interventions. For example, you can use Socratic questioning to assess whether the patient thinks she is manic. It might be necessary to do an evidence for/evidence against evaluation of the presence of mania or ask the patient to review her summary list of symptoms. If still unconvinced that mania is present, the patient should be asked for an alternative explanation for her symptoms. If possible, it is best for patients to draw their own conclusions about mania rather than for the therapist to simply tell them that they are manic. Table 8–7 includes a list of questions that might help patients conclude what is obvious to others—that a manic episode has begun.

It is reasonable for a therapist to share an opinion about whether the patient is demonstrating manic symptoms. However, it is better for the therapeutic alliance if the patient is given the benefit of the doubt and allowed to explore the facts and draw a conclusion. In Video Illustration 2 (first shown in Chapter 2, "Engaging and Assessing"), Dr. Basco helps Angela to consider the possibility that she may have bipolar disorder by using Socratic questioning. This collaborative approach promotes a positive therapeutic alliance while still addressing Angela's denial.

Engaging in overstimulating activities, moving from task to task, getting excited about new ventures, and talking to others about these ideas all seem to increase mental stimulation and escalate manic symptoms; therefore, limits should be set on these activities during the onset of mania. However, when manic symptoms are present, even in their mildest form, implementing behavioral interventions to control symptoms is more challenging. The goal of behavioral interventions is to contain activity while manic symptoms urge the patient to increase activity. Limit

---

Table 8–7. Socratic questions regarding the presence of mania

Do you think you are manic?

If not, what do you think is happening to you?

If not, why do other people seem to think you are manic?

How is mania different from how you feel now?

Is it possible that you are getting manic and just don't want to see it?

How do you explain your change in mood?

Have you ever felt this way before?

How could you tell if this was mania or something else?

What would have to happen to convince you that this is mania?

---

setting may be the most therapeutic strategy, but to the person with manic symptoms, it is counterintuitive. What makes this process even more challenging is that the emphasis in CBT is to encourage the patient to take charge, make decisions about the best way to cope with symptoms, and be responsible for executing those plans. If the urge for stimulation, change, risk, or challenge exists, a patient's decision making is impaired by racing thoughts and impaired concentration; follow-through is compromised by distractibility and poor judgment; and it is difficult to make the changes that will control mania. What makes behavioral interventions most effective once manic symptoms have started is that the plan has been previously developed and obstacles to adherence have been anticipated and worked out. It is also critical that the patient and therapist have a good working relationship. At times, therapists will have to leverage their alliance with the patient to counteract the patient's manic ideas. If trust has been established, the patient is more likely to listen to the therapist's warnings and follow instructions.

If behavior is disorganized—for example, with many activities started and abandoned before completion—limit setting might best be accomplished by helping the patient to select a few daily behavioral goals and complete one task before initiating the next. Described in Basco and Rush (2005), the A list/B list exercise helps patients set such goals. The A list requires patients to choose only one or two high-priority activities to do each day. These activities have a deadline or consequences for failing to complete them. The B list includes one or two lower-priority items. The goal is to complete the A list before attempting the B list items. This exercise can be completed at the end of the day in preparation for the next or can be done first thing each morning. The list should be prominently displayed so that the patient can refer to it when distractibility or the urge to do more threatens to take the patient off track.

More traditional activity scheduling interventions can be used. Examples of activity scheduling can be found in Basco and Rush (2005) and Wright et al. (2006). Stimulus control interventions may be the most useful behavioral interventions for reducing risk during mania. These strategies were described in the previous section, "Plan Ahead for Future Recurrences." If that preparatory work has not been completed, simplify the procedures by asking patients what things, if done today, would be likely to worsen manic symptoms. If the patient has difficulty generating ideas, describe the items that could escalate mania from Table 8–6. Identify the situations that would be most likely to occur and make a plan to avoid those experiences. Create a backup plan to escape or limit them if those sources of stimulation are unavoidable.

Another strategy is to enlist the help of family members in controlling mania. Improving medication adherence, for example, might require the assistance of a family member to monitor use of medications until the patient can manage it alone. Informing the family helps them to know what is happening to the patient and allows them the opportunity to avoid contributing to the problem. For example, if a wife is told that her husband is becoming manic, she can rearrange schedules to not put him in stressful or overstimulating situations. She can also avoid conflict and help to keep the environment calm.

Some patients benefit from burning off the excess energy when mania begins by redirecting it toward exercise or physical work, assuming these activities are done early in the day so as not to delay sleep onset. Psychomotor agitation can increase anxiety and irritability if there are no outlets for this feeling. Movements such as walking, household chores, or washing the car can ease tension and tire the person, which can reduce restless feelings. Engaging in these types of activities can also help to redirect the person away from overstimulating activities or activities with a high risk of negative consequences. It is best if the activities are those within the behavioral repertoire of the patient. Mania is not the time to begin a new behavior or activity.

Cognitive Interventions

The cognitions that might require intervention early in a manic episode are those related to acknowledgment of mania and the need for treatment (as described previously) and cognitions that have the potential for leading to problematic behaviors. Reluctance to acknowledge manic symptoms may be because of denial, but may also be related to changes in self-perception. It is common for people to mistake mania for normalcy, especially if they have previously been in a depressive episode. They lose their frame of reference for "normal." They assume that hypomania is "being at their best." If denial is the problem, use the Socratic questions regarding the presence of mania (see Table 8–7). If self-perception is the problem, refer the patient back to the mania symptoms worksheet (see Table 8–4).

To keep manic cognitions from leading patients to problematic behaviors, use the Catch—Control—Correct method described in *The Bipolar Workbook: Tools for Controlling Your Mood Swings* (Basco 2006). The general strategy is to become aware that manic thoughts are occurring and to know that they can be inaccurate or can lead a person toward making matters worse. This awareness allows for a pause between getting a manic idea and acting on it. During that pause, the person can consider whether the thought is true and the pros and cons of taking action on it. For example, when Angela is becoming manic, she thinks that others are disagreeing with her because they are jealous of her wonderful ideas. If she were to act on that thought, she might become angry or defensive or reject useful feedback. If she could recognize that she often thinks others are jealous of her when she is manic, she could pause and consider their feedback more objectively before reacting.

Other examples of distorted cognitions in mania that have been reported by some of our patients include the following: "I'm invincible"; "This investment [business plan, bet on stock market, marketing strategy, etc.] can't lose"; "I am sure to win"; and "Others are always going too slowly." The following steps can be taken to help patients modify these types of cognitions:

1. Catch the thought that is occurring.
2. Control reactions to the distorted cognition until there has been time to think it through.
3. Evaluate the accuracy of the thought using standard CBT logical analysis methods, such as examining the evidence, spotting cognitive distortions, or thought recording.

In Video Illustration 13, Angela explores and modifies a grandiose idea by examining the evidence. This exploration allows her to draw the conclusion that her symptoms of mania might be responsible for her belief that her coworkers are in love with her. After examining the evidence, Angela works on planning precautions to reduce her risky behavior. This video example shows how CBT can be directed at modifying grandiose thinking in mania and limiting the potential damage from these types of beliefs.

> **Video Illustration 13.**   Reducing Grandiosity:
>   Dr. Basco and Angela

Emotion-Focused Interventions

Just as in depression, the emotional shifts caused by the onset of mania can stimulate thoughts and behaviors consistent with those emotions. Distortions in logic caused by the emotion are difficult to capture and analyze because thoughts are racing, distractibility makes it difficult to focus, and grandiosity or paranoia biases perceptions. Sometimes it is easier to control emotional shifts than to logically analyze manic thoughts. Therefore, emotionally focused strategies might be the place to start until the patient is able to slow and focus thoughts.

Relaxation methods used in the treatment of anxiety disorders can be helpful in controlling irritability, agitation, and anxiety produced during mania. Active relaxation methods may be more helpful than passive exercises because it is easier to redirect the energy behind these emotions than to try to make them stop. Likewise, as mania begins, it is easier to redirect thoughts than to try to clear the mind of thoughts. For these reasons, relaxation may be best achieved by walking, stretching, swimming, tai chi, or other physical activities that allow the patient to expend energy without becoming further stimulated.

Mental relaxation may be achieved through inductions that redirect thought, such as with guided imagery or sensory-focus exercises where attention is directed to increase awareness of physical sensations and mental images. Progressive muscle relaxation methods, especially those that alternate between tensing and relaxing muscle groups, can help to lessen physical tension as well as emotional tension. These exercises may be difficult for patients to do on their own without prompts from therapists, instructors, or audiotaped instructions.

Euphoria is not usually the focus of emotional control in CBT. Most patients could not be convinced that the feeling of euphoria should be contained or limited, and efforts to do so by therapists might be perceived as cruel. However, patients who have experienced euphoric mania in the past might be frightened by the occurrence of euphoria even when it is the result of good news or good fortune rather than a symptom. In fact, patients who have learned to identify early symptoms of mania might overreact to positive feelings by assuming they are becoming manic rather than exploring the circumstances and any concurrent symptoms. Some patients are afraid to be too joyful even when they have reason to be, because they assume that too much happiness will inevitably lead to mania or is a sure sign that mania has already started. These individuals might downplay the impact of good news and not take pleasure from positive life events. Therapists can help in these circumstances by reviewing manic symptoms, considering the circumstances that led to the mood shift, and providing reassurance that the euphoria is a normal reaction or confirming the need to take precautions to stop mania from more fully emerging.

Emotional distress such as anger at having to deal with the illness, frustration with medication, hopelessness about the future, and sadness for missed opportunities in life can precipitate medication nonadherence that leads to increased symptoms. Or, these emotions can be the early signs that a manic or mixed state is beginning. In either case, the traditional CBT methods for coping with negative automatic thoughts (see Wright et al. 2006) can be used to help work through these thoughts and

emotions. Lessening anger, frustration, and sadness can increase the likelihood that the patient is willing to continue to use lifestyle management
strategies. Believing that change is possible and that if the illness can be
managed, life goals can be achieved, all serve to increase hopefulness
about the future. Sometimes, direct intervention to lessen these emotions
is not needed. Allowing patients to explore these feelings and providing
an empathic response can ease the acceptance of losses and allow patients
to make peace with their illness.

Learn From the Experience

The final step in the mania prevention plan is to try to learn from each
manic or hypomanic episode. Although the presentation of each manic
episode might be somewhat different, patterns usually emerge from precipitating factors, early symptoms, and strategies that help to contain
symptoms. Each episode is an opportunity to refine the mania prevention
plan. Rather than portraying new episodes as treatment failures, therapists can reframe them as learning experiences. Take inventory of the
cognitive, behavioral, physical, and emotional changes that occurred. Examine what happened during the course of the episode with the advantage of hindsight. Revise the prevention plan by incorporating these new
observations. Troubleshoot problems and identify actions that could
have been taken to avert a full episode. Reaffirm medication adherence
and lifestyle management plans. Table 8–8 is a checklist of common factors in the development of mania. Review them when your patient relapses to determine where therapeutic efforts can be targeted to prepare
for the next episode.

Some of the principal features of developing and implementing a relapse prevention plan for bipolar disorder are demonstrated in Video Illustration 14. In this vignette from a session with Angela, a symptom
summary worksheet produced in an earlier session was used effectively
to spot early warning signs of a possible relapse into mania. As the session
opens, Angela tells Dr. Basco that she was tempted over the weekend to
ride her motorcycle very fast. She got excited at the prospect of doing
this and also began to lament that she was missing all the fun in her life.
When they review the symptom summary worksheet, Angela recognizes
several other possible signs of impending mania (i.e., sleeping only 5
hours a night, exercising more, increased caffeine intake, a restless feeling
that she can do more, playing music loudly). Angela is showing increased
insight at this point in her therapy, and she is able to commit to some
changes that will limit the chances of symptom escalation and to keep
herself from potentially dangerous behavior in riding her motorcycle too

---

Table 8–8. Factors in the recurrence of mania

Behavior changes
Sleep disruptions
Late nights on the Internet or TV or engaged in new relationships
Alcohol and drug use
Medication nonadherence
Stimulation seeking and finding

Cognitive changes
Desire for change
Missing the highs
Reemergence of denial
Increased interest in socializing
Increased interest in sex—not wanting medication to interfere
Thinking that you are doing well and don't need the medications
Making a conscious decision to live on the edge

Mood changes
Anger at having the illness leads to decreased medication usage
Frustration with the side effects of medications
Hopelessness about the future
Sadness—missing the highs, missing the way life used to be, regrets

---

fast. An interesting feature of their plan is to work on ways to still have fun, despite putting controls on hypomanic and manic symptoms.

> ▶ **Video Illustration 14.** Using an Early Warning
> System: Dr. Basco and Angela

After you have viewed the video illustrations for this chapter, we recommend some practice in using CBT for bipolar disorder. Learning Exercise 8–1 draws together some key elements of bipolar disorder relapse prevention plans.

> **Learning Exercise 8–1.** A Prevention Plan for
> Mania
>
> 1. Make copies of Table 8–4 ("Mild, moderate, and severe symptoms of mania") and Figure 8–1 ("Symptom summary worksheet").
>
> 2. Use these worksheets, either with one of your patients with bipolar disorder or in a role-play with a

colleague, to develop a customized list for this patient
of the early warning signs of mood shifts into mania
or depression. If possible, involve a trusted family
member or friend of the patient to add detail to the
worksheet.

3. Now, brainstorm with the patient about possible
strategies for interrupting an escalation into mania.
Write these ideas down.

4. Choose two to four of the most promising ideas
and encourage your patient to use them.

Summary

Key Points for Clinicians

- Recurrences of mania and depression can be decreased through life-style management and early action to control symptoms of relapse.
- Commonly used cognitive restructuring methods can help patients accept and manage bipolar disorder.
- Each patient has a unique presentation of symptoms of mania. They can be identified using the symptom summary worksheet and monitored using mood graphs.
- The more patients understand about the factors that contribute to mania, the more empowered they are to take action to prevent its recurrence.

Concepts and Skills for Patients to Learn

- Lifestyle management, including good sleep hygiene and avoiding overstimulation, is needed to help prevent relapse.
- Development of an early warning system can help to detect mild symptoms of mania.
- Factors that precipitate mania can be identified and necessary behavioral adjustments can be made to avoid relapse.
- Cognitive and behavioral skills typically applied to depressive symptoms can be used to control manic symptoms.

References

Backhaus J, Hohagen F, Voderholzer U, et al: Long-term effectiveness of a short-term cognitive-behavioral group treatment for primary insomnia. Eur Arch Psychiatry Clin Neurosci 251:35–41, 2001

Basco MR: The Bipolar Workbook: Tools for Controlling Your Mood Swings. New York, Guilford, 2006

Basco MR, Rush AJ: Cognitive-Behavioral Therapy for Bipolar Disorder, 2nd Edition. New York, Guilford, 2005

Brady K, Casto S, Lydiard RB, et al: Substance abuse in an inpatient psychiatric sample. Am J Drug Alcohol Abuse 17:389–397, 1991

D'Mello DA, McNeil JA, Msibi B: Seasons and bipolar disorder. Ann Clin Psychiatry 7:11–18, 1995

Goodwin FK, Jamison KR: Manic-Depressive Illness. New York, Oxford University Press, 1990

Hallam KT, Olver JS, Chambers V, et al: The heritability of melatonin secretion and sensitivity to bright nocturnal light in twins. Psychoneuroendocrinology 31:867–875, 2006

Keck PE, McElroy SL, Strakowski SM, et al: Factors associated with pharmacologic noncompliance in patients with mania. J Clin Psychiatry 57:292–297, 1996

Kerr-Corrêa F, Souza LB, Calil HM: Affective disorders, hospital admissions, and seasonal variation of mania in a subtropical area, southern hemisphere. Psychopathology 31:265–269, 1998

Peden AR, Rayens MK, Hall LA, et al: Testing an intervention to reduce negative thinking, depressive symptoms, and chronic stressors in low-income single mothers. J Nurs Scholarsh 37:268–274, 2005

Strakowski SM, Tohen N, Stoll AL, et al: Comorbidity in mania at first hospitalization. Am J Psychiatry 149:554–556, 1992

Volpe FM, Del Porto JA: Seasonality of admissions for mania in a psychiatric hospital of Belo Horizonte, Brazil. J Affect Disord 94(1–3):243–248, 2006

Weiss RD: Treating patients with bipolar disorder and substance dependence: lessons learned. J Subst Abuse Treat 27:307–312, 2004

Weiss RD, Griffin ML, Kolodziej ME, et al: A randomized trial of integrated group therapy versus group drug counseling for patients with bipolar disorder and substance dependence. Am J Psychiatry 164:100–107, 2007

Weissman MM, Johnson J: Drug use and abuse in five US communities. N Y State J Med 91(11 Suppl):19S–23S, 1991

Wright JH, Basco MR, Thase ME: Learning Cognitive-Behavior Therapy: An Illustrated Guide. Washington, DC, American Psychiatric Publishing, 2006

9

Interpersonal Problems

Interpersonal relationships are difficult to develop, manage, and sustain for most people. For those who must battle a chronic psychiatric illness, the challenges are greater. This chapter discusses the interpersonal issues faced by people with severe or chronic depression; bipolar disorder; and schizophrenia and gives suggestions for helping patients cope with these types of problems. Because the focus of this book is on individual CBT, not marital or family CBT, we do not describe methods for conjoint therapy. The reader is referred to excellent books on marital and family CBT for guidelines on how to implement these types of therapies (Baucom and Epstein 1990; Beck 1988; Dattilio and Padesky 1990; Epstein and Baucom 2002; Epstein et al. 1988).

The support of family and friends can go a long way in helping people cope with severe and chronic mental illnesses. When that support is lacking, the patient has no choice but to cope alone. Even worse, when patients' relationships are strained, the added stress can worsen symptoms and precipitate relapses. Learning CBT skills can improve coping in people who lack social support or who deal with family dysfunction.

Common Interpersonal Difficulties

There are several interpersonal problems that can negatively impact the well-being of psychiatric patients across disorders. Some of the major problem areas are 1) skill deficits in forming and maintaining relationships, 2) symptom intrusions, 3) loss, 4) boundary issues, 5) lack of social

211

support, and 6) making the decision to disclose the presence of a mental disorder. These specific problem areas will be discussed before reviewing interpersonal problems that are more specific to depression, bipolar disorder, and schizophrenia.

Relationship Skills

Several predisposing factors may interfere with the ability to establish or maintain relationships and cope with interpersonal problems. One is the unavailability of role models for forming lasting relationships or for coping well with conflict or loss. If a patient's parents were not very good at handling their interpersonal lives, then skills training and modeling would have been lacking. Another predisposing family factor is mental illness in parents that impacted their parenting behaviors. Parents who struggled with the same mental illnesses might have been too preoccupied with their own problems to help their children acquire relationship skills during their childhood and adolescent years. As these children grow up and begin to form relationships, they can be ill equipped for these challenges.

Within the patient, a predisposing factor may have been the early onset of symptoms. Even if instruction and modeling had been available, those patients whose illnesses began in childhood and adolescence may have missed important opportunities to learn about relationships while they were preoccupied with managing their symptoms and regaining stability. Early symptoms may not have been obvious to others who would have been in a position to help. Instead, these youth had to cope internally with thoughts and feelings that were unusual and unfamiliar while trying to get along with family members, establish friendships, begin dating, and deal with issues of sexuality. A frequent end result of feeling deficient in interpersonal skills is using avoidance as a coping strategy (Barrett and Barber 2007).

Role-playing in session is a simple intervention that can help patients gain skills for a variety of social interactions. Preparation for role-play should include definition of the goal of the interaction. Angela wanted to handle day-to-day interactions without showing the irritability and suspiciousness she was feeling. Mary wanted to find a way to explain to others that she was depressed and not angry. People can't always identify a specific improvement they would like to make in their communication with others, but if they can imagine an ideal interaction (e.g., a respectful listener, no interruptions, an ability to control emotions), they can usually explain why such a conversation is not possible. At the mention of trying to talk to others about their feelings, patients will often recall the difficulties encountered in the past and may overgeneralize to future conversations. Unfortunately, they may be correct in assuming that interactions will usually be difficult with key people in their lives—unless there is a way to change the manner with which they interact. Any negative automatic thoughts about communication can be addressed using standard cognitive restructuring interventions before beginning the role-play exercise.

Role-playing to improve interpersonal communication skills generally includes the following steps:

1. The patient describes what he would like to be able to say. This is most easily accomplished if the patient is encouraged to speak aloud as if talking with the targeted individual. This script is modified and rehearsed through the role-play exercise.
2. Feedback is given to the patient, including any needed modifications in wording or nonverbal behavior.
3. The patient is encouraged to modify the statements based on the feedback and then to try again to verbalize the message aloud. This can be a frustrating experience for patients if too much feedback is given at one time. For example, refinements or clarification in wording might be suggested and practiced first before critiquing nonverbal behaviors such as eye contact or voice tone. The prepared statements do not have to be delivered perfectly, so feedback should be limited to only essential elements. The statements should always be in the patient's words and not the therapist's.
4. Encouragement and positive reinforcement from therapists can increase patients' confidence with their efforts at communication.
5. When the plan has been finalized, the patient should write out his statements on an index card or in a notebook. Reminders will aid rehearsal and will help when anxiety interferes with recall or when an unexpected response from the listener distracts the patient from his point.
6. After the patient has clearly stated what is to be communicated, the therapist can practice the interaction by playing the role of the listener. To prepare for this element of the role-play the patient should describe the listener and the listener's likely reactions to the interaction.
7. The interaction should be rehearsed by allowing the patient to first make her prepared statement without the therapist challenging the content or style. This will build confidence.
8. This initial practice run can be distressing for the patient. Therefore it is helpful to debrief the interaction, assessing automatic thoughts and emotional reactions.

9. During subsequent rehearsals of the role-play, the therapist can make the interaction more challenging, reacting in the manner the patient anticipates from the intended listener. It is best to avoid overacting the part—a mistake that can discourage the patient by representing a situation as too complicated or challenging.
10. These subsequent role-plays should be debriefed as well. Additional statements may need to be prepared in anticipation of other possible responses from the listener. These statements can be added to the patient's notes.
11. As with any homework assignment, it is best to anticipate obstacles to implementation of the plan and develop strategies to avoid these obstacles or to cope when them as they occur. For example, task-interfering cognitions (TICs; Burns 1999)—such as "I can't do it"; "It won't do any good"; "I don't know what to say"—might flood the patient's mind causing her to avoid the interaction altogether. If the patient is likely to lose her nerve in attempting the planned interaction, a list of task-orienting cognitions (TOCs; Burns 1999) can be prepared in session to counter these negative thoughts, such as "I want to speak my mind"; "I need to stick up for myself"; "I can handle this."

If the obstacles are more practical in nature, such as finding time, privacy, or cooperation from the listener, problem solving can be used to develop a backup plan. If the patient makes a negative prediction about the interaction, the exercise can be framed as an experiment to test this prediction. If the negative prediction turns out to be valid, other communication strategies may be needed to accomplish the goal intended by the interaction exercise. If the prediction was proved invalid, the therapist can explore how the experience changed the patient's belief about self, others, and future interactions. Inquiring about changes in emotion resulting from the experience and how any changes in cognitions might affect future interactions with others can help to reinforce the patient's understanding of basic CBT concepts.

Sometimes avoidance of interpersonal situations is appropriate when symptoms can color the interaction in a negative way. Some interactions with others that are highly emotional can exacerbate symptoms. To determine whether approach or avoidance strategies should be used, the patient can be helped to weigh the advantages and disadvantages of interactions when symptoms are present. If the patient determines that the interaction is worth the risk, a plan can be made for coping with any symptom exacerbations that might occur.

Learning Exercise 9–1. Advantages and Disadvantages of Assertive Communication

1. Think of a situation in which it might be appropriate for your patient to communicate directly with another person on a topic that has been avoided. If you do not have a patient in this situation, you may use yourself as an example.

2. Write out a script that a patient might use to communicate with another person on an avoided topic. Try to put yourself in the patient's situation and use words that reflect the patient's voice.

3. Troubleshoot your script by evaluating the language used, making sure that it is the patient's sentiment and choice of words and not yours.

4. Try to anticipate how the message will be received and write out several counterresponses that the patient might use.

5. Practice the script with someone other than the patient and elicit feedback on your words.

Symptom Intrusions

Severe mental illnesses produce a variety of symptoms that affect interactions with others. For example, mood changes, such as irritability, can color tone of voice and make a person less tolerant of the actions of others, thereby producing conflict. Anxiety can lead to fearfulness of abandonment and suspiciousness of the motivations of others, thereby causing the person to withdraw from people. Although seemingly protective, these types of responses may interfere with receiving support from others. Paranoid ideation and mind reading of others has the same effect. Rapid speech, tangentiality, poor concentration, and distractibility all impair communication. Others may not understand what the patient is trying to say. Not being understood is frustrating and can lead to either an unpleasant escalation in the communication or an avoidance of interaction.

The CBT interventions that can be most useful are those that help patients gain some self-awareness of how their symptoms affect their interpersonal behaviors and teach them how to make adjustments. For example, when a patient is highly irritable and difficult conversations are not avoidable, differential relaxation and assertiveness skills can be taught to help the patient slow down and verbalize ideas in an assertive and un-aggressive manner.

Symptom recognition and awareness can be facilitated by using the symptom summary worksheet from Chapter 8 ("Mania") and adapting it for use with psychosis and depression. The symptoms that are most likely to interfere with interpersonal functioning can be identified. Then the occurrence of those symptoms can be monitored using a mood or symptom graph like the one in Chapter 8. When a particular symptom is reemerging, the patient is alerted to the possibility that it could impair communication or cause relationship stress. Efforts are made to minimize the impact of the symptom until it has remitted. Angela, for example, can become critical of others when manic symptoms are returning. The irritability and mistrust of others that emerges during mania makes her suspicious without justification and colors her tone of voice and choice of words. As Angela has become more aware of her manic symptoms, she has learned to take precautions not to lash out at others while in a manic or hypomanic state. To keep herself from saying the wrong things, she measures her words, takes time to think before reacting, and discusses her assumptions with others before responding in an angry or defensive manner.

When Majir talks with his parents about his daily activities, he often feels ashamed and senses that he is a failure in their eyes. He also becomes very suspicious about what they are thinking and saying about him. Thus, he keeps his head down, speaks in a very soft voice, and says little. This behavior tends to make his parents more frustrated by Majir's problems. To help reverse this cycle of dysfunctional communication, Majir applies what he is learning in his sessions with Dr. Kingdon. He uses a coping card that lists the following items:

1. Remind myself of my strengths: I know computers really well, I am a good uncle, I am trying very hard to overcome my problems.
2. Try not to jump to conclusions about what my parents are thinking—I know that they are disappointed, but they are also pulling for me to do better.
3. Hanging my head and mumbling just makes people think I don't have any confidence—practice speaking up and telling them about a couple of positive things that I am doing.

Loss

Grief work can be accomplished in CBT with some modification of basic strategies to allow for a longer elicitation phase before specific interventions, so that patients have time to express and process feelings of loss. It is not necessary or even useful to rush the grief process by moving too quickly to identify and correct negative automatic thoughts, to reduce emotion, or to advance to more active coping strategies. A general rule of thumb is that normal bereavement takes 3–6 months to resolve depending on the severity of the loss, the degree to which the patient processes the loss, and the psychosocial consequences that follow, such as loss of financial support. People with chronic and severe mental illnesses may need more time to process a loss, particularly if a symptomatic relapse followed the loss and prevented the person from focusing on grief.

Because grief generally follows a predictable course and diminishes over time, it may be not be necessary to use cognitive restructuring methods initially. As the sadness diminishes, the negative thinking usually lessens. Discussion of the loss may be the major agenda item for a session and can consume most of the therapy time. Patients should be allowed to talk about the loss, express emotions, replay the events that occurred, and discuss what the loss means for the future. Residual negative thoughts that appear to be distortions of reality can become targets of intervention and can be addressed briefly at the end of a session using Socratic questioning. However, it may be more useful to allow the patient to express himself fully within a session, eliciting automatic thoughts as well as feelings, and not intervene with cognitive-behavioral methods until the next session. This delay allows the patient time to think about what was said in session. Negative thoughts about losses can resolve on their own or with the patient's own effort and may not require intervention.

After expression of grief, many patients can benefit from discussing active coping strategies such as problem solving, behavioral activation, or a balanced amount of diversion. For example, Peggy, a 57-year-old woman with schizoaffective disorder had just lost her daughter to cancer. Peggy was devastated by this loss and was very worried about the impact of the illness and death on her grandchildren. After following the guidelines discussed above for providing an empathic sounding board for grief, the therapist inquired about methods Peggy was using to cope with the pain. At first, Peggy struggled to describe any helpful strategies other than writing thank-you notes, which she found difficult but somehow comforting. However, over the next two sessions, they were able to work out a plan that included these elements: 1) allow time for grieving, but try to do at least one diverting activity a day (e.g., try a new recipe for a dessert or some other food, work on a crafts project, accept friends' invitations to dinner); 2) resume walking on a daily basis (had stopped all exercise in past 3 months); and 3) discuss with son-in-law how family can best work together to help grandchildren. Peggy and her therapist worked on building this coping plan over the next few sessions.

Boundary Issues

People who have had mental illnesses for many years can sometimes find that the assistance and support of family and friends can become intrusive over time. This assistance takes many forms, from invading the privacy of the patient by asking too many questions about symptoms and treatment, to telling the patient how to manage her life. The patient is caught between being grateful for the assistance and feeling angry about the boundary violations, especially when family or friends push too hard, threaten to withdraw support, or become angry when the patient does not comply with their wishes.

Some people cope with these situations by giving in. Some passively resist or ignore the intrusions. Others take a more aggressive approach by arguing, pushing people away, and resisting what they perceive as efforts to control them. This aggressive approach usually leads first to intensification of supporters' efforts to assert influence, followed by giving up and withdrawing support and communication.

If patients' frustrations with boundary violations are communicated angrily, the message can be misinterpreted as a lack of gratitude. Supporters often do not understand why the patient is "turning on them" or why he doesn't realize that they are "only trying to help." Their defensive statements fall on the deaf ears of the patient who no longer has tolerance for the intrusions. Instead of being helpful, family and friends become another source of stress than can exacerbate symptoms.

A possible solution for this problem is to help patients communicate their concerns about boundary violations in a way that respectfully sets limits and does not antagonize their supporters. Assertive statements of this nature communicate appreciation for support and state the problem in a calm and positive way. Negative feedback regarding boundary violations should be delivered after an expression of gratitude and then followed by another positive statement, including a plan for how the problem will be solved in the future. Supporters need guidance on when to help and when not to help. That information has to come from the patient, as shown in the example below:

> Jim was grateful for his parents' support, but they violated his boundaries by calling his boss to let him know that he was not doing well. Their intention was to get Jim's boss to be more lenient and not fire him for missing work or for coming in late. Jim, however, did not think it was their place to talk to his boss. After calming down and carefully selecting his words, Jim called his parents and raised the issue by saying, "Mom and Dad, I know you care a lot about me and want to help, but it caused a problem for me when you called my boss. I need to handle my problems

> on my own. You have shown me how to do it and I am grateful for that. I promise to let you know when I can't handle things and need your help."

In this example, Jim expressed gratitude, behaved respectfully, and gave a specific instruction for how the problem would be handled in the future. This type of assertive interaction can be planned out and practiced in session using role-playing. The planned statements should be written down by the patient and reviewed before the interaction.

Not all family members or friends will accept negative feedback graciously. They may initially behave in a defensive manner. The patient should be prepared for this possibility by having another response ready that reinforces the original message but is not defensive in return. For example, Jim's mother was upset when he asked her not to call his boss. Calling him had been her idea, and she did not like being told that she was wrong. When she began to defend herself, Jim handled it by allowing her to speak her mind. He then reiterated his acknowledgment of her good intentions, even though he had some doubts that her intentions were completely altruistic. He elaborated on his plan to handle things himself by framing it as a positive and not as a negative. In other words, it was not that he didn't want her help—but that he needed to learn to handle things on his own and the only way he could learn was by trying. If he failed, he would learn from the experience.

It may be necessary to troubleshoot assertive statements about boundary violations by anticipating the responses of others and helping the patient to practice a response. Given how stressful it can be to behave in an assertive manner when not accustomed to doing so, the patient is likely to have negative automatic thoughts about it. Cognitive restructuring to address any negative automatic thoughts or dysfunctional beliefs about being assertive can be an important element in preparation for this new style of interaction.

Lack of Social Support

For many different reasons, people with severe mental illnesses often can find themselves alone and lacking in support from family or friends. For example, symptoms can keep people from forming attachments with others. They may not feel "normal" and therefore withdraw from contact with those who could provide support in times of need. Sometimes support is lacking because of strains or conflicts in relationships. In some cases, support from other people might be available, but not accessed by the patient because of distorted beliefs about those relationships, lack of interpersonal skills, shame or embarrassment about being ill, or lack of awareness by potential supporters that their assistance is needed.

Increasing social support begins by assessing patients' beliefs about accepting help from others. Schemas about the value of being self-reliant or independent may keep a person from accessing helping resources. Negative automatic thoughts, including predictions about the harmful intentions of others or the potential for rejection, might also keep a person from seeking out or accepting support from others. Standard logical analysis methods can be used to evaluate the accuracy of these thoughts or weigh the advantages and disadvantages of retaining schemas about self-reliance that preclude reaching out to others.

When family support is unavailable, seeking support from friends, self-help groups, faith-based organizations, or group therapy members might be alternatives to consider. Behavioral activation or activity planning interventions can assist patients in planning contact with others. Activities that could lead to increased social support can be assigned as homework. Identification of obstacles to participating in social activities and creating a plan to avoid or cope with them will increase the chance that the patient will follow through with the plan.

Disclosing the Disorder to Others

Another common dilemma across mental disorders is the question of self-disclosure regarding psychiatric illnesses. Some people want to "be honest" with others by disclosing this information early in a relationship. The hope is that the honesty will be appreciated and the relationship will proceed undisturbed. Unfortunately, in personal, work, or school relationships, disclosure about psychiatric illness is not often received positively (Michalak et al. 2007). Although there is more understanding of mental illnesses, social stigma and rejection because of mental illness are still a reality.

In some social situations, disclosure may be appropriate, for example, when forming a new romantic attachment that has potential for marriage. In this case, nondisclosure may be perceived as dishonesty. In a work environment, disclosure may be necessary if the illness requires a modification in usual work schedule or performance—for example, if time is needed during working hours to attend appointments or if sick leave must be taken to control symptom recurrence. Before providing information about mental illness or its treatment to coworkers, employers, or social acquaintances, the patient should weigh the advantages and disadvantages of disclosure. As shown in Table 9–1, this can be done by using a two-by-two matrix, where the patient lists the advantages and disadvantages of disclosure along with the advantages and disadvantages of not disclosing the mental illness. Although this task can be accomplished through Socratic questioning as well, it may be easier for the patient to complete the exercise and reason through the options in a written format. Once the four squares are completed, the patient can be asked to identify the most important or compelling advantages and disadvantages, one from each box. These items should represent the most important factors in the patient's decision to self-disclose illness information. The final step is to generate ways in which the patient could experience the advantages of self-disclosure in a way that minimizes the likelihood that the disadvantages will occur. In the example in Table 9–1, the primary advantages of disclosure were honesty and prevention of rejection at a later time. The primary disadvantage was also rejection from others. With these themes in mind, the therapist can help the patient find a way to be honest in a way that lessens the chance of rejection.

After some discussion, the patient decided that there was less chance of rejection if the disclosure was made when she was less symptomatic. If she waited until she was in the midst of a relapse, she would not be able to explain her problem as well and her partner would also have to deal with her symptoms without having any warning and without knowing how to respond. She believed that the risk of rejection would be higher if the person was caught off guard. Role-playing was used to practice how the disclosure would be made. The patient planned to offer to provide additional information about the illness and her treatment if the disclosure did not lead to immediate rejection.

Table 9–1. Advantages and disadvantages of self-disclosure

	Advantages	Disadvantages
Self-disclosure	✓ Being honest Avoids later rejection Others might be sympathetic and supportive.	Others will think I'm weird. ✓ I will be rejected.
Nondisclosure	No one will think badly of me. I will seem normal. ✓ I will not be rejected. I can act like nothing is wrong.	They might find out later and be angry that I didn't tell them. I will have to hide my medicines and my symptoms. ✓ I will feel dishonest.

Note. ✓ = most important or compelling reasons.

In a work scenario, an evaluation of the advantages and disadvantages of disclosure might lead to a decision not to disclose or to wait until disclosure is absolutely necessary, for example, if the patient is being shifted to a work schedule that would interrupt sleep and precipitate relapse. The key advantages at work might be the assumption that the information would help others understand and that some allowances might be made, whereas the disadvantages are the same as those for social situations (i.e., that rejection would occur). Instead of making the decision to share information about their illness, patients might decide to find other ways to cope.

Interpersonal Problems in Specific Disorders

Severe and Chronic Depression

The most common interpersonal dilemma for people with severe and chronic depression is social isolation. Sometimes the isolation stems from avoidance of contact with others and sometimes it is the result of the withdrawal of support when family and friends tire from the unrelenting negativity that comes with depression. The irritability that accompanies depression can stimulate negative automatic thoughts about others. Negative mind reading, personalization, jumping to conclusions, and magnification of the negative actions of others can result in hurt feelings that are acted out against others. The resulting strains might not be resolved by either party. When confidence is lost in the ability to form and maintain attachments, new relationships are likely to be avoided. The end result is the same: the support, encouragement, and distraction provided by interpersonal relationships is unavailable when patients need it the most.

Assumptions

Negative automatic thoughts and cognitive errors in depression can lead to inaccurate assumptions about the intentions of others. Also, the helplessness that is characteristic of depression can ready the person to perceive others as unwilling or unable to help, and a sense of hopelessness can make relationships seem destined to fail. The perception of worthlessness that accompanies depression can have negative consequences as well. For example, seeing oneself as unworthy of being treated well or incapable of being loved might increase tolerance to being abused or neglected. This perception can also lessen confidence in finding friends, building alliances, or asking for assistance. Some people who have had depression for much of their lives develop a schema of worthlessness that is resistant to change.

Negative automatic thoughts about relationships can be monitored and analyzed using cognitive restructuring strategies. Setting up experiments to test negative automatic thoughts about other people is particularly useful. Negative predictions about others can become self-fulfilling prophecies when the patient's avoidance creates a negative response or reduces attention from others. Experiments not only help gather information about negative automatic thoughts, but create an opportunity for an exposure exercise if the experiment includes interacting with others. This allows for both a cognitive intervention and a behavioral intervention to be done simultaneously.

Experiments to test negative thoughts pertaining to relationships might include gathering information about a person's ability to interact with others. When depression has persisted for some time and social isolation has been an issue, the patient may have forgotten how to initiate an interaction, engage in casual conversation, or make requests of others. Their prediction is often that they "can't do it anymore." The patient can be helped to test this prediction by selecting an easily achievable goal, practicing the interaction, selecting a specific time and place to conduct the experiment, and developing a plan for monitoring the outcome. The outcome should be something immediately observable to the patient, such as the ability to speak the words as practiced, a positive nonverbal response from the target of the experiment, or a verbal interaction that generally went well. Before selecting a social experiment of this nature, patients can be helped to create a hierarchy of social interactions from the simplest and most easily accomplished, like saying "hello" to a grocery store clerk who is paid to be friendly and polite, to more complicated or difficult goals such as reconnecting with a family member who has been distant for some time or asking someone out on a date. The first experiment should be easier than the patient is capable of accomplishing so that success can be guaranteed. Encourage patients not to try to do too much in their first effort. An early failure can thwart plans to increase social contact.

Perspective-taking exercises can also be effective in testing negative automatic thoughts about interactions with others. One such intervention is to generate alternative explanations for events that may have been distorted by personalization. Distancing methods are also useful, such as asking the patient to take the role of adviser and generate ideas for how someone else might view a troublesome interpersonal situation. Another perspective-taking exercise is to ask the patient to try to imagine how he might have viewed the issue in question at a time in life when depression was not present. Reacting as if not depressed allows the patient to use his own prior experience as a guide.

The simplest experiment to test negative automatic thoughts about others is to ask for feedback from the person who is the target of mind reading or whose action may be misinterpreted. This can be accomplished by having the patient state his negative automatic thought as a hypothesis and then ask for verification of this idea. For example, when Stan did not return Emma's telephone call one evening, she assumed that Stan was angry at her for something she had said about his mother the day before. Emma's experiment was to call Stan and ask if he had been bothered by what she had said and to ask if that had been the reason he had not returned her call. When Stan talked with her, he said that he had been bothered by her comment about his mother, but that the reason he had not called her back was that he worked late and was too tired by the time he got home. In this case, Emma's assumption was partially correct. The experiment allowed her to adjust her negative thinking and to apologize for what she said about Stan's mother, thereby resolving the tension between them.

Another example of work on automatic thoughts that influence interpersonal relationships comes from the treatment of Mary, the woman with chronic depression featured in the video illustrations. You may recall from Chapter 4 ("Case Formulation and Treatment Planning") that one of the examples of automatic thoughts in Mary's case conceptualization concerned her maladaptive response to an invitation from a friend (Table 9–2).

In a therapy session not shown in the video illustrations, the impact of these automatic thoughts was explored, and an attempt was made to help Mary break her pattern of social isolation:

Dr. Wright: How do you feel now about turning down this invitation?

Mary: Bad. I know that I need to get serious about doing things to get out of the house. I don't get many invitations like this.

Dr. Wright: Could we take a look at your automatic thoughts? They seemed to set you up to say no.

Mary: I just feel like a failure when I compare myself to her.

(They then identify cognitive errors [e.g., magnifying friend's successes and minimizing Mary's strengths, disqualifying the positive nature of friend's invitation, ignoring Mary's skills to be a friend and to participate in social activities] and write out a rational response on a thought change record).

Dr. Wright: Let's review the work that we did with this thought change record. What were the rational responses that you wrote out on the sheet?

Mary: She does have a very good job and probably hasn't been depressed like me—but she may have had problems in life that I don't know about. If I think about the past, there were times when I did things with friends. I know how to socialize….I just haven't been doing

---

Table 9–2. Automatic thoughts: Mary's example

Event

I get a call from an old friend from school. She asks me to join a women's bowling league with her.

Automatic Thoughts

She's been a big success.
She has a great job and all kinds of friends.
I don't know why she asked me to join the league.
I've messed up my life and don't deserve to be around people like that.

Emotions

Depressed
Tense

Behaviors

Politely told her no. Made an excuse about being too busy.

> any of this. The bowling league would be a good chance for me to meet new people.
>
> Dr. Wright: That sounds like a more reasonable way to see things. What would you like to do about this situation?
>
> Mary: I guess I missed my chance. They probably have filled the team by now.
>
> Dr. Wright: It could be that the team is filled, but could there be any positive opportunities in giving your friend a call?
>
> Mary: Maybe it isn't filled....Or, I guess I could offer to be a sub.
>
> Dr. Wright: Any other opportunities?
>
> Mary: Well, I suppose I might be able to tell her that I would be interested in doing other things with her if anything pops up.
>
> Dr. Wright: Good idea. Can we role-play having this conversation?

This intervention with Mary shows how core CBT methods for modifying automatic thoughts can be directed at interpersonal problems or deficits. Schemas of worthlessness, failure, and unlovability that impact interpersonal functioning are more difficult to change and may require extensive use of methods described in Chapter 7 ("Depression"). If proven inaccurate or dysfunctional, a replacement schema must be generated that acknowledges the valid elements of the old schema and eliminates the distortions. New experiments will be needed to verify the accuracy of the modified schema and to practice methods of proceeding in life following the precepts of the revised schema. Further modifications may be needed until the new schema accurately characterizes the patient. Chapter 7 contains an illustration of schema change techniques that have the potential to improve self-concept and enhance interpersonal relationships.

Burned Bridges

In his cognitive behavioral analysis system of psychotherapy, James Mc-Cullough (2000) describes the impact that complaints of chronic depression can have on social relationships. Over time, the person with depression burns out her social support networks when perceived by others as not making sufficient efforts to overcome symptoms. The depressed person returns to the well of support until the well runs dry. Those who might have felt compassion at one time run out of patience when they believe the patient is not doing enough to change his fate, when advice seems to fall on deaf ears, or when actions appear to be more self-defeating than helpful. Supporters can get the impression that the patient is too passive when efforts that could be made or opportunities that could be pursued are ignored. Responses vary from avoidance to verbalized anger or frustration. Patients do not always understand these reactions but perceive the negativity, which leaves them feeling hurt and rejected.

McCullough's approach is to help patients draw connections from their actions toward others, the attitudes that guide those actions, and the outcomes they experience. For example, when they feel hopeless to change their fate and complain to others about it, they may not receive assistance, encouragement, understanding, or support in response. Through diary exercises and discussion, the patient is encouraged to contrast the desired re-action from others and the actual response. When the desired response is not achieved, the patient is encouraged to examine how her mind-set and actions might have been responsible. In a proactive manner, the patient is encouraged to identify an attitude and behavioral response that would more likely achieve the desired outcome. For example, if the patient wanted support from a friend in dealing with loneliness, rather than complaining, a more proactive behavior might be to invite the friend to go to the movies. Instead of an attitude of helplessness, an attitude of determination might be adopted to achieve this goal. With this approach, patients are encouraged to select a course of action and accompanying attitude to help improve social interactions rather than relying on the emotions of depression to stimulate thoughts and actions.

Bipolar Disorder

The interpersonal problems that occur during the depressive phase of bipolar disorder are the same that occur in chronic major depression. In mania, hypomania, and mixed states, the most common relationship problems stem from conflict due to irritability, impulsivity, and impaired judgment. In the video illustrations of Angela's CBT sessions, she provided examples of how impulsivity led her to marry a man after knowing him for only a few weeks. Her irritability caused her to behave too aggressively with customers at work. Her poor judgment led her to send sexually inappropriate photographs to men at work. In all of these instances, she was not aware that her behavior was being influenced by her symptoms of bipolar disorder. For people like Angela, self-awareness can be enhanced through Socratic questioning and self-monitoring of symptom changes. When awareness is increased, patients with bipolar disorder can be encouraged to intentionally make different choices in behavior. For example, if Angela had realized that she was in a manic episode, she could have postponed her wedding until she was more certain about the decision. If she was aware that she was irritable as a result of mania or hypomania, she might be able to reason through a stressful work situation rather than blame the client or her coworkers. If she was aware that her sex drive had increased due to mania, she could have tried to keep herself from giving in to urges to act impulsively.

The symptom-recognition methods presented in Chapter 8 ("Mania") can help patients to gain more self-awareness and track the course of key symptoms such as irritability. When early detection is missed and symptoms can't be easily controlled, the methods described in the following sections can help people to more effectively cope with the manifestations of mania, hypomania, and mixed states.

Irritability and Conflict

Conflict can be so stimulating, especially when irritability is present, that the person does not realize that his symptoms contributed to the argument until long after the conflict is over. With perfect hindsight, people realize that the topic of discussion was not worthy of the amount of emotion that was expressed. By this time, it is usually too late to prevent the damage caused by hurtful words and actions. Therefore, the best way to deal with irritability and conflict is prevention.

Although irritability is an emotion, it may not be detectable as such. The consequences of irritability, such as physical sensations of stress, discomfort, or agitation, may be easier to recognize. There may be difficulty with concentration, an urge to move around, muscle tension, or fatigue. Irritability can make noises seem loud or unpleasant and can draw a person's attention to repetitive sounds or actions of others that would normally be outside awareness or easily ignored. Irritability can also show itself in choice of words when interacting with others, as well as in tone of voice and body language. When Angela is irritable, she speaks with a harsh tone, uses sarcasm to make her points, and is critical of others. She had not been able to hear the irritability in her speech until her therapist pointed it out.

When people are unaware of feeling irritable, they can sometimes learn to tune into 1) physical sensations, such as muscle tightening or jaw clenching; 2) communication changes, such as altered tone of voice; or 3) behavior changes. For example, Angela notices that when she is irritable, she rubs her face and forehead like she is trying to wipe away the irritation. She also catches herself holding her breath and pursing her lips. These behaviors are easier for her to identify than the feeling of irritability. A symptom-detection plan can include monitoring physical sensations or behavioral cues. When patients have these physical symptoms, they can ask themselves if they are feeling irritable and rate intensity on a simple 0–10 scale, with 10 indicating maximum irritability. A personal irritability scale can be developed where physical indicators of various intensity levels are noted. This exercise teaches people to self-monitor levels of irritability so they know when it is reaching a level that can cause interpersonal problems. Figure 9–1 shows an example of Angela's personal irritability scale.

To use a personalized irritability scale to avoid interpersonal problems, the patient sets a number at which it is time to avoid contact with others that could lead to conflict. In Angela's case, there were certain people with whom she often had conflict when she was feeling irritable, such as her mother or her boyfriend. Her personal rule was to avoid conflict when she reached a score of 6 or greater. When she was at a level of 4 or 5, she knew she had to make efforts at lessening her irritability, such as reducing stimulation, taking time to rest, and making sure she tended to her basic needs such as eating. A third column can be added to the personal irritability scale for the action to be taken at each level. In Angela's example, no protective action may be needed until reaching a level of 3, at which point it would be helpful to take a few deep breaths and walk away from stressful situations.

Learning Exercise 9–2.   Emotion Intensity Scale

1. Construct a symptom severity scale for a patient who has had difficulties with irritability or anger, or construct a scale for yourself. Use a simple scale of 0 to 10, with 0 meaning that the emotion is absent and 10 indicating the highest intensity of the emotion.

2. Label each level of emotion with a word that describes its intensity.

Rating	Symptoms
10—Can't stand my own skin	Pacing, scratching at myself, can't sleep, angry
9	
8—Want to shout at someone	Lose temper, argue, accuse people of being annoying
7	
6—Edgy	Snap at people for being too slow
5—Annoyed	Sarcastic when talking to people
4	
3—People bug me	Complain more about people
2	
1—A little bothered	Notice annoying people but ignore them easily
0—Not irritable	Nothing bothers me

Figure 9–1. Angela's irritability scale.

3. Identify a behavior, physical sensation, or thought that would be present at each level of intensity.

4. Create a plan of what should be done to manage each level of intensity. Keep in mind that no action may be required at level 0 or 1 and only a mental note may be needed at level 2 or 3.

Although using avoidance as a coping mechanism is generally frowned upon by therapists, there is a place for it in the management of bipolar disorder. When manic symptoms such as irritability are beginning to emerge, the person is vulnerable to showing this emotion in her interactions with others. Rather than run the risk of being in a situation that will prove irritating and could lead to conflict, it may be more useful to avoid these risky situations until the irritability has subsided. Coping strategies can be taught to help manage irritating situations when avoidance is not possible. These strategies could include relaxation training or using role-play to script responses to stressful situations.

For example, Alex inevitably got into arguments with his father when he was feeling irritable. In fact, Alex found his father to be annoying even when he was not irritable, especially when his father had been drinking heavily. Alex did not want to avoid visiting his parents altogether just because he was experiencing irritability, so he had to learn how to manage his reactions to his father so that they did not end up in an argument. Alex learned several skills including differential relaxation, response prevention, and assertiveness to help him cope with his father (Table 9–3).

Differential relaxation is the ability to physically relax muscle groups when engaging in activity. When Alex was able to relax the muscles in his body not needed for interaction, he could lower his irritability enough to make it through dinner with his parents. Sitting at the dinner table, Alex released the tension in his lower body, his shoulders, and some of the muscles in his face. He would note his breathing pattern and take a few calming breaths to slow his respiration. With each breath, he said the word "calm" in his mind.

Response prevention was also helpful in controlling his irritability when visiting his parents. Alex found that irritability made him hypersensitive to the things his father said and did, particularly his father's unkind comments to Alex's mother. Alex kept himself from overreacting to his father, but focused more of his attention on his mother. He helped her prepare dinner while his father watched TV and drank beer. During meals, Alex engaged

---

Table 9–3. Alex's plan for coping with irritability

Avoid potential conflict situations when possible.

Use differential relaxation.

Focus on nonirritating aspects of the situation or less irritating people.

Ignore the comments or make light of the situation.

Acknowledge first, then change the subject.

Agree, and then ask to change the subject.

Challenge the intention of the comment and discontinue the conversation.

Remove self from the situation.

his mother in conversation, which kept him from focusing too intently on his father and overreacting to his behavior. A secondary component of response prevention was used when Alex's irritability made it difficult for him to ignore his father or to keep his comments to himself. In those situations, rather than risk an argument, Alex politely excused himself and left his parents' home. While he was not concerned about the impact of his departure on his father, he did not want to hurt his mother's feelings, especially given her efforts at preparing a meal. So Alex informed his mother of his response prevention plan before his visit. Together they came up with a cue that would let his mother know that his irritability was becoming difficult to control, and it was time for him to leave.

Another preventive strategy was to come up with several standard assertive responses to the types of things his father would say that Alex found irritating and difficult to ignore. Examples include statements that implied criticism of Alex, recalled his prior failures, or demeaned his mother. Alex's father did not seem to know how to initiate a positive or even neutral conversation, although he clearly wanted to interact with his son. Provoking an argument had become a common way to get Alex's attention. When he was not irritable, Alex could ignore the comments, laugh them off, or join his father by making fun of himself. These methods all seemed to diffuse the situation and allowed for an interaction that was tolerable, although not enjoyable for Alex. When Alex was irritable, however, these coping strategies were too difficult for him. So, he and his therapist developed standard phrases that were direct but did not counterattack his father and lead to an argument. One type of response was to acknowledge his father's statement and then change the subject altogether, such as "I'm afraid I'm not up to joking about that today, Dad. How are things going at work?" Another type of statement was to first agree with his father and then ask to change the subject, such as "You're right. I haven't done so well in that area. Do you mind if we focus on something else today?" A more assertive statement was to challenge the intention of the father's comment and discontinue the conversation: "Dad, I know you are trying to get a rise out me, but I'm not up for it today. Let's just watch TV." If his father would not comply, then Alex would have to decide whether he could ignore his father's comments, and if not, he would politely leave his parents' home.

Changing Relationships

Irritability coupled with impulsivity and a fluctuating sex drive can make people believe that they want to end an existing relationship and begin a new one. In addition, long-standing relationship difficulties can set the stage for hasty decisions and impulsive behaviors such as sexual indiscretions. Conflict, communication problems, and dissatisfaction with the relationship, especially an unsatisfying sex life, are often used as justifications to seek out romantic encounters with new partners. If mania or hypomania is fueling these decisions, the outcome is usually problematic. Marriages are strained; risky sexual behaviors create health problems; and the end result may be the exchange of one set of relationship difficulties for another.

Similarly, in the depressive phase of bipolar disorder, the prevailing negative attitude can make relationship difficulties seem insurmountable and the situation hopeless. Just as people have passive suicidal thoughts about escaping life's problems, depression can stimulate fantasies of an improved life after escaping a bad relationship. Sometimes there are real problems that the person does not have the ability to address during a depressive episode, but which may be solvable when the episode remits. To keep bipolar disorder from disrupting relationships, the patient must learn to know how to differentiate real relationship problems from misperceptions stimulated by depression or mania. The time to make relationship changes is not during a manic or depressive episode, when mistakes in judgment are too easily made. When emotions make the relationship seem unbearable, strategies are needed to delay making changes until the episode is over or until the patient can rationally evaluate the evidence for and against the intolerability and the hopelessness of the relationship problems. If after careful evaluation and attempts to remedy the situation it appears that it is time to end the relationship, it should be done in a manner that minimizes distress for all parties involved.

An increased sex drive may be the motivating factor for wanting to begin a new romantic encounter, even when the person is not currently in a committed relationship. Sally, for example, picks up men in bars and gets involved sexually when she is hypomanic. She has some awareness that this may not always be a good idea, but her increased libido, overly positive thinking that comes with hypomania, and the availability of a willing partner make it hard for her to resist. There have been times when Sally suffered the negative consequences of unprotected sex and when her partner wanted more intimacy from her than she desired. She considered herself lucky, however, that she had not experienced any serious harm from these casual sexual encounters thus far.

Sally wanted to gain more control over her bipolar disorder, which included curbing her sexual activities. To do so, she used response prevention and the 24-hour rule (Basco 2006). Response prevention for Sally meant avoiding high-risk situations. For her, that meant avoiding hotel bars at night when she was traveling alone and suspected that she might be hypomanic. She kept a short list of common symptoms of hypomania in her wallet, which she reviewed whenever she had doubt. If she had more than one symptom, she made different plans for her evening, which might include having dinner with a girlfriend or female colleague, watching a movie, or exercising. When she was uncertain that symptoms of mania or hypomania were driving her sexual interest, she imposed a 24-hour rule. She avoided sexual contact or romantic involvement for 24 hours after first having the desire. When her symptoms were stimulating her interest, she generally forgot about the man by the next day. If he was worth pursuing, the delay gave her time to think about ways to develop a relationship rather than rush into sex.

Overall, the strategies for preventing interpersonal problems in bipolar disorder require self-monitoring of symptoms to determine when they are coloring perceptions of the positive and negative aspects of relationships. When symptoms may be present, precautions are needed to prevent the symptoms from controlling actions in a negative way. These interventions might include evaluating automatic thoughts about relationship difficulties and weighing the advantages and disadvantages of making any changes in the status of a relationship. Until it is clear that taking action is the right thing to do, strategies must be used to prevent inappropriate actions, including removing oneself from risky circumstances that could lead to words or behaviors that the patient might later regret.

Schizophrenia

It is often assumed that relationship problems are inevitable in schizophrenia and that significant deficits in communication and development of intimate relationships will surely increase as the illness progresses. However, this unfortunate overgeneralization can become self-fulfilling as people with schizophrenia pull back from engaging with others because of fear, low expectations, and stigmatization. People with schizophrenia vary greatly in their abilities to form relationships. Some develop the illness later in life—as paranoid states or delusional disorders are molded by anxiety-provoking circumstances. Relationships with others have often developed earlier in life; patients may have married and held responsible jobs, but these relationships now are affected by the interference of delusional beliefs. It is crucial to minimize this effect by intervening early and using techniques to understand and work with these delusional beliefs. Efforts should be made to try to keep others on the patient's side—that is, sympathetic and understanding—even when the paranoia may be directed at them.

When the illness develops earlier, it may follow a period of stimulant or hallucinogenic drug use during which the initial psychotic episode occurs and after which it persists. These patients with a drug-related psychosis often have had sufficient social skills to make friends—some of whom may provide opportunities for ongoing positive relationships. But other relationships may have been formed with persons who have introduced them to the illicit drugs.

Experiences of prior traumatic events will also shape relationship formation. The capacity to build trust may be significantly impaired by such damaging incidents. Nevertheless, some patients with a trauma-related psychosis can be personable and socially competent and are able to effectively develop friendships.

Then there are some schizophrenia patients who do appear to be shy and stress-sensitive, who have avoided social contact throughout childhood, who may have been bullied, and who find developing adult relationships particularly difficult. They can easily misinterpret nonverbal messages (e.g., develop ideas of reference) and have social anxiety that leads to increased social withdrawal. Although this withdrawal is often for perceived self-preservation, it is distressing for family members who might wish to provide support (Quinn et al. 2003).

Individuals with schizophrenia who have relationship problems require approaches tailored to their needs. If drug or alcohol abuse remains an issue, therapists need to help the patient find alternative social outlets to those perpetuating the habit. Where trauma has been an issue, therapeutic work will be needed to enable the person to see beyond the trauma and reach out to those who can be trusted. Initially, the treatment may need to focus on developing acquaintances. As patients build relationship skills, cautious movement can occur to develop friendships and, lastly, intimate relationships.

Where relationships are intact, their preservation may be possible over the acute episode. However, providing necessary explanations and support to families and friends can easily be overlooked. Where relationships are troubled, the general methods for specific problems described earlier in this chapter become relevant. Also, basic social skills training may be required. Short- and long-term goals for relationship building can be set. A common long-term goal may be to have at least one close relationship outside the family—a boyfriend or girlfriend. This relationship may often be with someone of like mind and personality, quite frequently another patient, because most of the patient's social circle may be from his contacts within mental health services. As long as this relationship is not exploitative, it can be very successful. Family and staff can sometimes be wary of these relationships, but it is worth noting that the relationships patients form with each other can be often more lasting than the relationships formed with professional caregivers.

Gradual persistence in increasing social contacts is often needed. As in Majir's case in the video illustrations, the first step simply may be leaving the house to go to a shop where the only contact is with the shop assistant. However, success with these types of activities can be gradually built on.

Living with stigma is a major issue with schizophrenia. It can affect relationships with family, friends, and coworkers because of their negative views and fears. Patients can retreat from relationships because they want to hide away from those who may see them inappropriately as alien, unapproachable, or dangerous. Although effective public education and destigmatization programs are needed to overcome this problem, patients and their families can still take some actions that may possibly reduce the negative effects of stigma on relationships.

When someone is asked, "What's wrong with you?" or a parent is asked, "What's your son's problem?" providing an explanation can be difficult. Unfortunately, saying that the problem is schizophrenia can lead to misunderstanding and social distancing. We have been increasingly advocating that individuals develop a credible explanation to use in such circumstances (e.g., "I had some problems as a child that came back to haunt me"; "I'm a bit sensitive to stress and going to college got to me"; or "I had a lot of stress at work and thought people were ganging up on me"). It also helps to say that one is now on the road to recovery. As relationships deepen, more information may be given but sometimes it needs to be released gradually. Sudden outflows of revelation can occur, perhaps because the person is being listened to sympathetically by a friend for the first time. These revelations can run the risk of being counterproductive.

There are now many patients with schizophrenia who are developing and sustaining relationships in a way that goes against the stereotype of the isolated, awkward, and disheveled individual. Encouragement and support from the therapist, with increased but realistically timed expectations, can do a great deal to help.

Summary

Key Points for Clinicians

- Social support is needed by people with severe mental illnesses.
- People with severe mental illnesses may be lacking in basic interpersonal skills. These skills can be taught in CBT.
- Negative automatic thoughts about social interactions can keep people from communicating with others.

- Honest self-disclosure of psychiatric disorders or assertive statements to others are not always worth the risks. The pros and cons should be objectively evaluated for such communications.

Concepts and Skills for Patients to Learn

- Communication skills training can help people become more assertive, form social contacts, and resolve problems with others.
- Role-playing in therapy sessions is a good way to learn social skills.
- Evaluation of negative automatic thoughts about social interaction can facilitate formation of new relationships.
- Learning to recognize the presence of symptoms can help people in making appropriate adjustments in social interactions, including decisions to temporarily avoid interactions or to implement an active response.

References

Barrett MS, Barber JP: Interpersonal profiles in major depressive disorder. J Clin Psychol 63:247–266, 2007

Basco MR: The Bipolar Workbook: Tools for Controlling Your Mood Swings. New York, Guilford, 2006

Baucom DH, Epstein NB: Cognitive Behavioral Marital Therapy. New York, Brunner/Mazel, 1990

Beck AT: Love Is Never Enough: How Couples Can Overcome Misunderstandings, Resolve Conflicts, and Solve Relationship Problems Through Cognitive Therapy. New York, Harper & Row, 1988

Burns DD: Feeling Good: The New Mood Therapy, Revised and Updated. New York, Avon Books, 1999

Dattilio FM, Padesky CA: Cognitive Therapy with Couples. Sarasota, FL, Professional Resource Exchange, 1990

Epstein NB, Baucom DH: Enhanced Cognitive Behavioral Therapy for Couples: A Contextual Approach. Washington, DC, American Psychological Association, 2002

Epstein NB, Schlesinger SE, Dryden W: Cognitive-Behavior Therapy With Families. New York, Brunner/Mazel, 1988

McCullough JP Jr: Treatment for Chronic Depression: Cognitive Behavioral Analysis System of Psychotherapy. New York, Guilford, 2000

Michalak EE, Yatham LN, Maxwell V: The impact of bipolar disorder upon work functioning: a qualitative analysis. Bipolar Disord 9:126–143, 2007

Quinn J, Barrowclough C, Tarrier N: The Family Questionnaire (FQ): a scale for measuring symptom appraisal in relatives of schizophrenic patients. Acta Psychiatr Scand 108:290–296, 2003

10

Impaired Cognitive Functioning

This chapter describes the CBT techniques used to work with cognitive dysfunction in patients with severe mental illness. The most challenging situation is often found in individuals who exhibit schizophrenic thought disorder, such as "knight's move thinking" (see the section "Major Thought Disorder" later in this chapter). Classically, no form of psychological treatment has been able to make much progress with seemingly incomprehensible dialogue. However, research on the emotional salience of disordered thinking has led to the description of a viable CBT model and the development of potentially useful intervention strategies. This approach is demonstrated here with video illustrations of the treatment of Daniel, a young man with rather severe disorganization of thought. In addition, methods are described for milder forms of schizophrenic thought disorder, such as pseudophilosophical thinking, concrete thinking, and thought blocking. Because cognitive impairment is a common manifestation of mood disorders, we also provide guidelines for using CBT to enhance cognitive functioning in bipolar disorder and severe or treatment-resistant depression.

Efforts to address cognitive deficits in schizophrenia (e.g., impaired attention, working memory, and executive functioning; see Goldberg et al. 2003 for information on these deficits) with cognitive remediation or rehabilitation interventions are not discussed here because these procedures are not typically a component of CBT for severe mental illness.

Readers who are interested in these methods are referred to publications by McGurk et al. (2007), Penades et al. (2006), Velligan et al. (2006), and Wykes et al. (2007).

Thought Disorder in Schizophrenia

Mild to Moderate Thought Disorder

Thought disorder in schizophrenia lies on a continuum between normality and word salad. The more severe manifestations are usually seen in acute hebephrenia and in chronic patients who have been institutionalized for many years. However, the milder forms need specific attention because they are commonly present and can lead to increasing alienation and social avoidance. The milder forms of thought disorder are listed in Table 10–1 and described further below:

- **Pseudophilosophical thinking** can lead clinician and patient to never really getting to know each other. Examples include patients who quickly resort to discussion of the tarot, esoteric religions, science fiction, chakras, the crucial importance of prime numbers, and so forth. The clinician needs to decide whether the patient is frantically searching for meaning in life or whether such thinking is basically a form of avoidance of discussion of more painful matters. If the former is the situation, then the clinician can normalize the search for meaning as something that is fundamental to everyone. The search for meaning then becomes a joint endeavor as part of the problem list. The end result of such work can be to accept a philosophy for life that does not run counter to attempts to work toward recovery. The avoidant patient with pseudophilosophical thinking tends to jump from one area to the next rather than staying focused on one explanation (e.g., numerology). In such a case, therapists can attempt to cull the core issues and main emotions that the patient is avoiding and gradually help him to develop methods to manage these problems.

- **Wooliness of thought** is a problem where the patient's flow of thought isn't frankly incomprehensible but is just vague and imprecise. Here the crucial anchor for each meeting is the agreed target. The clinician and patient need to come to agreement on what they might be trying to achieve (e.g., use an activity schedule). The clinician should speak in brief concise sentences and model this for the patient. Every sentence should relate specifically to the target and the patient should be gently encouraged to clarify any specific queries or criticisms.

Table 10–1. Mild to moderate thought disorder in schizophrenia

Pseudophilosophical thinking

Wooliness of thought

Talking past the point

Concrete thinking

Tangential thoughts

Loosening of associations

Thought blocking

- **Talking past the point** occurs when a patient loses the benefit of clear communication by consistently elaborating in a different but related area. The clinician should explain that he is very interested in some specific points that the patient is making and ask for permission to "press the buzzer" or "ring the bell" once such an interesting comment is made. The patient can also be given the right to "press the buzzer" to stop the clinician. This strategy introduces humor, which is usually appreciated by the patient.

- **Concrete thinking** is a common form of mild to moderate thought disorder that needs to be detected early in the establishment of a collaborative CBT approach. Because therapists tend to use speech forms that are illustrative and representative, patients with concrete thinking may misunderstand the intent of the communication. For example, when the clinician informs the concretely thinking patient that she needs to decide on a target, the patient may look puzzled. A target seen concretely may be a board with colored rings for shooting practice. Similarly, when the clinician asks the patient to "catch" his automatic thoughts, the patient may be thinking about attempting to set a trap for them. Clinicians need to be aware of the potential for concrete thinking and thus clearly describe the elements of each concept. It can be useful to ask for regular feedback to ensure understanding and to draw out key points on paper or a whiteboard.

- **Tangential thoughts** are of intermediate severity compared with wooliness of thought, loosening of associations, and knight's move thinking (the last two items are described later). Tangential thoughts are similar to a slow flight of ideas, as seen in hypomania and mania. To help explain tangential thoughts to patients, clinicians can diagram this style of thinking on paper or a whiteboard as a series of zigzagging lines that never achieve their goal. In contrast, normal thinking and speech are portrayed as a series of straight lines leading to a clear endpoint. We therefore ask patients to state their communication goal at the start and then describe how their tangential thoughts get them nearer or further away from this goal. The important questions here are "What is the main thing you want to communicate?" and "Can you slow down and explain how one point leads to another?"

• **Loosening of associations** is more problematic than tangential thoughts because the links in thought are more difficult to understand. The clinician can struggle to keep track of concepts that seemingly have some underlying connection but have no clear direction. Here the underlying links between ideas need to be identified with the patient, and she should be gently brought back to the focus of the work on specific targets.

• **Thought blocking** is described to patients as sudden gaps or stoppages in their train of thought and their interaction with others. These blockages can be normalized by commenting that anyone can lose his train of thought, particularly if he is anxious or stressed. This phenomenon can be addressed by asking patients to identify the thoughts that were going through their mind at the time just before the block. Often an anxious automatic thought or an unpleasant obsessional image can be detected. Help can be offered for these types of upsetting thoughts with rational responding, mindfulness, or other techniques for positive symptoms described in Chapters 5 ("Delusions") and 6 ("Hallucinations"). In situations where patients cannot identify any interfering thoughts or state that they "just went blank," therapists can help patients find the thread of their thought by reflecting back on the previous conversation and then linking this to a communication goal.

The symptoms in Table 10–1 may not dominate the clinical picture, especially when patients are describing florid delusions and hallucinations, but efforts to improve the organization of thought and communication style can often yield benefits. The techniques described above for mild to moderate forms of thought disorder may have applicability across a variety of conditions in which patients are having difficulty organizing and communicating their thoughts. These methods are summarized in Table 10–2.

Major Thought Disorder

Patients who have more severe disorganization of thought processing present greater obstacles for implementation of CBT. For some patients

---

Table 10–2. CBT methods for mild to moderate thought disorder

---

Normalize problems with thinking clearly.

Cull the core issues and main emotions that patients are trying to communicate.

Set clear targets for sessions.

Model clear and precise communication for patients.

Gently encourage patients to clarify what they are trying to communicate.

Introduce idea of "pressing the buzzer" to let patients know when they are getting off track.

Use diagrams to demonstrate disruptions in the flow of thinking—contrast these with diagrams of effective patterns of communication.

Ask patients to clearly state their communication goal.

Help patients identify the links between ideas.

Ask patients to slow down and explain how one point leads to another.

Identify automatic thoughts or obsessive images that precede thought blocks.

---

with very severe disorganization of thought, it may be quite difficult or impossible to form a therapeutic relationship and to communicate effectively until symptoms are reduced with antipsychotic medications. However, CBT methods can be quite useful in many situations where severe manifestations of thought disorder are present. The major forms of thought disorder in schizophrenia are listed in Table 10–3 and discussed below:

- A knight's move in chess is a horizontal or vertical move followed by a jump along a diagonal. **Knight's move thinking** is used to describe thought disorder when there is a sudden and incomprehensible jump from one concept to another. The effect on hearers is to leave them perplexed by the communication. In the face of this type of thinking, many people disengage and attempt little in the way of further conversation. However, it is usually possible to ask the patient to explain why this jump in the flow of thoughts occurred.

- **Derailment** is less overt than knight's move thinking, but again a shift in topics occurs without completion of the initial point. Patients don't seem to notice that they aren't completing the train of thought and can become frustrated by the lack of comprehension and interest

Table 10–3. Major thought disorder in schizophrenia

Knight's move thinking

Derailment

Fusion

Neologisms

Word salad

of the listener. To help with this type of thought disorder, therapists can stop the patient each time the derailment happens to ask her to complete the previous point.

- **Fusion** is a more disconcerting problem in thinking: the patient intermingles two or more topics within one conversation in a manner that makes it extremely difficult to discern the message he is trying to convey. When patients are communicating in this manner, therapists can attempt to identify the main theme or themes in the conversation and then shape the interview to keep the focus on this content area.

- The more pronounced manifestations of thought disorder, neologisms and word salad (described next) will present steep barriers to effective communication. If a **neologism** is produced by a patient, we attempt to discover why the two apparently unrelated sections of words have been put together. Patients can sometimes explain their neologisms, and this information can be used to help discover the underlying theme.

- If **word salad** is present, thought linkage is often impossible due to the marked degree of thought fragmentation. Often caregivers and key workers who know the patient well can identify fluctuations in the severity of the word salad in relation to particular situations and stressors. One such patient became much more agitated and thought disordered when the news came on the TV. The linked affect here appeared to be of anxiety worsened by news of war, weather disruption, and famine.

Additional CBT methods drawn from Table 10–2, such as giving patients direct feedback when they are getting off track and asking patients to clearly state their communication goal can be helpful. Also, it may sometimes be useful to identify and reduce dysphoric emotions that are intertwined with the disorganized pattern of thought. Methods for addressing severe thought disorder are demonstrated in the next video illustration of a man who has some of the major features of schizophrenic thought disorder, such as knight's move thinking, derailment, and fusion:

> Daniel is a 30-year-old man who had a first episode of psychosis at age 18. There were no clear precipitants or traumas. However, the illness appeared very shortly after he left home for his first year of college. The first episode was characterized by paranoia toward roommates and other students, isolation, and aggressive behavior. He shouted at others, became agitated, tore up a TV because he thought it was talking especially to him, and went through roommates' belongings looking for proof that they were tape-recording him. He didn't attend class, eat meals regularly, or blend into the social activities at the college. There was no pattern of substance abuse.
>
> After about 2 months at college, Daniel's parents were called to take him home. He was hospitalized briefly and placed on risperidone. This helped modestly, but he has not taken medications regularly because he believes that they make him feel like a robot. Long-acting risperidone shots were recommended, but he refused. His illness has been chronic since that time. There have been no periods of sustained recovery. Daniel has been unable to work and was asked to leave a halfway house because he did not follow rules for cleanliness and did not help with cooking and other chores.
>
> His parents are very supportive and have advocated that he take medication and attend a day center. Unfortunately, Daniel has deteriorated further. His current hospitalization was ordered by the court after his parents filed a warrant. Daniel has been trying to live on his own, but he has been extremely paranoid and reclusive, and he has not been bathing or eating regularly. His refrigerator was found to have spoiled food, and his personal hygiene and care of the apartment showed disregard for cleanliness. He had stopped all medication at least 3 months ago.

> ▶ **Video Illustration 15.** Helping With Thought
> Disorder: Dr. Turkington and Daniel

Daniel tells a disjointed story about his family trying to control him, problems with world conditions and politics, and his paranoid beliefs about neighbors. He believes that his neighbors modified his TV to listen in on him. He can hear them talking about him. He plots out the building plans for electrical wires, plumbing, and heating ducts in the apartment complex and thinks that neighbors are controlling him through these conduits. Thus, he has determined the places he can safely stand in the apartment and has tried to block various ducts and openings.

The interview is marked by Daniel's knight's move thinking and derailments, in addition to elements of milder thought disorder, such as talking past the point. Dr. Turkington demonstrates how to engage a person with this type of psychosis and to shape the communication to decrease the thought disorder. A variety of techniques are used to help Daniel communicate his key concerns and generate a problem list. Several CBT methods for major thought disorder in schizophrenia are listed in Table 10–4. Some of these methods are drawn from the interventions described earlier for less severe types of thought disorder (Table 10–2) that may have applicability across the continuum of thought disorder severity.

It can be very difficult for both therapist and patient when the patient's train of thought appears to be incomprehensibly muddled. However, there is evidence that most thought-disordered content has meaning to the individual (Harrow and Prosen 1978). In Daniel's case, Dr. Turkington initially finds it very difficult to understand Daniel's knight's move jumps. An apparent complete loss of associations proceeds from Daniel's comments about his parents being angry with him, to a description of vents in his apartment being covered, to a rambling account of his dislike for using credit cards in the local shops. Dr. Turkington's first attempt to unravel this apparently confused pattern of thought was to use *thought linkage*. This technique involves taking the patient back to the knight's move and saying, "You seem to jump from A to C—can you put in the B for me? What is the link between these thoughts?" Daniel is eventually able to respond to this request and to link his parents' being angry over his apparent untidiness to the fact that he was using his clothes to cover the vents, through which he thought his persecutors were spying on him. Daniel said that his parents were also angry that he wasn't eating and not even doing his shopping. He explains this link as related to his belief that his persecutors could monitor his activities by checking on his credit card records. The underlying theme here was therefore a delusional one—he believed he was being persecuted by people who could track his activities and potentially harm him.

Daniel's disintegration of thought also appeared to be influenced by emotional arousal—anxiety about his perceived persecution and some anger toward his parents for not understanding him. The sessions were therefore directed toward goals of fully understanding his delusions, reducing his anxiety, and then developing alternative explanations that could be checked out using reality testing.

The process of making sense of Daniel's speech seemed to help him begin to communicate more clearly. His frustration about not being understood also diminished. Daniel was then introduced to anxiety reduction methods, and a homework assignment was devised for him to practice clearer communication with his parents by using a role-play exercise with one of the nurses playing the part of his mother.

Another step in Daniel's treatment was to use reality testing to attempt to reduce his delusional convictions. The goals of this intervention

Table 10–4. CBT techniques for major thought disorder

Use thought linkage.

Focus on the key underlying theme.

Identify the main affect linked to the thought disorder.

Employ CBT techniques, including homework assignments, to work with irrational thinking within the main theme.

Practice structuring, summarizing, and feedback methods.

Review audiotape or videotape to clarify the main themes.

were not only to modify the delusional belief, but also to improve the thought disorganization that appeared to be aggravated by the intensity of the delusions and the fear that was associated with the persecutory beliefs. The next video illustration shows a brief segment of the interview in which Dr. Turkington helps Daniel check out the validity of his perceptions about being spied on and controlled in the inpatient unit.

> ▶ **Video Illustration 16.**   Investigating a Delusion:
> Dr. Turkington and Daniel

Dr. Turkington begins this intervention by summarizing the previous work of helping Daniel communicate more clearly. Daniel notes that he believed himself to be under surveillance and to be a victim of persecution in his apartment. Dr. Turkington then asks if this fear has transferred to the surroundings of the inpatient unit. Daniel confirms that he still believes that there are miniature cameras in the vents and sprinklers and that he has spotted something that appears to be a surveillance device.

Next, Dr. Turkington proposes a reality-testing homework exercise—he suggests that Daniel investigate the vents and sprinklers with the help of the ward nurse in an attempt to discern the nature of the "silver thing" that he thought he saw in his room. It is agreed that if they can't come to a conclusion on whether it is a surveillance device or not, the nurse will request that the hospital engineer give a technical opinion. Daniel is asked to keep an open mind until they can gather this information. He agrees to work on his delusions of persecution in the hope that doing so might reduce his anxiety. It was expected that relief of anxiety would have a positive effect on his thought disorder.

Throughout the two sessions shown in Video Illustrations 15 and 16, Dr. Turkington heavily uses standard CBT methods of structuring, summarizing, and providing and asking for feedback. With patients who have significant thought disorder, these basic techniques are a mainstay of therapeutic efforts. The only method listed in Table 10–4 not demonstrated in the videos is the use of audio or video recordings to assist patients with thought disorder. Such recordings can help patients recognize the main themes in their conversations and also better understand the difficulties that others may have in understanding them. However, recordings need to be used with caution in patients who are very disorganized and paranoid. The intent of the recordings can be misunderstood and can increase anxiety, especially if the patient perceives that she is being experimented on as a "guinea pig." Thus, when recording techniques are used, therapists should carefully assess the patient's readiness for this approach and also give a detailed explanation of why the technique is being suggested.

The CBT approach to thought disorder in schizophrenia, as summarized in Tables 10–2 and 10–4 and shown in the video illustrations with Daniel, is less well developed and has received less empirical study than the methods described in this book for delusions, hallucinations, and negative symptoms. However, we have included suggestions for addressing thought disorder because it is such a common manifestation of psychoses. CBT interventions for thought disorder can be more demanding and more tiring for patients and clinicians than techniques for other problems. Thus, we recommend working in this way for only 10–15 minutes at a time.

Learning Exercise 10–1.   Practicing CBT Methods for Thought Disorder

1. For this exercise, ask a colleague to view the video illustrations of Daniel and to then attempt to simulate a case of moderate to severe thought disorder. To construct a case that will present challenges but not impossibilities, ask your colleague to play a patient who has some loose associations or other significant problems. However, this "patient" should not have so much fragmentation of thought that CBT methods are unlikely to be of benefit.

2. Now practice some of these techniques: structuring, summarizing, and providing feedback; "pressing the buzzer"; thought linkage; finding the main theme; reducing intense emotion related to the main theme; and reality testing to reduce confusion and intense emotion.

3. Ask your colleague for feedback. Do either of you have ideas for improving the interaction or of doing further work with this patient?

Racing Thoughts, Distractibility, and Disorganization in Mania and Hypomania

In bipolar disorder, cognitive impairment can include problems with the amount, speed, and quality of thought, as well as mental disorganization (Table 10–5). These difficulties can be present in both the depressed and manic state. In mania, there is a heightened speed and volume of thoughts, with too many ideas for the patient to fully process before others take their place. Distractibility can move the focus from one thought to the next before the former is fully formulated. Also, Tai et al. (2004) showed that the speech of manic patients was more affectively responsive than the speech of remitted bipolar depressed and normal participants. In depression, the speed is slow, clarity may be low, and the volume of thoughts is lessened as a result. The interventions for improving cognitive processing in the depressive phase of bipolar disorder are the same as in unipolar depression, which will be discussed later in this chapter.

Many people with bipolar disorder report an improvement in cognitive clarity and in the quality of their ideas and analytic abilities when hypomanic, particularly in the early stages of manic evolution. Creative ideas appear to be more prevalent and there is a freedom of thought that allows the person to think "outside the box." Those who have experienced hypomania in this manner look forward to its recurrence. Unfortunately, enhanced cognitive abilities may be short-lived as mania continues to escalate. In addition, the subjective sense of creativity may be a misperception because the ability to evaluate the quality of ideas is often impaired. The relevance of all these points in the treatment of bipolar

---

Table 10–5. Cognitive difficulties in mania and hypomania

Racing thoughts

Distractibility

Disorganized thoughts

Tangentiality

Grandiosity

Impaired judgment

---

disorder is that patients may be motivated to reexperience this enhanced, although temporary, state rather than limit or control it. In Chapter 8 ("Mania"), we discuss ways to manage denial and to motivate people to control their symptoms.

People who want assistance with improving their cognitive processing are those who find it troubling or annoying. They report frustrations with their inability to formulate clear ideas and hold on to them long enough to solve a problem or reach a conclusion. The three-step process described in *The Bipolar Workbook: Tools for Controlling Your Mood Swings* (Basco 2006) is to slow thoughts, focus on one at a time, and use an organizational structure for reasoning through a problem. This "Slow It, Focus It, Structure It" strategy uses behavioral relaxation strategies to reduce tension, which in turn helps to slow racing thoughts. Racing thoughts can, of course, be treated pharmacologically. Alternative strategies to manage racing thoughts are breathing training, differential relaxation, or any other commonly used relaxation technique. Active relaxation, such as taking a walk or a shower, may be preferable for some patients. Quieting a noisy external environment full of distractions can also help to lessen internal stimulation that fuels racing thoughts.

The second step is to select a topic on which the patient needs to focus. This might include making a decision or solving a problem. The target could also be something less complicated like organizing daily activities or deciding what to do first. Once the target has been selected, the third step is to use written step-by-step methods to work through the idea. Focusing on a written sequence of steps helps the patient to keep on track until a conclusion is reached. Tables 10–6 through 10–8 include some common cognitive structuring strategies for problem solving, decision making, and organizing daily activities.

Slowing, focusing, and structuring thoughts can decrease impulsivity and allow for a more objective evaluation of ideas. This objectivity lessens the chance that grandiosity or impaired judgment will govern behavior. As with all cognitive-behavioral strategies, it is useful to practice the steps in session

Table 10–6. Problem solving: step-by-step

1. State the problem.
2. Generate solutions.
3. Select a solution.
4. Implement the plan.
5. Evaluate the outcome.

and to ask the patient to write out the instructions on a coping card or in a therapy notebook. Adherence can be increased by taking time to determine where the instructions will be kept for future use. Also, patients can be helped to identify the cues that their cognitive processing is becoming less efficient. This problem is not always obvious to patients because their thoughts can be too muddled to figure out what to do about them. The cue can be cognitive, such as recognizing that thoughts are developing in rapid succession. An emotional cue might be anxiety or feeling overwhelmed. A behavioral cue might be starting tasks but not completing them, losing one's train of thought in the middle of a task, or inactivity due to indecision.

Angela enjoys the challenges and excitement of her work. Once she gets started on a project, she has difficulty letting go. Her thoughts race

---

Table 10–7. Decision making: step-by-step

---

1. Identify the problem (e.g., behind in paying cell phone bill).

2. List the available options (e.g., get a job, borrow money from parents, pawn something).

3. Select a subset of options that appear to be the most viable (e.g., get a job, pawn guitar).

4. List the advantages and disadvantages of each option in a table format:

	Advantages		Disadvantages
Job:	Money; **make parents happy;** feel better about self	*Job:*	**Stress;** people may not like me; don't know what to do
Pawn:	Quick money; **easy to do**	*Pawn:*	**Mom will be mad;** have to give up something I like

5. Select the most important advantage and disadvantage for each option and identify the key factors involved in the decision (e.g., most important are in bold type; key factors to consider are the stress or effort required and parents' response).

6. Weigh the key factors on importance (0–10, 10 being most important—e.g., stress/effort=10; parents' response=5).

7. Make a selection and implement the plan (e.g., pawning something will solve the immediate problem with minimal stress). Get feedback from others as needed (e.g., talk to parents about this plan before going to the pawnshop).

Table 10–8. Organizing daily activities: step-by-step

---

1. Make a list of activities that are high in priority for the day (i.e., there is a consequence for noncompletion).

2. Select a number of activities for completion that match the time availability and energy level of the patient. This selection of tasks is completed daily. Whatever is not completed can be added to the next day.

3. Set a reasonable limit on the number of tasks completed. Do not allow mania to drive overestimation of what can be completed.

4. Identify times of day to accomplish each task.

5. Repeat this process daily as needed.

---

to all the things that need to be completed on a project. It is not unusual for her to work late into the night and not be able to fall asleep as her mind swims with new ideas. Because Angela has bipolar disorder, sleep loss brings on symptoms of mania. In the short run, the mania seems to help her to do her job, which is highly creative. If she does not set limits on her sleep loss, however, and allows manic symptoms to worsen, her performance disintegrates as she describes in Video Illustration 2. There seems to be a reciprocal relationship between her creativity and her mania. It often begins with sleep loss when involved in a project at work. She is naturally creative and hardworking. The sleep loss stimulates hypomania, which increases her flow of thoughts, especially creative ideas. The internal stimulation she experiences from working on projects also seems to fuel her symptoms. Manic symptoms worsen and eventually her thoughts become disorganized and confused, making it difficult to complete tasks. It is to Angela's advantage to use her creative abilities and, at the same time, to control her work behavior and overstimulation so that she does not become hypomanic or manic in the process.

Angela was new to the management of bipolar disorder. In fact, she had just recently begun to believe that she had a mental illness. For her, the first step was to recognize the process described above. She learned the methods for mania described in Chapter 8 ("Mania"). Highly motivated to be successful, Angela agreed to try to slow, focus, and structure her thinking when she realized that she was at risk for mania. The times she needed to slow down were at bedtime and when she felt anxious at work. She had learned how to meditate when she was in college, so she used a brief exercise to clear her mind and release the tension from her body before bedtime and occasionally during her lunch hour at work. At work, she knew it was time to focus her thoughts when she was overwhelmed, stuck, and uncertain about what to do next. She knew that in the middle of a project with many steps yet to complete, it was better to complete any one component than to waste time worrying about what to do first. When uncertain how to proceed, her default position was to do the easiest task first. Although she knew how to do her job, the steps to problem solving provided by her therapist helped her to stay organized. Working through a task step-by-step helped Angela to focus her mind and made her feel confident in her ability to manage the job along with her illness.

Problems With Cognitive Functioning in Depression

Depression frequently has an adverse effect on learning and memory functioning, especially when symptoms are severe. Studies of performance on memory tasks have shown that people who are depressed are likely to have a decrement in ability to perform memory functions that require significant effort or sustained concentration (Cohen et al. 1982; Weingartner et al. 1981). Thus, it may be unrealistic to expect that persons with severe depression will quickly grasp therapy concepts or be able to have excellent recall of the material from therapy sessions. And, of course they often have problems with school, work, and home functioning because of cognitive deficits. Some of the common problems with cognitive functioning are listed in Table 10–9.

In working with patients with significant depression, therapists may need to pay special attention to some of the basic features of CBT (e.g., structuring, feedback, psychoeducation, rehearsal, homework exercises) that can help with concentration and successful performance in cognitive

Table 10–9. Problems with cognitive functioning in depression

Poor concentration and attention

Slowed thinking

Difficulty performing effortful or complex cognitive tasks

Distraction by ruminative, negative automatic thoughts

Disorganization

Reduced effort at performing cognitive tasks because of hopelessness and helplessness

Procrastination in performing cognitive tasks

functions. For example, structuring procedures may be particularly useful when patients are disorganized and having difficulty keeping an effective focus on problem solving. Often the simple procedure of setting a practical agenda for the session and limiting the discussion to a few salient topics can be beneficial. Also, choosing and sticking with some reasonable goals for treatment can help focus the patient's cognitive efforts and reduce distraction from the myriad worries and concerns that may be interfering with concentration.

Effective use of feedback is another core CBT method that can help with cognitive functioning deficits in depression and other severe mental disorders. Therapists need to check for understanding by asking questions, such as "We've covered some important ground in the last 15 minutes or so. Can you sum up the main points?" Or at the end of the session the therapist may ask, "Let's review the things we covered today. Can you tell me what you want to remember from today's session?" When depression is severe and concentration problems are quite significant, the therapist may want to take more responsibility for reinforcing learning by stopping at multiple intervals to repeat or rephrase points.

Psychoeducation is discussed in detail in Chapter 3 ("Normalizing and Educating"). When learning and memory functioning appears to be significantly impacted by depression, the therapist may need to reduce the complexity of the teaching element of CBT by assigning short or easily understood readings or to ask patients to only try to read a small section of a pamphlet or self-help book at a time. Computer-assisted CBT programs such as *Good Days Ahead* and *Beating the Blues* (both described in Chapter 3) can be used with patients with moderate to severe depression, but the therapist may need to regulate the pace of the experience so patients do not feel overwhelmed by the computerized training. Typically these programs are designed to be used by persons with depression-induced cognitive impairment and thus contain learning enhancement features such as video and audio explanations, repetition of main themes, and interactive learning exercises.

Another basic CBT method that can help with learning and memory is *cognitive rehearsal*. The therapist may present a concept in a session and then practice putting it into action with a role-play or another CBT rehearsal exercise. An important principle is reinforced by practicing it in an emotionally relevant situation, which should heighten the patient's grasp of the material and his ability to recall and use the information in the future. For example, Thad, a 57-year-old salesman with deep depression, was struggling with attempts to make contacts for potential business, despite being preoccupied with very negative automatic thoughts and a pervasive sense that he would fail. His therapist was attempting to help him better prioritize and organize his sales efforts so that Thad could counter his view that he was totally overwhelmed and floundering, and so that he would start to have some successful experiences:

> Therapist: So, we have sketched out a plan for you to revise the way you are making your sales calls. Can you put the plan into words? What will you actually do tomorrow when you make your calls? (Therapist asks for feedback from patient to reinforce learning.)
>
> Thad: Well, you recommended that I remind myself in advance that I have had a good track record selling insurance and that I actually know how to do this. Basically, I need to pump myself up and boost my confidence by remembering the things I can do instead of continually putting myself down.
>
> Therapist: Good…What's next?
>
> Thad: Rehearse giving a clear message on the call….Think in advance of the main things I want to get across….Try to keep it short so my attention doesn't wander.
>
> Therapist: Anything else?
>
> Thad: Yes. Focus only on this single call, instead of letting my mind jump ahead to all of the other calls that I think I should be making.
>
> Therapist: Great…Now can you rehearse this here in the session? I want to be sure that you remember all of the key things that you will do.

Rehearsal was then used to practice calls to potential customers: one who would likely be interested in buying insurance and one who would likely reject the offer. Then, the therapist asked Thad to write out the plan to further reinforce learning. Finally, a homework assignment was arranged to use the written plan. As noted in Chapter 3 ("Normalizing and Educating"), writing down the main lessons of treatment sessions in a therapy notebook, on coping cards, or in other documents can be very helpful in promoting acquisition and retention of CBT concepts and skills. And, homework assignments are a fundamental component of the learning enhancement features of CBT.

The strategies described earlier for improving cognitive functioning in mania—such as the step-by-step plans for problem solving, decision making, and organizing daily activities, in addition to relaxation exercises—can also be helpful in patients with severe or chronic depression. Generally, any method that can help patients who are distracted and overwhelmed to better focus their mental energies is worth trying. Other techniques that might be useful include setting aside a specific time for worry so that the patient may have other times of the day when her mind is less troubled by interfering cognitions; memory aids, such as daily organizers or computerized schedules; and CBT interventions for sleep. The last intervention can be very important when insomnia is playing a major role in producing concentration and attention problems.

The CBT techniques that are used to improve cognitive functioning in therapy sessions can serve as models for patients with a range of severe mental illnesses to improve cognitive functioning in everyday life. Thus, if a patient learns structuring methods, the usefulness of summarizing key points, or the utility of written instructions in sessions, he may be able to generalize these lessons to daily activities outside therapy. Table 10–10 provides a summary of CBT methods that can be helpful in promoting improved cognitive functioning.

Summary

Key Points for Clinicians

- Because impairments in cognitive functioning are such common manifestations of severe mental illness, CBT methods need to be modified to address these problems.
- An accurate assessment of the nature of the cognitive impairment (e.g., type of thought disorder or cognitive deficit, learning and memory dysfunction, degree of distractibility, amount of interference by disturbing or ruminative thoughts) is the first step in designing interventions.
- Therapists should model clear and precise communication for patients.
- Structuring, summarization, and feedback are good general techniques for helping patients with cognitive impairments.
- Written instructions, coping cards, and other reminder systems can also be useful.
- For some patients who are struggling with thought disorder, a beneficial approach can be to 1) identify the main theme in their thinking, 2) address this concern, and 3) perform reality testing for delusions that are linked to the main theme.
- Patients with manic or hypomanic hyperactivity and distractibility can often be helped with instruction on and practice with problem solving, decision making, and daily organization skills.
- The CBT approach for depression includes a variety of methods to reduce the ruminative, negative thoughts that can interfere with concentration.

Concepts and Skills for Patients to Learn

- Difficulties with concentration, memory, or communicating clearly are experienced by most people. Thus, these problems are a part of normal life.

Table 10–10. CBT methods for improving cognitive functioning in depression

---

Structuring

Feedback

Psychoeducation

Rehearsal

Homework exercises

Writing down key points in notebooks or coping cards

Using step-by-step methods for problem solving

Relaxation exercises

Strategies for reducing ruminative, negative thoughts

Memory aids

CBT interventions for improving sleep

- Therapists can help people learn how to reduce confusion in their thinking and to improve concentration.
- If it seems that other people are not understanding you, it may be useful to try to slow down the communication and to only discuss one main idea at a time.
- Reminder systems can be very beneficial—some of the best methods are writing key ideas down on paper, listening to a tape of important points discussed in therapy sessions, and using a coping card.
- Sometimes a troubling fear or worry can interfere with concentration. If this seems to be the case, a therapist can help find ways to cope with the fear or concern.

References

Basco MR: The Bipolar Workbook: Tools for Controlling Your Mood Swings. New York, Guilford, 2006

Cohen RM, Weingartner H, Smallberg SA, et al: Effort and cognition in depression. Arch Gen Psychiatry 39:593–597, 1982

Goldberg TE, David A, Gold JM: Neurocognitive deficits in schizophrenia, in Schizophrenia, 2nd Edition. Edited by Hirsch SR, Weinberger DR. Oxford, England, Blackwell, 2003, pp 168–186

Harrow M, Prosen M: Intermingling and disordered logic as influences on schizophrenic "thought disorders." Arch Gen Psychiatry 35:1213–1218, 1978

McGurk SR, Mueser KT, Feldman K, et al: Cognitive training for supported employment: 2–3 year outcomes of a randomized controlled trial. Am J Psychiatry 164:437–441, 2007

Penades R, Catalan R, Salamero M, et al: Cognitive remediation therapy for outpatients with chronic schizophrenia: a controlled and randomized study. Schizophr Res 87:323–331, 2006

Tai S, Haddock G, Bentall RP: The effects of emotional salience on thought disorder in patients with bipolar affective disorder. Psych Med 34:803–809, 2004

Turkington D, Kingdon D: Ordering thoughts in thought disorder. Br J Psychiatry 159:160–161, 1991

Velligan DI, Kern RS, Gold JM: Cognitive rehabilitation for schizophrenia and the putative role of motivation and expectancies. Schizophr Bull 32:474–485, 2006

Weingartner H, Cohen RM, Murphy DL, et al: Cognitive processes in depression. Arch Gen Psychiatry 38:42–47, 1981

Wykes T, Reeder C, Landau S, et al: Cognitive remediation therapy in schizophrenia: randomized, controlled trial. Br J Psychiatry 190:421–427, 2007

11

Negative Symptoms

The need for treatment of the positive symptoms and the mood disturbances encountered in severe mental illness is quite obvious. The distress these problems cause and their impact on functioning contribute significantly to the impairment of quality of life that patients experience. What can be less obvious and less of a priority in the treatment of schizophrenia are the insidious effects of negative symptoms. These difficulties may concern caregivers to a greater extent than clinicians who are focusing on the more dramatic symptoms of psychotic illnesses. Yet in many studies of schizophrenia, negative symptoms have been shown to have greater deleterious effects than positive symptoms such as hallucinations and delusions (Provencher and Mueser 1997).

In Chapter 7 ("Depression"), we describe classic CBT methods for managing depressive demotivation and anhedonia. These techniques (e.g., behavioral activation, activity scheduling, graded task assignments, modifying beliefs that contribute to states of low motivation and interest) can also be applicable in schizophrenia where such problems manifest as negative symptoms, especially when depression and hopelessness are predominant features of the illness. However, the timing and pacing of these techniques may differ. We give a brief illustration of this type of work later in the chapter. First, we offer a broad CBT conceptualization for negative symptoms that can help therapists, patients, and caregivers better understand and cope with this difficult-to-treat element of schizophrenia and other chronic psychoses.

What Are Negative Symptoms?

Negative symptoms include phenomena that suggest the relative absence of the key components of thinking, feeling, and doing:

- *Alogia:* lack of thoughts
- *Attention deficit:* inability to focus and concentrate
- *Anhedonia:* absence of feeling
- *Amotivation:* limited level of activity—particularly demonstrated in social withdrawal

These types of symptoms suggest that fundamental neurobiological changes may be responsible for these impairments. There is evidence from imaging studies that schizophrenia is associated with structural changes that could explain negative symptoms. However, a conclusion that the only help for these problems would need to come from a treatment that directly reverses the pathology seems unwarranted. Such a conclusion underestimates the potential that people have to adapt to an injury or disease. For example, individuals with the assistance of physiotherapists and speech and occupational therapists can adapt to brain damage from accidents or strokes. With the help of rehabilitation experts, these patients can learn to compensate for brain damage and maximize their potential. Enabling individuals to cope with disability from negative symptoms of schizophrenia can be a key step in recovery, whether from overt or more subtle cognitive impairment.

There may be multiple causes of negative symptoms. Institutionalization is well recognized for its deleterious effects. Negative symptoms may be a reaction to a range of other circumstances:

- Alogia: This problem may occur because of a lack of thoughts, but it also can stem from the inability to express thoughts or even not wishing to do so (because of paranoia, experiences of persistent criticism, or simply a wish for privacy).
- Attention deficit: Competing stimuli from hallucinations or paranoid fears can be an important factor. Voices may be commanding the person not to cooperate or simply may be distracting the patient. Patients' beliefs that they are under threat may also preoccupy them to the detriment of their focus on the tasks they need to complete. Increasing anxiety may also divert their attention and impair concentration.
- Anhedonia: When patients have been traumatized, they can become withdrawn and disinterested in engaging with people or in other pleasurable activities. Demoralization, hopelessness, and depression can

lead to a numbed expressionless presentation to others. Medication side effects can also cause a masklike appearance.

- Amotivation: Frequently patients will describe situations where they have attempted to achieve goals but have become frustrated and demoralized ("driven themselves to a standstill") and so have given up. Trying harder may increase frustration and concentration problems, so eventually patients stop trying and sink into demoralization, apathy, and inactivity.

The CBT Conceptualization

The CBT method for working with negative symptoms is built on an understanding of possible influences on these phenomena. For example, these CBT strategies could help clinicians offer useful interventions for negative symptoms:

- Alogia: Focusing on improving communication—even when speech may be slow, hesitant, and thought disordered—can build bridges to understanding and have a favorable influence on thought disorder (see Chapter 10, "Impaired Cognitive Functioning").
- Attention deficit: Direct work on the distracting influences of voices, delusional beliefs, and anxiety can improve alertness either by reducing the intensity of the experiences or by persuading patients that they need not focus on the voices or delusional beliefs. Helping patients regain control of their thoughts and actions can assist them in focusing on tasks.
- Anhedonia: If lack of emotional reactivity is related to past traumatic experiences, CBT work may be needed to help with maladaptive beliefs about those experiences and patterns of avoidance (see treatment of Majir in video illustrations). A slow implementation of strategies described in Chapter 7 ("Depression") can also be tried. Discussion of areas that interest the patient often can lead to increased emotional reactivity as he begins to enjoy the conversation and interact more.
- Amotivation: When patients feel exhausted from trying too hard and not succeeding, additional pressure may only worsen the situation. Patients may become more discouraged instead of more motivated. A different approach may be needed.

Motivation comes from wanting to achieve personal goals and believing that it is possible to do so. Motivation recedes if the following occur:

- The goals are set too high for the individual's current capabilities.

- Goals are set too distant in the future, and sustained effort is unrewarded along the way.
- Repeated attempts have been made to reach goals, and these efforts have met with obstacles or failure.

Many patients and their families have experienced great frustration in their attempts to meet the ordinary goals that most people set for themselves in education, work, or relationships. These negative experiences may then be followed by an inability to achieve lowered goals for jobs or daily activities. Sometimes, the more patients try, the more frustrated and impotent they become. A vicious circle of nonachievement can develop, which eventually leads to nihilistic withdrawal and pervasive hopelessness.

Additional symptoms such as voices, delusions, anxiety, and depression can seriously interfere with functioning and hasten the descent to states of demotivation. These positive symptoms and mood disturbances can also increase when patients try to overcome their limited level of activity. Because leaving the house leads to contact with other people and an increase in paranoia, thought broadcasting, or voices, it can feel safer to remain withdrawn. Even when positive symptoms are not precipitated, an increase in anxiety to the extent of experiencing panic symptoms can lead patients to seek safe, nonstimulating environments.

Demotivation in Schizophrenia

When motivation existed, perhaps years before, but demoralization has now set in, the key objective is to enable patients to return to feeling competent, capable, and in control—and most of all, not under undue pressure to achieve. To realize this objective, therapists may often need to help patients lower their goals to a level that is within their current capacity. Often this means collaborating with patients to set very simple goals (e.g., get out of bed by 2 P.M. and make a cup of tea). Reductions in activity levels may be needed at first, even for patients who are rather inactive. This process of backing off on expectations may seem alien to therapists who themselves are very self-motivated and hardworking. However, once patients are able to achieve simple goals consistently, they then can be ready to move to the next step. The reduction in activity may include advocating taking time off (i.e., a time of readjustment and rest) for several months or more to work on the voices, beliefs, and depressive symptoms that are interfering with patients' functioning. A suggestion of this kind can noticeably relax patients and, far from making them less motivated, enable them to take back control of their lives and begin to hope for the future.

Development of a shared understanding of this strategy with family or other caregivers is vital. They may have tried to provide motivation for the patient by encouraging, prompting, or cajoling. Unfortunately, these efforts may have been perceived as being overly critical and pressuring to the patient, despite the good intentions of the family or other caregivers. It can be a challenge to effectively explain the rationale for standing back and allowing the patient to take the lead. We have found that the analogy of treating a broken leg can be useful.

A broken leg is rested and immobilized in a plaster cast in order to heal. Without immobilization, the leg fails to heal properly, and the person cannot walk on it. However, with proper immobilization, the leg is healed, the cast is removed, and there is a gradual process with physical therapy of beginning to use the leg again—gently and not putting too much pressure on it.

Likewise, when someone has experienced a "broken mind"—a psychotic episode—they also need time to heal. People need unpressured time to come to terms with these experiences and to learn how to cope. Without this period of healing, they can be stuck for years until healing can occur and they can get back to life at their own pace.

Families and other caregivers often feel inappropriate guilt about their son or daughter becoming ill. They have thoughts such as "We should have been better parents and this wouldn't have happened." It may be worth reminding them that there is no specific advice that we, as "experts," can give parents to prevent severe mental illness from developing. Thus, they are being very hard on themselves in taking blame for these circumstances.

This tendency to self-blame can make caregivers very sensitive to anything resembling criticism of their actions. It is therefore very important to ensure that the family understands that the therapist recognizes their good intentions and is not attributing blame, but is providing advice on tactics for managing a distressing and difficult situation. Such tactics tend to focus on reinforcing positive behavior, rather than commenting directly on negative symptoms, and gradually—when the patient is ready— building up her ability to cope as independently as possible.

Ideally, collaboration with the therapist, patient, and caregivers can lower short-term expectations to achievable levels and then reinforce attempts to achieve these goals. Longer-term goals for 5–10 years need to be set collaboratively. These more far-reaching goals usually involve development of meaningful activity (e.g., a job, independent living arrangements, and confiding relationships). These types of goals can provide hope for the future, as long as a realistic plan can be made for taking small steps to reach them.

Sometimes long-term goals, even with a substantial timescale, can seem unrealistic (e.g., to become a professional football player or a film star). Generally, it is better to not immediately dash patients' hopes with reality-testing exercises but to use gradual, guided discovery as time progresses. Sometimes patients can surprise you, caregivers, and themselves with goals that they can accomplish. Working toward their goals can be motivating even if those goals need readjustment at a later stage. For example, the therapist could say, "If you are going to become a film star, what would be the first thing you need to do?" "Well, how about taking a shower and dressing in some fresh clothes?" Sometimes it is possible to identify and use individual motivators to increase activity (e.g., a particular interest or hobby that requires activity). Processes and procedures for improving motivation in patients with negative symptoms are summarized in Table 11–1.

The action plan involves initially reviewing potential blocks to progress (e.g., suboptimal medication levels) and identifying motivating interests. Setting long-term goals is done initially to provide overall direction and hope. If a period of readjustment and rest seems appropriate while work is done on positive symptoms, this strategy can also provide hope for the future. Nothing much may seem to be happening now, but this is still a period of preparation for the future. The short-term goals may also seem almost inconsequential to the patient and caregivers, but if the goals are seen as being the first steps on the road to recovery, they are much more acceptable.

As short-term goals are set and achieved sequentially, the patient will reach a point at which more challenging goals present themselves (e.g., finding work, restarting education). This is a time to be particularly careful about pressuring patients with goals or expectations. Allowing patients to lead at their pace, but with continued support, can help them find opportunities that may not be predictable. For example, a family friend might offer a work placement or the patient may see an opportunity on the Internet or at a local college to develop a specific skill. One of our patients capitalized on an interest in craft projects to build a very small business making grapevine wreaths to sell at craft shows. Goals may have combined functions (e.g., work may provide money and socialization), but the patient may be only able to cope with one pressure at a time. Thus, an unpaid job or developing social contacts through the Internet may be the single and most appropriate step to be taken. Use of the Internet or mobile phone for nonthreatening initial contact can be an interim step toward social goals, although supplementing these efforts with face-to-face contacts in the longer term is clearly desirable.

A very gradual effort to set goals and engage the patient in a collaborative process to break out of a pattern of withdrawal and apathy is dem-

Table 11–1. Building motivation

1. Assess initial and current reasons for demotivation.

2. Review medication levels. Are they interfering with functioning rather than facilitating it?

3. Discuss and set long-term goals, such as living independently or getting a job or a girlfriend or a boyfriend.

4. Decide with the patient if time off (i.e., a time of readjustment and rest) is needed to unwind and get back in control again.

5. Identify individual motivators (e.g., interests, hobbies, sports, relationships, spiritual activities).

6. Plan work on current positive symptoms and mood disturbances that may be needed to improve motivation and concentration.

7. Plan work on positive symptoms and mood disturbances that may emerge once the patient starts to reengage in activities.

8. Discuss when to start setting short-term goals.

9. Engage family and other caregivers in the collaboration.

10. When the patient is ready, set short-term goals that are easily and consistently achievable.

11. If goals are not achieved consistently, identify why not. Review the steps above and set goals that are achievable.

12. When goals are achieved, review and set new ones in a similar way, gradually building toward long-term objectives.

onstrated in Video Illustration 17. In this vignette from a session with Majir, Dr. Kingdon has already established a fairly good working relationship and has made it clear that he does not want to exert any pressure to change. Instead, he simply wants Majir to be able to enjoy himself more and to begin to feel more comfortable about being in public places.

> ▶ **Video Illustration 17.** Treating Negative Symptoms:
> Dr. Kingdon and Majir

Dr. Kingdon: I am just wondering if there was any particular thing that maybe you had done in the past or have thought of doing that we could set as one little thing that we could aim for over the next week or two—that might be of interest to you, that you might be able to do?

Majir: I spend a lot of time in my room, so it is hard for me to see that I could do that.

> Dr. Kingdon: You tell me how you go down to the computer shop and you go to see your sister....Is there anywhere else that you have been going out to in the last few years?
>
> Majir: I think I had a hobby of bird-watching quite a few years ago, and I used to go to the park—especially early in the morning—and I watched the birds....I used to enjoy that very much, but I haven't done that for a number of years now.
>
> (Dr. Kingdon picks up on this opening and asks questions that may help Majir overcome barriers to reactivation.)
>
> Dr. Kingdon: So what sort of time did you get up to do that?
>
> Majir: It was fairly early. Six o'clock in the morning...I wasn't comfortable having a lot of people around.

They then discuss potential problems that could interfere with Majir resuming this pleasurable activity (e.g., getting up early in the morning, coping with paranoid beliefs about people that he could see in the park) and agree that he can set an alarm clock, use the coping strategies for paranoia he had learned in earlier sessions, and go to the park to bird-watch on a Sunday at 6 A.M. when he would probably not encounter many other people. In a way, this type of work with negative symptoms uses the hierarchical methods of graded task assignments for depression described in Chapter 7 ("Depression"). However, the pace is considerably slower—only one or a few steps may be outlined at a time—and the overall plan may be less organized.

After they settle on a simple plan for Majir to try a trip to the park for some bird-watching, Dr. Kingdon follows up by asking if there are any other things Majir might look forward to in the future. Interestingly, Majir starts to talk about being good with computers and hoping that someday he could get a job working in this field. Although this suggestion was a positive step for Majir to take, Dr. Kingdon assures Majir that there is no need to put too much pressure on himself now. The current goal is to take a small step toward getting out of the house and participating in pleasurable activities.

Socialization

The level of optimal socialization for any patient varies considerably with his temperament and life circumstances. Many patients with severe mental illness have developed relatively limited social skills before onset of their disorder. These social limitations may be part of the buildup to becoming unwell. For other patients, the circumstances of the development of their illness have led to social withdrawal because of shame at being ill, loss of social contacts and confidence, and stigmatization. Some patients become, or already are, quite socially anxious. For these persons, social avoidance is used as a coping mechanism. This avoidance can become quite dysfunctional but may have protective qualities in reducing anxiety, ideas of reference, and paranoia. For therapists working with patients' negative symptoms, it may be necessary to support, at least in part, avoidance strategies until patients build the ability to be involved in social situations. For example, the strategy with Majir in Video Illustration 17 involved going out early in the morning when fewer people would be encountered.

Each of the factors in Table 11–2 needs to be considered in evaluating and treating social withdrawal in schizophrenia and other chronic psychoses. Because premorbid factors may be quite ingrained, the target may be learning to cope with them. However, social skills training can assist patients in a sequential process of developing acquaintances and building friendships. Social skills groups are particularly powerful at modeling and developing relationships between group members and therapists. Such groups are an excellent and efficient vehicle for providing basic information about developing listening and conversation skills and identifying opportunities to meet people and eventually make friendships. These groups can also provide encouragement by setting and completing homework tasks. However, many patients, at least initially, are too socially anxious, paranoid, or poorly motivated to attend groups. In these circumstances, it is still possible to provide individualized social skills training. Discussing perceived obstacles to social interaction (e.g., not knowing where to go, what to do, or what to say) can lead to coping solutions.

Table 11–2. Causes of social withdrawal in schizophrenia

Premorbid personality

Adverse childhood experiences (e.g., bullying, abuse, or repeated moves to different schools)

Adverse adult experiences (e.g., breaking of trust by close friends, divorce, estrangement from family)

Consequences of illness (e.g., paranoia or command hallucinations)

Consequences of hospitalization (e.g., disconnection from social network, alienation from health care providers because of involuntary commitment)

Withdrawal used as a coping strategy to manage anxiety and psychotic symptoms

Stigmatization

Working directly with CBT methods for social anxiety and psychotic symptoms can also lead to productive changes (see Wright et al. 2006 for methods for treating social anxiety). For example, the therapist might teach patients to use breathing retraining, relaxation, or other behavioral methods to manage social anxiety. The "befriending" and collaborative nature of the therapeutic relationship offers another opportunity to influence social functioning. Sometimes positive changes may happen because a rewarding social relationship is developed with the therapist and other members of the mental health team. Improved socialization becomes an "added bonus," resulting from incidental relationships developed with staff as patients spend time with them in hospital units, day centers, or other outpatient treatment programs.

Applying Standard Behavioral Methods

Chapter 7 ("Depression") details the classic CBT methods (e.g., behavioral activation, activity scheduling, and graded task assignments) typically used for treating anhedonia, low energy, and lack of motivation in depression. As we have noted in this chapter, work with negative symptoms in schizophrenia typically requires modification of these procedures so that patients can participate in assignments that they can actually carry out. Video Illustration 17 shows a behavioral activation exercise that could be built into a more extensive graded task assignment, depending on Majir's response to the first homework effort. If the attempt to get out of the house to enjoy some bird-watching at 6 A.M. on a Sunday morning was successful, subsequent steps that Dr. Kingdon might suggest to Majir could be to 1) try to go bird-watching early in the morning at least once every 2 weeks, 2) go to a library to check out some bird-watching books, 3) pick up a notebook at the corner store to record his observations of birds, 4) choose one more activity he could enjoy that would get him out of the house, and so forth. Of course, the therapist would be alert to possible problems in carrying out these assignments and would try to help Majir overcome obstacles that would be encountered.

For some patients who are less symptomatic than Majir, or who appear more motivated and capable of change, the pace can be a bit faster in using behavioral methods for negative symptoms. The treatment of Helen, a 45-year-old woman with schizophrenia, demonstrates this type of approach. Helen had experienced paranoia, hallucinations, and negative symptoms (e.g., apathy and social withdrawal) for many years. She had been recently admitted to a psychiatric hospital after telling her outpatient therapist that she was hearing voices telling her to kill herself. Helen was quite depressed and was feeling defeated by her illness. She was living alone and appeared to have little or no interests other than having a meal with her family once a week and spending time reading magazines at a library.

During the first few days of her hospitalization, the treatment focus with CBT was primarily on reducing suicidality (see Chapter 7, "Depression") and coping with hallucinations (see Chapter 6, "Hallucinations"). Fortunately, these approaches along with medication adjustment led to significant improvement. Yet, pronounced negative symptoms, such as apathy, anhedonia, and social withdrawal, remained largely unchanged. As the therapist and staff were preparing Helen to leave the hospital, they suggested that she try to use a daily activity schedule with ratings for mastery and pleasure. With patients who are experiencing psychotic symptoms, it is often best to assign only a daily activity schedule instead of asking them to log an entire week of activities at a time. Patients can record only a portion of a day, if a full day's record would be too challenging.

With the assistance of one of the nurses who was trained in how to use activity scheduling, Helen completed a schedule for the afternoon and early evening hours of 1 day. The goals were to determine if her negative symptoms could be reactive to any variation in daily activities and to gather information that could be used in planning further outpatient treatment. Despite Helen's comments that "I never feel like doing anything" and "I'm better off staying to myself," her daily activity schedule showed a variety of items (Table 11–3).

As can be seen from Helen's activity schedule, there were variations in her ratings of both mastery and pleasure that gave clues for further treatment planning. Part of the session with her doctor the next day went as follows:

Doctor: Can you take a look at the schedule you made yesterday and tell me what you think of it?

Helen: The day wasn't as bad as I thought it might be.

Doctor: What things did you enjoy the most?

Helen: Actually, it was the game we played last night. I wouldn't usually do anything like that, but the nurse was very nice and talked me into it. After we got going, it was sort of fun (laughing just a bit). And I came in second. At least I wasn't last.

Doctor: Good, I'm glad you enjoyed it. I know that you haven't been doing many things that are fun lately. Anything else that stands out as a good experience when you look at the schedule?

Helen: Well, the craft project was another thing. We made some cards to send to our families. I hadn't done anything with painting or crafts for years. Having something to do, instead of just sitting around, was a good idea.

Table 11–3. Daily activity schedule: Helen's example

Time	Activity	Mastery[a]	Pleasure[a]
12–1 P.M.	Lunch and watched TV	2	1
1–2 P.M.	Session with doctor	5	6
2–3 P.M.	Craft project	4	7
3–4 P.M.	Rested and looked at magazines in room	3	4
4–5 P.M.	Recreational therapy meeting	2	3
5–6 P.M.	Exercise group	2	3
6–7 P.M.	Dinner and time in room	3	2
7–8 P.M.	Played a board game with nurse and another patient	7	7

[a]Rated on a scale of 0–10, with 10 being the highest.

Doctor: Yes, I noticed that the time in your room was OK, but it didn't seem to be as enjoyable as some of the other things. And you didn't rate it very high on mastery—the rating of how well you think you did the activity. I know that you have been spending almost all of your time alone at home. What do you think this activity schedule might tell us (holding the schedule for both of them to see)?

Helen: Maybe it isn't so good for me to stay by myself all the time...but I usually feel uncomfortable going out. And I never really want to do it.

Doctor: Could we spend some time talking about ways to make it easier for you to have the kinds of enjoyable experiences you reported here?

Helen: OK.

The psychiatrist then used this opportunity to brainstorm with the patient about other activities that she might find enjoyable and would involve being out of her house and around at least a few people. They also discussed an option to start attending a day treatment program that had some of the programmatic elements Helen liked in the hospital (e.g., "meetings with nurses or therapists that are interested and want to do things with me," crafts, games, and so forth), but the psychiatrist did not push her to do intensive group therapy, which she found upsetting.

The discharge plan collaboratively developed with Helen included these elements geared toward negative symptoms: 1) follow a very gradual program to increase pleasurable activities, some of which involve participation with others (i.e., "Go see a movie once a week and be around people without having to speak to them"; "Try to attend the free concert next month, even if I sit in the back and don't socialize with others"; "If I feel up to it, take a class that starts at the craft center next month"); 2) continue CBT with an outpatient therapist; 3) start attending the day treatment program two times a week for a half day.

The work with Helen in using an activity schedule, followed by a graded task assignment, was possible only because she was ready for this intervention. Also, she had a fair amount of secondary depression associated with the positive and negative symptoms of her disorder. The activating aspects of the behavioral methods appeared to help relieve some of the depression, and thus gave her encouragement to continue to work with the CBT approach. Helen's path away from negative symptoms was just beginning, but there appeared to be good prospects for further change.

Selection and use of the standard behavioral methods discussed here should be based on a careful assessment of the patient's readiness for change, degree of thought disorder, level of positive symptoms, ability to engage, and cognitive capacity. The decision on how much pressure to put on patients is a critical one. Any time a specific behavioral plan is suggested, there is at least a small amount of expectation for carrying out the plan. If a reasonably strong therapeutic relationship has been forged so that the patient knows that the therapist is on his side, and if the intervention is carefully designed to match the patient's needs and capacities, classic behavioral methods can play a valuable role in relieving negative symptoms.

Learning Exercise 11–1. Working With Negative Symptoms

1. Think of a patient you have that has significant negative symptoms. If you can't think of a specific case, imagine a patient, or use the material from the treatment of Majir for this exercise.

2. To better understand the impact of negative symptoms for this patient, write out a list of symptoms. Then make a list of advantages (if any) and disadvantages of negative symptoms for this individual.

3. Now make a list of efforts that you have made (if any) to help with negative symptoms. Also, list influences of caregivers (if known). How much pressure

has been on this patient? Is there a good balance between support and appropriate expectations? Or is the patient feeling more defeated because of inability to meet the expectations of others?

4. Write out a brief treatment plan. Could this patient benefit from reduced pressure and some time off before fully engaging in the process of modifying negative symptoms? Or is the patient ready to use CBT methods to tackle these symptoms?

5. Identify at least two specific CBT interventions that might eventually be helpful in relieving negative symptoms in this patient.

6. Ask a colleague to help you role-play therapeutic work with this patient, or imagine how the therapy might work out if you followed this treatment plan. Obstacles or barriers will probably be encountered. Think ahead to plan possible methods for overcoming these obstacles.

Summary

Key Points for Clinicians

- Develop an understanding of the cognitive-behavioral conceptualization of negative symptoms.
- Focus on enabling patients to regain control of their lives, even when this may mean taking an initial step back.
- Collaborate with caregivers.
- Set long-term goals that give hope. Revise these goals as therapy proceeds.
- Set short-term goals that ideally come from the patient's suggestions and that are specific but readily achievable.
- Modify standard behavioral methods—such as behavioral activation, graded task assignments, and activity scheduling—to match the capacities of patients with negative symptoms.

Concepts and Skills for Patients to Learn

- Long-term and short-term goals need to be meaningful and achievable.
- Rest and relaxation may be important steps in preparing to achieve goals consistently.
- Learn ways of coping with voices, paranoia, and anxiety.
- Social contact can begin gradually and build successfully if you do it at your own pace.
- Developing resilience to the pressures of life takes time. As you become able to control and cope with the pressures around you, it will be possible to move toward recovery and achieve your long-term goals.

References

Provencher HL, Mueser KT: Positive and negative symptom behaviors and caregiver burden in the relatives of persons with schizophrenia. Schizophr Res 26:71–80, 1997

Wright JH, Basco MR, Thase ME: Learning Cognitive-Behavior Therapy: An Illustrated Guide. Washington, DC, American Psychiatric Publishing, 2006

12

Promoting Adherence

The medical literature is full of reports of studies aimed at predicting and improving adherence to medications and other treatment interventions (Akincigil et al. 2007; Basco and Rush 1995; Cochran 1984; Keck et al. 1997; Kemp et al. 1996; Lecompte 1995; Meichenbaum and Turk 1988; Perris and Skagerlind 1994; Rosa et al. 2005; Weiden et al. 2007). It is clear from reading this literature that knowing medications will control symptoms, improve outcomes, increase quality of life, and avoid morbidity and mortality is not always enough to make people use medications as prescribed. For people who have the good fortune to be without chronic illness or for people who require continuous medication treatment for a less severe health problem, this lack of adherence may appear completely illogical. Common sense would dictate that if a drug could make someone feel better he would take it. Yet people don't always take their medication even when it could improve their lives.

One of the particularly appealing features of CBT for severe mental illness is its usefulness in enhancing treatment adherence. For example, Cochran (1984) noted that patients with bipolar disorder who received a CBT intervention had improved adherence to lithium, reduced rates of rehospitalization, and fewer noncompliance-related relapses. Lam et al. (2000) and Ball et al. (2006) had similar results with more lengthy CBT interventions (12–20 sessions) delivered over a 6 month period. In both cases, CBT was superior to standard treatment in improving medication adherence.

In treatment of schizophrenia, several groups of investigators have reported positive effects of CBT on medication adherence (Kemp et al. 1996, 1998; Lecompte 1995; Perris and Skagerlind 1994; Weiden et al. 2007). Kemp et al. (1996, 1998) developed a brief CBT intervention for adherence that consisted of 4–6 sessions, each lasting 10–60 minutes. This research group found long-lasting effects in medication adherence, global functioning, and reduced hospitalization rates. Another research group (Weiden et al. 2007) has reported that the collaborative approach of CBT almost doubled the adherence to antipsychotic medications in schizophrenia and also encouraged patients to be more open about their concerns about medication.

Before starting to explain CBT strategies, we want to make a brief note about the use of the terms *adherence, compliance,* and *collaborative medication management.* Some clinicians prefer not to use the words compliance or adherence because these terms might carry meanings associated with a proscriptive versus collaborative approach. However, we use these terms interchangeably in this chapter. It would be tedious to always use the term *collaborative medication management* throughout, and we believe that the highly collaborative style of CBT trumps any possible misinterpretations of terms such as adherence or compliance. CBT certainly does not seek to have a passively "compliant" patient who is not actively engaged as a partner in the treatment process.

To illustrate the CBT approach to adherence, we begin with the story of Angela:

> Angela has had bipolar I disorder for more than 15 years, including several episodes of mania and of major depression. Her life has been altered by these experiences, which continue to threaten her well-being. She has known about bipolar disorder for many years because she watched her uncle go through similar phases throughout her childhood.
>
> Angela's mood swings started in high school. Her uncle was living with her family when she became severely depressed. He knew what was happening to Angela and warned her of what could happen if she didn't get help. But, she didn't listen. When she had her first manic episode, her uncle begged her to not follow in his footsteps, but to stick with her treatment. Again, she didn't listen. She had access to doctors and medications. Money was not a problem. Her unwillingness to participate was the major obstacle.

When Angela sought treatment recently, it was only because her employer forced her to do it. Although in the back of her mind, she knew she had an illness that required treatment, she was fixated on the idea that she could go it alone. Her first therapy visit (see Video Illustration 2) focused on Angela's reluctance to admit that she had a psychiatric illness. The therapist had to be certain that she and Angela were in agreement about the need for treatment before they could proceed. Rather than insist on the diagnosis, a more Socratic approach was initiated to help Angela come to terms with her illness. Coming to a shared understanding of the nature of the problem is an essential element of therapeutic work that leads to better adherence to treatment (Becker 1974). Video Illustration 2 demonstrates that establishing a good therapeutic relationship and providing effective psychoeducation provide an essential base for the more specific CBT methods of improving adherence.

Types of Nonadherence to Treatment

Either partial or full noncompliance with medication regimens is a very common occurrence in treatment of severe mental disorders (Akincigil et al. 2007; Keck et al. 1997; Rosa et al. 2005; Scott and Pope 2002; Weiss et al. 1998). For example, individual studies have reported nonadherence rates of 48% for schizophrenia (Rosa et al. 2005); 51% for bipolar disorder (Keck et al. 1997); and 49% for depression (Akincigil et al. 2007). Consistency with medications varies over time, with greater adherence expected when symptoms are more troubling (Meichenbaum and Turk 1987). The amount of adherence or nonadherence is not static but will fluctuate over the course of treatment. Rather than labeling a patient as noncompliant, it may be more accurate to describe the amount of nonadherence as in the list below:

- *Full*—refuses treatments of any kind
- *Partial*—will take some, but not all treatments
- *Never*—full compliance at all times
- *Periodic*—from time to time skips doses, runs out of medication

Common Reasons for Nonadherence: Possible Solutions

Reasons for nonadherence vary greatly across patients and within patients. There can be many reasons why people are inconsistent in their approach to treatment, and sometimes more than one explanation is applicable at a given point in time. Table 12–1 lists some of the more common reasons. The approach to improving adherence will depend on the amount of nonadherence and the reasons given. Using the items in Table 12–1 as a guide, we will discuss further the reasons for nonadherence and some possible solutions for each item.

Table 12–1. Common reasons for nonadherence

1. Has not accepted the illness
2. Symptoms are not perceived as severe and medication seems unnecessary
3. Prefers to tough it out
4. Does not want to be controlled by medications
5. Does not believe in medication or doctors or rejects medication for religious reasons
6. Uses alcohol or street drugs to control symptoms
7. Has had negative experiences with medications and/or with the health care system
8. Does not like or can't tolerate the side effects of medication
9. Medications have not seemed to help
10. Has seen friends or relatives have negative experiences
11. Does not have the resources to pay for care
12. Forgetfulness
13. Disorganization
14. Family has negative attitudes toward psychiatric illness and treatment
15. Interpersonal relationships are creating barriers to medication adherence

The first two items listed in Table 12–1 indicate that the patient is probably in denial. Acceptance and denial are two end points on a continuum according to the stages of adjustment to loss described by Kubler-Ross (1974). In this case, the transition is to the loss of mental health. Like the process of grieving any other loss, people with psychiatric illnesses often experience anger in response to a diagnosis of mental illness. They engage in the process of bargaining when they promise to make other changes in order to avoid having to take psychiatric medications. And it is not unusual for people to feel depressed when they have the full realization that they have a mental illness that will require a lifetime of treatment. These stages—denial, anger, bargaining, depression, and acceptance (Kubler-Ross 1974)—might be reflected in the level of adherence maintained. In these cases, the intervention might be to ease the transition toward acceptance of the diagnosis and the treatment. Standard methods for helping people cope with grief or loss would apply, with care taken not to rush the person toward premature acceptance by insisting that the diagnosis is valid.

Providing education about symptoms, diagnosis, and treatment is a good start in aiding adjustment, but information alone is usually insufficient in helping a person accept the idea of having a chronic mental illness. Use Socratic questions to explore thoughts about having a mental illness, listen for cognitive distortions, and use standard logical analysis methods to work through any of these distortions. Time spent with the patient exploring these thoughts will be well spent and will improve adherence in the long run.

Items 3–5 in Table 12–1 constitute rejection of treatment. Some clinicians would call this another form of denial, but it is not any different than nonpsychiatric patients expressing a preference to not take medication for other health problems. Some people just do not like taking medications. In these cases, a conscious decision to decline the offer of medication is based on preference or attitudes toward medical treatment in general. The reason these ideas are considered manifestations of denial is because clinicians assume that if a diagnosis is rendered and its treatment adequately described, a logically minded person who understands that she is ill would not decline treatment. Refusal is seen as pathology rather than preference. To satisfy the clinician's concerns and respectfully address patients' preferences, the advantages and disadvantages can be weighed of participating in treatment versus handling the illness and its treatment on their own. If the conclusion is that there are too many disadvantages of treatments and not enough advantages, the patient may well exert her right to decline medication or other treatments. In cases where medication is believed to be absolutely mandatory for the safety and welfare of the patient, court-ordered treatment might be necessary. When the patient is less symptomatic and better able to reason through treatment choices, the issue of medication can be revisited.

Item 6 in Table 12–1 is influenced by 1) personal factors such as addiction, preference, lack of understanding of medical treatments, or denial; 2) social factors such as acceptability of alcohol consumption versus the stigma attached to mental illness; 3) family factors such as family use of substances or attitudes toward the health care profession; and 4) practical factors such as not having health insurance, not realizing that health care is needed, availability of substances, and the fact that alcohol and street drugs can make the person feel better, albeit temporarily. Depending on the source of interference, the required intervention might be to address substance abuse issues or stigma. It might be useful to involve the family if their concerns are impeding treatment. Providing information about the illness and its treatment and addressing objections to treatment might remove that roadblock. If addiction is a problem, specific substance abuse treatment should be provided. The substance abuse treatment can be based on CBT principles (see Appendix 2 for resources to learn about these methods), traditional 12-step models, or a combination of these two approaches.

Items 7–10 in Table 12–1 are based on personal experiences with the illness and its treatment. In these situations, the care-seeking process has left a negative impression on the patient or his significant others. Patients may be using cognitive errors, such as overgeneralization, when they assume that bad experiences will repeat themselves if treatment is sought again. These patients also may be magnifying the negative aspects of treatment and minimizing the positive effects. Socratic questions and examining the evidence can be used to explore the occurrence of less negative treatment experiences as a way of overcoming these cognitive errors.

It may also be helpful to frame seeking treatment as an experiment to test the overgeneralization hypothesis. The patient monitors the aspects of treatment encounters for those factors that she finds most important such as the behavior of the health care team, the hassle involved in following treatment recommendations, and the difficulties in navigating through the health care system. If the experiment confirms the patient's negative view, strategies can be developed for coping with each of the elements of the encounter that was problematic.

Items 11–13 in Table 12–1 are all practical in nature and affect both psychiatric and nonpsychiatric services. If resources are not available (item 11), treatment cannot be sought even if the patient is fully aware that medication is needed to control symptoms. In countries without universal health coverage, or in any health care system where patients are having difficulty accessing resources, clinicians may need to make special efforts to assist patients with receiving needed medication or other care.

Forgetfulness (item 12) and disorganization (item 13) about medication dosing are also common problems. Complex dosing regimens and multidose daily schedules combined with poor concentration and a lack of a consistent schedule for meals, sleep, or activity all make medication adherence a challenge. Problem-solving strategies should be employed to define the nature of the difficulty, identify possible solutions, and select interventions that may be most likely to help.

Some simple behavioral strategies to improve patients' adherence to prescribed treatment are listed in Table 12–2. Suggestions include providing clearly understood written instructions, including dose times and amounts. Computerized medical records can be very helpful for this purpose, because the dosing schedule can be printed out and given to the patient whenever needed. To assist patients in remembering to take their medication, therapists can suggest a variety of reminder strategies. For ex-

Table 12–2. Behavioral reminder strategies

Devise uncomplicated dosing strategies.

Clearly explain medication regimen.

Give printed instructions.

Place medication in a place that is viewed routinely each day.

Use pillboxes or other reminder systems.

Pair medication taking with other daily activity.

ample, the therapist and patient can work out a plan for the patient to store the medication in a place that will be seen routinely each day. Our experiences with asking patients about where they typically store their medication have revealed some rather "out of the way" places (e.g., in the bottom drawer of a clothes chest behind a stack of shirts) or a habit of just putting the pills "anywhere." A safe, but easily accessed, daily storage place that will serve as a good reminder to take the medication may help promote adherence (e.g., in the medicine chest in the bathroom right beside the toothbrush and toothpaste).

Pillboxes can be used help to organize medications, particularly if several different types are used daily. This device can make it easy for people to verify whether or not they have taken a given dose, thus helping to avoid the problem of missing doses or taking double the dose because of impaired short-term memory. Also checklists, placing a mark on a daily calendar after medication is taken, or using computerized alarm systems on cell phones or other devices can help remind patients to take their medication. Another particularly useful behavioral strategy is to pair the medication taking with some other daily routine, such as drinking their morning coffee, brushing their teeth, or eating a meal that occurs most regularly. Taking medication often can be easier to add to an existing routine than creating a new one.

CBT interventions for negative attitudes of family toward psychiatric illness and treatment (item 14, Table 12–1) and interpersonal relationships creating barriers to medication adherence (item 15) may require the therapist to schedule family sessions or devise other methods to help patients and their significant others better understand the illness and its treatment. Some relationship factors that can interfere with compliance include the following:

• Unhelpful attitudes of significant others toward the patient, the illness, taking medication, or participating in therapy (e.g., "You should be

able to do this on your own"; "Don't you have any willpower?"; "I don't believe that you have bipolar disorder"; "You can't trust doctors"; "Medications are too dangerous"; "You should stick with natural remedies"; "Therapy is just a bunch of talking, it could never help")
- Interpersonal conflicts, strains, or ruptures that undermine adherence

Psychoeducational efforts can be helpful, but therapeutic work on developing rapport with the family and gentle exploration of absolutistic, maladaptive beliefs may be needed. The strategies for assertive communication described in Chapter 9 ("Interpersonal Problems") can help prepare the patient to discuss medication concerns with family members or significant others. If this discussion proves too difficult for the patient, a conjoint therapy session can be arranged so that the therapist or psychiatrist can explain the need for medication and field any questions or concerns.

Video Illustration 18 shows an adherence intervention with Angela, the woman with bipolar disorder. In this session, Angela describes an interpersonal situation that is a barrier to full compliance with her medication regimen.

▶ **Video Illustration 18.**   Promoting Adherence:
Dr. Basco and Angela

The session opens with a review of some of the behavioral targets of Angela's treatment plan—to limit coffee to three cups a day, to keep her medications on schedule, and to promote sleep by reducing activity close to bedtime and exercising only in the morning. After Angela and Dr. Basco decide to focus first on medication adherence, Angela notes that one of her problems is waking up late, being in a hurry, and then forgetting her medication. She also tells Dr. Basco about a problem with her boyfriend that is having a major effect on her medication-taking habits:

> Dr. Basco: What else can interfere with your plan?
> Angela: Sometimes my boyfriend—he doesn't like the idea that I have bipolar disorder—that I need to take medicines…then I feel uncomfortable taking the medicines when he is there.
> Dr. Basco: Does he actually say, "Don't take it?"
> Angela: Sometimes he does.…And then I try not to make a huge problem of that…so I just don't take the medicine.

The remainder of this therapy vignette demonstrates a problem-solving strategy for overcoming the interpersonal obstacle to adherence. Angela identifies one possible solution that she has already tried—taking the medication before he arrives in the evening. Although this is a reasonable idea, it doesn't directly address the problem with her boyfriend's apparent negative attitudes about her diagnosis and use of mood stabilizing medication. Because Angela reveals that she has had trouble talking about her illness, and it is likely that her boyfriend is not well educated about bipolar disorder, Dr. Basco and Angela develop the following plan: 1) use role-play to rehearse ways for Angela to talk effectively with her boyfriend about her illness, 2) ask the boyfriend to accompany her to a session with Dr. Basco, 3) try to schedule a session with Angela's psychiatrist that the boyfriend can attend.

Angela also agrees to a homework assignment to build a plan for her problem of getting up late, being in a hurry, and missing her morning medication dose. The general strategy used in this session was to first identify obstacles to adherence and then to figure out possible solutions to overcome these barriers. We highly recommend this solution-focused method—or any of the CBT methods for adherence described in this chapter—for tackling the problems listed in Table 12–1.

Working With Cognitions

The cognitive-behavioral model (see Chapter 1, "Introduction") can be used to help explain problems with adherence to treatment. The thoughts a person has about his mental illness can have a major effect on treatment-related behaviors such as taking medication, keeping appointments with health care providers, or doing CBT homework. As with many things, the meaning a person places on his psychiatric diagnosis and treatment strongly influences emotional and behavioral reactions. Using the CBT model as a guide, therapists should explore the thoughts that patients have about themselves, about others in their world or the world in general, and about their future regarding the illness. Table 12–3 provides some sample questions the therapist might ask to elicit patients' thoughts about their diagnosis and treatment. The meanings attached to having a mental illness will be directly related to the amount of effort a person puts toward controlling symptoms, the level of anxiety about the future, and the degree to which he cooperates with health care professionals.

Standard cognitive restructuring methods can be used to examine any negative or dysfunctional thoughts. These procedures could include Socratic questioning, examining the evidence for and against the thoughts, considering the advantages and disadvantages of keeping or changing an attitude, and generating alternative explanations. Once a conclusion has been made, the patient can be asked to write out the original negative thought and the alternative, rational thought on an index card—one thought on each side. These cards can be kept for review during times

---

Table 12–3. Inquiring about the meaning of illness and treatment

Questions about self
  What does having an illness mean to you?
  How has having this diagnosis affected your self-image?
  What kinds of people have illnesses like yours?

Questions about others and the world
  How do you think other people see you?
  What does your family think about your illness, your treatment?
  How does having this illness affect how other people feel about you?
  How does the world treat people who have problems like yours?
  What do you think of other people who struggle with an illness
    like yours?

Questions about the future
  When you look ahead in your life, what do you see?
  How does this illness fit in with your plans for the future?
  Do you think that change is possible?
  Where do you go from here?
  Can you imagine your treatment fitting in with your plans for
    the future?

---

when commitment to treatment wanes. Figure 12–1 provides an example of using a coping card to improve adherence.

There are some common themes—helplessness, hopelessness, and worthlessness—that are often found in the automatic thoughts patients express about their illnesses and the treatments they must undergo.

Helplessness

Themes of control or lack of control can be heard in patients' resistance to treatment. Patients sometimes perceive medication as a vehicle of control—that they will be controlled by the drug itself, by health care providers, and/or by other elements of the health care system.

Taking medication can change a person's perceptions and sensations. Even if these are positive changes, it is not uncommon for people to feel as if they are succumbing to the control of drugs, and therefore to feel that they have little control over what is happening to them. The emotions elicited by these thoughts are anxiety and fear. Depending on the strength of these helpless feelings, which fuel negative thoughts about treatment, the result may be a decision to suffer with symptoms rather than relinquish control to the medicine or to others.

Side 1 The Problem	Side 2 The Solution
Thinking that taking medication means that I am a loser.	Remember that I take medications because I have an illness. I am a good person in many ways. Having an illness doesn't have to define who I am.

Figure 12–1. Coping card on adherence to medication.

To follow the recommendations of doctors or therapists requires the patient to trust in other's motives and abilities. This level of trust is a lot to ask of someone who is fearful, does not fully understand what is happening, and may be suspicious of the intentions of others.

Another way the theme of helplessness emerges is in thoughts about self-control. Symptoms may seem to emerge randomly and not at the will of the individual. When symptoms are present, few people have the ability to suppress them through a sheer act of will. Thus, patients come to believe that they cannot trust themselves. They lose confidence in their abilities and feel "out of control."

No one likes the feeling of being out of control. It elicits an instinctual reaction to grab hold of things that are constants, things that can be counted on, things that seem more real to the individual. If patients have had a mental illness for some time, the daily experiences of living with and coping with the symptoms may be one of those constants in their life that ground them in reality. Medications alter those experiences. Discontinuing medication can bring back what is familiar and bring with it a sense of control.

For patients who associate treatment with relinquishing control, full adherence will be difficult to maintain unless this attitude can be changed. Therapists must help patients find a way to exercise control over their illness, their treatment, and their lives in a proactive way so that their actions improve symptoms and increase the quality of their lives. Laying the groundwork for establishing a plan that patients are willing to follow should begin by openly acknowledging to them that they have ultimate control over the decision to utilize treatments. Participating in their own care by choosing to take medications or complete home-work assignments is their exercise of control over the illness. They are making a decision to use available tools and to take action.

The interventions best suited to this process are Socratic questioning and generating alternative explanations. Exploring the logic behind the sense of losing control can be accomplished by asking the patient to ex-plain what is meant by control and how she experiences control at present. Gently challenge the logic that taking medication is the same as losing control. Inquire if the patient has had any life experiences of construc-tively gaining control and ask the patient to consider how those strategies might apply to the current situation. The goal is to help the patient recall ways in which she has been able to take control of problems and resolve them and then apply those strategies to the current dilemma of needing treatment to control symptoms.

Another related strategy is to generate alternative explanations. In this exercise, the therapist encourages the patient to consider other ways to conceptualize or explain the circumstances surrounding treatment. For example, instead of viewing treatment as relinquishing control, what else could it indicate? Examples of alternative views might be self-care, being proactive, using available resources, allowing others to help, trying to feel better, or relieving distress. It can also be useful to help the patient ex-plore strategies for taking control other than refusing treatment.

Hopelessness

In the process of gaining acceptance, people realize that they have a chronic mental illness that will probably need lifelong treatment. When this awareness reaches its height of clarity, there can be a sense of defeat, despair, and hopelessness about the future. Patients say things like "There is nothing I can do about it"; "My fate is sealed"; "I will never escape this"; or "I will never be the same as I used to be." These thoughts do not always affect adherence to treatment in the short run, but when combined with other obstacles such as unpleasant side effects, the expenses associated with care, or the fatigue that comes from fighting the illness for many years, people sometimes relax their efforts at controlling symptoms or give up altogether. They become discouraged and think, "Why bother?" "Nothing is going to help anyway"; "I'm tired of trying"; or "I can't fight it anymore."

Sometimes therapists have to function like coaches, providing encour-agement and support when patients are losing their ability to persevere. Caution must be taken to avoid statements that appear insincere or that do not show appreciation for the amount of effort required to stick with treatment year after year. Expressions of empathy for the patients' plight let them know that you understand what they must live through each day. Pep talks and the use of platitudes, such as "Hang in there," are likely to backfire.

As patients verbalize their unhappiness about their lot in life, therapists should not move too quickly to intervene unless there is a risk of suicide (see Chapter 7, "Depression"). As patients talk through their distress and express their desire to stop trying, they often talk themselves out of this frame of mind if given the opportunity to air their feelings. It often helps to allow sufficient time to explore the discouragement that is rightly theirs and use basic reflecting, paraphrasing, empathy, and validation skills before moving to problem solving. When sufficient discussion has occurred, ask, "So what do we do now?" Gently use Socratic questioning to explore the available options. A brainstorming list of options might look like the one presented in Table 12–4. Help the patient to evaluate the pros and cons of each option and select a short-term strategy with the promise to reevaluate it at the next visit and modify the plan if needed.

Worthlessness

Having a chronic mental illness and all the problems that accompany it often has a negative impact on self-esteem. Examples of negative self-statements that individuals may develop in response to having a severe mental illness are as follows: "People who have schizophrenia [or bipolar disorder or chronic depression] are weak"; "I'm broken"; "I will never be

Table 12–4. Treatment alternatives

Change a medication that is causing the most side effects.

Learn to cope with side effects better.

Change something else besides treatment.

Join a support group.

Talk to friends about how they keep going when they want to give up.

Learn a new way to cope.

Keep taking the medications as prescribed and reevaluate the options next month.

Make a list of the pros and cons of sticking with treatment.

Make a list of the pros and cons of stopping treatment.

accepted by people again." When patients develop this type of thinking, they may not see the use of taking medication, doing CBT homework, or following other treatment recommendations. The normalizing and de-stigmatizing strategies described in Chapter 3 ("Normalizing and Educating") can be very useful in helping patients continue to value themselves in the face of a severe mental illness. Also, Socratic questioning can be used to detune the absolutistic, overgeneralized, and self-condemning nature of these types of cognitions. However, therapists need to be careful not to move too quickly to dismiss all of the patient's conclusions. The reality is that having any of the psychiatric disorders described in this book is not a good thing. Therapists should express appropriate empathy for the patient's bad fortune and not be too aggressive in "looking at the bright side." A realistic assessment of the problems, along with judicious efforts to reverse true cognitive distortions, will enhance the clinician's credibility and promote adherence.

Developing a Written Adherence Plan

As noted earlier in this chapter (in the section "Types of Nonadherence to Treatment"), there are different levels of nonadherence ranging from total refusal to take medication to full compliance, in which patients take all doses on the schedule unless collaborative decisions are made to alter the regimen. For some patients who have only minor problems with adherence, rather brief interventions may suffice to get them back on track. For others with more significant compliance issues, histories of chronic difficulties following treatment recommendations, frequent relapses associated with noncompliance, or other reasons for the therapist to suspect high risk for adherence lapses (e.g., patient is denying illness, has disorganized thinking, is admitted to hospital with first episode of psychosis), a more comprehensive and structured plan may be needed. We usually recommend that a written plan be developed for these more challenging situations. For example, written adherence plans are a common feature of our work with patients who have been hospitalized and are preparing for discharge.

Treatment of Daniel, the man with schizophrenia featured in Video Illustrations 15 and 16, provides an example of this type of work. Daniel had been admitted to the hospital because of severe deterioration in functioning. He had been so fixated on his delusional beliefs about being watched, and had became so thought disordered, that he was not eating or bathing regularly. Even when his parents brought food to his house, he had trouble eating it because he was paranoid and disorganized. An antipsychotic medication had been prescribed, and he had told his outpatient psychiatrist that he would take it. However, most doses had been missed in the several weeks before his admission to the hospital.

You may recall that Daniel didn't want to accept any dose increases or changes in medication when Dr. Turkington talked with him in Video Illustration 15 (first shown in Chapter 10, "Impaired Cognitive Functioning"). Because noncompliance was a major factor in Daniel's deterioration, a change in medication, or at least helping Daniel to take the medication already prescribed, was a highly appropriate goal of therapy. Yet Daniel wasn't ready at that point to accept the therapist's efforts to improve adherence. It was only after Dr. Turkington was able to forge a therapeutic relationship with Daniel and to have some success at helping him with other issues (see Video Illustrations 15 and 16) that productive work could be done on improving his ability to stick with a medication regimen. Subsequent sessions, not shown in the video illustrations, were directed at defining the obstacles to adherence, developing specific strategies to overcome the obstacles, and then helping Daniel write out a plan that he could follow after returning home.

Table 12–5 shows an analysis of barriers to adherence that was developed collaboratively with Daniel, Dr. Turkington, and inpatient nurses who were trained in CBT methods. Daniel's disorganized thinking improved substantially during the hospitalization so he was able to participate fully in this process. However, he still needed help from the staff to perform this analysis and to develop ideas for change. Daniel started out in early sessions saying he wouldn't accept any more medication than he was currently taking. He was actually refusing many doses, even in the hospital setting. By performing the following analysis and participating in other CBT activities, a clear change was noted in his thoughts about pharmacotherapy: "I need a different medication, one that I can tolerate better"; "The right medication could make me think more clearly and help me communicate better with people"; "Taking medication could keep me out of the hospital."

The analysis of barriers in Table 12–5 was developed over about a week of short daily visits by Dr. Turkington and several conversations with one of the nurses who worked on the inpatient unit. Socratic questions were used to help Daniel identify obstacles and explore ideas for managing each of the barriers to adherence. Daniel was able to generate many of the solutions shown in Table 12–5. But sometimes guidance was needed, as is demonstrated in this brief segment of dialogue with the nurse:

> Nurse: You said that you often forget to take your medication when you start thinking about being controlled. Can you come up with any ideas on how to remember to take the medication?

Table 12–5. Taking medication: obstacles and solutions—
        Daniel's example

Obstacles to taking medication	Solutions
Get side effects—I feel stiff and restless.	Talk with my doctor about switching medications or lowering the dose.
I start dwelling on all of my fears. Then I forget to take pills, eat, or do any other routine things.	Simplify medication schedule—take meds only once a day before I go to bed.
	When I go home, place pill bottle on bedside table so that I will see it every night when I go to bed. Get into habit of taking pill every night before I turn off the light.
I could get worried again about people being able to track me when I use credit cards. Then I wouldn't fill the prescription because of the copay that would get charged to my card.	Ask my mother to give me the $20 in cash that I would need for the copay each month. She would be happy to do this if it would help me get the prescription.
I start thinking that I would be better off not taking medication—I would feel more natural.	Remind myself that the medication actually makes me think more clearly and it keeps me out of the hospital.

Daniel: I don't know, maybe I could write myself a note.

Nurse: That's a good idea....Let's see if we can come up with any other suggestions. Is there anything you do every night before you go to bed? Sometimes if you get into the habit of taking the medicine when you brush your teeth, or something like that, you can always remember to take the medicine.

Daniel: Well...I should brush my teeth...but I don't always do that.

Nurse: Anything else that you do routinely before going to bed? I guess I should ask—do you sleep in a bed every night?

Daniel: Yeah...That is one thing that I actually do.

Nurse: So, where could you put your pills so that you would see them and would remember to take them before going off to sleep?

Daniel: I have a table right beside my bed.
Nurse: You live alone, don't you?
Daniel: Yes.
Nurse: So would it be safe to leave the pills on your bedside table, and
would that help remind you to take them?
Daniel: Sure, I could do that. It would probably work. There's nobody
around that would take the pills except me.

This interchange shows how therapists and staff members can involve
patients in generating adherence plans and can help shape the plans by
collaborative questioning. The written adherence plan that was developed by Daniel and the treatment team included the items in Table 12–
6. Daniel was asked to take a copy of the plan with him when he went
home, to post it on his refrigerator, and to bring a copy in his notebook
to each outpatient therapy session.

> **Learning Exercise 12–1.** Developing an
> Adherence Plan
>
> 1. Are you currently taking a prescription medicine
> or have you ever been prescribed a medication to take
> for more than a few days or weeks? If you haven't
> been prescribed such a medication, imagine that you
> have been diagnosed with some condition that will
> require long-term or lifelong treatment with one or
> more medicines.

Table 12–6. Daniel's adherence plan

Discuss medication at each visit with doctor. Report any
side effects or worries about medication. Negotiate
changes with doctor.

Take medications once a day as agreed with Dr. Turkington.

If I start thinking I would be more natural off medication,
remind myself that the medication keeps me out of the
hospital and makes me think more clearly.

Write myself a reminder note and place it on my mirror in the
bathroom.

Place pill bottle on bedside table. Take medication every
night before turning off light and going to sleep.

Always use cash for the copay for my prescriptions so
I don't have to worry about credit cards.

2. Write down some attitudes that you have or might have about having this illness and taking the medication.

3. Now, make a list of some obstacles to full adherence. Would you have negative or conflicted attitudes about taking the medicine? Would you be so busy that you might forget? Would there be other reasons you might miss doses?

4. Finally, draw up a plan for trying to achieve full adherence. Include both cognitive and behavioral strategies if possible.

CBT Homework

We have centered our discussion of adherence problems on taking medication because this is such an important part of CBT for severe mental illnesses. However, many of the same methods for improving medication compliance can also be used for helping patients follow through with homework assignments and other CBT exercises. As detailed in Wright et al. (2006), one of the best ways to troubleshoot problems with homework assignments is to identify obstacles and then devise solutions. This work can be done in advance of a homework assignment to help improve the chances of success, or it can be performed after difficulties have been encountered. In Video Illustration 18, Angela notes that she has been trying to cut down her coffee intake and to exercise earlier in the day so that her sleep improves. These types of lifestyle changes are ideal candidates for an obstacles/solutions analysis. Other examples might include dieting, cutting down on alcohol intake, and breaking patterns of procrastination.

Changing habits like Angela's can be difficult, and the first attempt at an obstacles/solutions analysis may be only the starting point in the process of assisting with change. Even with good intentions, patients may not be able to adhere to their homework plans. Some ideas to help with homework adherence are listed in Table 12–7. Of course, good collaboration is essential in designing homework assignments that are likely to be carried out. And it is critically important to ask about homework at each session. If the therapist forgets to check the homework, it sends a powerful message that the homework is not very important. The therapist needs to set an example that homework is a core part of CBT.

Another method that can help patients complete their assignments is to rehearse the planned actions in the therapy session or to ask them to

---

Table 12–7. Strategies for improving homework adherence

Collaboratively develop homework assignments. Always request the patient's input.

Always check the homework assignment at the next session.

Perform an obstacles/solutions analysis in advance of a homework assignment. Ask patients what would get in the way of their completing the assignment.

Rehearse homework assignments in sessions. Help prepare the patient for potential problems.

If the patient doesn't do the assignment or experiences difficulties, use the obstacles/solutions method to troubleshoot problems.

Be willing to recognize that you may have designed an assignment that is too difficult or is flawed in some way.

Make adjustments to the homework plans if necessary. Keep trying.

"walk through" assignments in advance. For example, if Angela had decided she would change to decaffeinated coffee after 10 A.M. in the morning, the therapist could ask her to imagine how she might feel drinking a cup of decaf and to think of some coping strategies (e.g., take a short break to go on a walk) if she felt like she had a sag in energy.

When patients have difficulty completing assignments, it is always a good idea to ask yourself if you could have been part of the problem. Was the assignment too hard or too easy? Was it meaningful to the patient? Or did it seem off target or inconsequential? Did you adequately prepare the patient? If the patient didn't follow through with the plan or an assignment didn't work out, all is not lost. In fact, difficulties with assignments can be viewed as excellent learning opportunities. Go back to the drawing board, and try again.

Summary

Key Points for Clinicians

- Research studies have documented the usefulness of CBT approaches for adherence.
- Common reasons for nonadherence can be denial of the illness, rejection of treatment, substance misuse or abuse, negative experiences with treatment, and practical issues (e.g., finances, availability of medication).

- Therapists can improve adherence by troubleshooting the reasons for nonadherence and working collaboratively to devise solutions.
- There are a number of behavioral reminder strategies (e.g., written instructions, pillboxes, pairing) that can be very helpful in improving adherence.
- Negative cognitions about the illness, the treatment, or the self can impair adherence. CBT methods can be effective in modifying these negative cognitions.
- Written adherence plans may be useful for patients who have particular difficulty in achieving treatment compliance.
- Adherence interventions can also be targeted toward helping patients carry out homework assignments.

Concepts and Skills for Patients to Learn

- It is normal to have problems in accepting a diagnosis and in following a treatment plan.
- Discussing the meaning of an illness and its treatments with a therapist can help people better understand and manage psychiatric disorders.
- Many influences can impact whether people take their medication. For example, families can be either for or against use of medication, side effects can be irritating or intolerable, or people can get so busy that they forget to take their medication. If you talk openly about these issues with your doctor or therapist, she will help you work out a plan for change.
- It is easy to forget to take medications. Simple reminder strategies, such as always taking the medication along with some other routine daily activity, can help people follow a treatment plan.
- If you can figure out the obstacles that are getting in the way of taking medication, solutions can usually be found.

References

Akincigil A, Bowblis JR, Levin C, et al: Adherence to antidepressant treatment among privately insured patients diagnosed with depression. Med Care 45:363–369, 2007

Ball JR, Mitchell PB, Corry JC, et al: A randomized controlled trial of cognitive therapy for bipolar disorder: focus on long-term change. J Clin Psychiatry 67:277–286, 2006

Basco MR, Rush AJ: Compliance with pharmacotherapy in mood disorders. Psychiatr Ann 25:269–279, 1995

Becker MH: The Health Belief Model and Personal Behavior. Thorofare, NJ, Charles B Slack, 1974

Cochran SD: Preventing medical noncompliance in the outpatient treatment of bipolar affective disorders. J Consult Clin Psychol 52:873–878, 1984

Keck PE, McElroy SL, Strakowski SM, et al: Compliance with maintenance treatment in bipolar disorder. Psychopharmacol Bull 33:87–91, 1997

Kemp R, Hayward P, Applewhaite G, et al: Compliance therapy in psychotic patients: randomised controlled trial. BMJ 312:345–349, 1996

Kemp R, Kirov G, Everitt B, et al: Randomised controlled trial of compliance therapy: 18-month follow-up. Br J Psychiatry 172:413–419, 1998

Kubler-Ross E: The languages of the dying patients. Humanitas 10:5–8, 1974

Lam DH, Bright J, Jones S, et al: Cognitive therapy for bipolar illness—a pilot study of relapse prevention. Cognit Ther Res 24:503–520, 2000

Lecompte D: Drug compliance and cognitive-behavioral therapy in schizophrenia. Acta Psychiat Belg 95:91–100, 1995

Meichenbaum D, Turk D: Facilitating Treatment Adherence: A Practitioner's Guidebook. New York, Plenum, 1988

Perris C, Skagerlind L: Cognitive therapy with schizophrenic patients. Acta Psychiatr Scand 89 (suppl 382):65–70, 1994

Rosa MA, Marcolin MA, Elkis H: Evaluation of the factors interfering with drug treatment compliance among Brazilian patients with schizophrenia. Rev Bras Psiquiatr 27:178–184, 2005

Scott J, Pope M: Nonadherence with mood stabilizers: prevalence and predictors. J Clin Psychiatry 63:384–390, 2002

Weiden P, Burkholder P, Schooler N, et al: Improving antipsychotic adherence in schizophrenia: a randomized pilot study of a brief CBT intervention. Poster presented at the 160th Annual Meeting of the American Psychiatric Association, San Diego, CA, May 19–24, 2007

Weiss RD, Greenfield SF, Najavits LM, et al: Medication compliance among patients with bipolar disorder and substance abuse. J Clin Psychiatry 59:172–174, 1998

Wright JH, Basco MR, Thase ME: Learning Cognitive-Behavior Therapy: An Illustrated Guide. Washington, DC, American Psychiatric Publishing, 2006

13

Maintaining Treatment Gains

Patients with severe mental illnesses can make substantial progress in reducing or eliminating distressing symptoms and can develop a much improved quality of life. Yet, most will have to contend with a risk for symptom worsening or relapse throughout their entire lives. Thus, CBT for severe mental illnesses needs to go beyond the typical courses of short-term treatment offered in uncomplicated cases of depression and anxiety disorders. In Chapter 8 ("Mania"), we introduced relapse prevention methods for bipolar disorder. We extend this discussion here by providing a basic framework for implementing CBT relapse prevention techniques across the range of severe mental illnesses. Suggestions are offered for helping patients use CBT skills to promote enduring treatment gains. We also discuss practical issues in designing long-term treatment plans and maintenance therapy regimens.

Relapse Prevention

The basic structure and methods of CBT are well suited for promoting long-term benefits of treatment because patients are taught skills that can be used over time to manage symptoms, cope with stress, and build self-efficacy. Although much more research needs to be done, studies on CBT for unipolar depression and bipolar disorder have usually, but not always, shown favorable long-term results (Ball et al. 2006; Bockting et al. 2005;

Hollon et al. 1992a, 1992b, 2005; Kovacs et al. 1981; Lam et al. 2003; Scott et al. 2006; and see review by Wright et al. 2008). Investigations of relapse prevention effects for CBT of bipolar disorder examined post-treatment follow-up over a period of 6 months (Scott et al. 2001), 18 months (Lam et al. 2000, 2003), and 30 months (Fava et al. 2001).

Several studies of CBT for schizophrenia have shown positive findings for relapse prevention and longer-term follow-up (Grawe et al. 2006; Gumley et al. 2003; Turkington et al. 2006, 2008). However, in a review of earlier research, Tarrier and Wykes (2004) observed that investigations of CBT dedicated to relapse prevention found superior results compared with treatment as usual, but other studies not directly geared to long-term results did not find an added benefit for CBT in forestalling relapse. With one exception (Grawe et al. 2006), these investigations have only examined short-term therapies instead of evaluating the potential of extended forms of delivering CBT to patients with chronic psychoses. Grawe et al. (2006) demonstrated that a 2-year program of CBT that was integrated with family work and crisis intervention did not reduce rehospitalization rates. However, this longer-term therapy doubled the number of excellent outcomes compared with treatment as usual (53% vs. 25%). Sessions were tapered after the first 2 months to a minimum of one session every 3 weeks. During the second year of treatment, patients received one session monthly.

The methods described in this chapter are intended to help make the effects of the acute phase of CBT as enduring as possible and also to provide useful ongoing treatment when needed. Table 13–1 summarizes relapse prevention strategies.

Teach and Practice Basic CBT Skills

If you wait until termination to consider relapse prevention strategies, you may have missed many opportunities to develop relapse prevention skills. All of the basic CBT methods that are used to control current symptoms (e.g., identifying automatic thoughts, spotting cognitive errors, examining the evidence, thought records, activity scheduling, graded task assignments, and so forth) can continue to be used during maintenance phase treatment and after therapy has ended. Helping patients to solidify these skills, practice them in multiple settings, and apply them to potential symptom triggers can significantly strengthen patients' abilities to respond to future challenges.

Table 13–1. Relapse prevention strategies

Teach and practice basic CBT skills.

Identify potential triggers for relapse or symptom worsening.

Develop relapse prevention plans.

Involve family in long-term treatment planning.

Use rehearsal techniques.

Reinforce learning with notebooks, coping cards, and other aids.

Use CBT adherence methods.

Identify Potential Triggers for Relapse or Symptom Worsening

For some patients with severe mental illnesses, it is possible to forecast future stresses or other influences that may aggravate symptoms or kindle a relapse. For others who have a more autonomous course of illness, identifying possible environmental influences may not be as relevant in designing relapse prevention strategies. However, even when symptomatic relapses seem to come out of the blue, it is useful to detail early warning signs that symptoms are worsening or recurring. If potential triggers or warning signals can be identified, then plans can be made to manage symptoms before they escalate.

The treatment of Mary, the woman with chronic depression featured in the video illustrations, demonstrates the value of spotting problems that can send patients into a downward spiral. In Chapter 7 ("Depression"), we showed how Mary was able to recognize that an argument with her husband would wound her self-esteem and stimulate suicidal thinking. A somewhat different approach was used with Angela, the patient with bipolar disorder. She completed a symptom summary worksheet that listed possible signs that she was shifting into a manic or depressed phase of her illness. Whether specific triggers can be projected, as in the treatment of Mary, or the signals of a rather endogenous pattern of symptom changes can be identified, as in the treatment of Angela, this information is a key element in devising plans to sustain treatment gains.

Develop Relapse Prevention Plans

Chapter 8 ("Mania") describes a system of developing specific strategies for specific symptom changes or problems that might be encountered in the future. After becoming more familiar with the symptoms of mania,

Angela came to realize when her symptoms were affecting her behavior and perceptions of others, as shown in Video Illustration 14. Not wanting to create difficulties for her child or in her work, Angela decided to reduce her caffeine intake, slow her activity, and avoid risky behaviors when a return of manic symptoms seemed possible. Other commonly used strategies for relapse prevention in bipolar disorder include maintaining good sleep hygiene, limiting overstimulation, and working with the psychiatrist to develop a plan for quickly addressing sleep loss and other manic symptoms if they return. The same strategy of identifying triggers or signs of potential relapse and then working out possible solutions can be used for patients with recurrent unipolar depression and for some individuals with schizophrenia who are able to collaborate on building relapse prevention plans.

An illustration of these techniques comes from the treatment of Brenda, the patient with schizophrenia featured in Video Illustrations 8 and 9. After Brenda learned basic coping strategies for hallucinations and was able to spend time with her new grandchild without difficulty, she and Dr. Turkington worked on relapse prevention. First, they identified any shifts in symptoms that might indicate that she would need to take action to forestall a worsening of voices. Then they detailed coping strategies to handle each of these potential problems (Table 13–2).

Brenda's efforts to plan ahead for potential problems were incorporated into a basic relapse prevention program. More elaborate or detailed plans can be built if needed and if patients are able to participate in the process. In Chapter 7 ("Depression"), we illustrated methods of building suicide prevention plans for patients with depression and schizophrenia. Methods of strengthening and maintaining adherence to pharmacological and psychotherapeutic methods were explained in Chapter 12 ("Promoting Adherence"). All of these types of intervention strategies can be incorporated into an overall relapse prevention plan. The therapist can then help patients hone their skills with additional practice.

Involve Family in Long-Term Treatment Planning

For conditions that are likely to require long-term treatment, the involvement of family (or caregivers or significant others) in developing and supporting the treatment plan can improve the quality of the plan and increase the chances of it being carried out. Thus, we often recommend that family members attend at least a few sessions during the acute phase of treatment so that the therapist can gather their input and enlist their help in developing the formulation and implementation strategies. And we may suggest an open-door policy of family attending maintenance ther-

Table 13–2. A coping plan: Brenda's example

Symptom or problem	Coping plan
If I sleep very poorly for four or five nights, the voices will get much worse.	Stay away from caffeine. Call the doctor to ask for sleeping medication if this problem goes on for more than two nights.
I could get caught up with worrying all the time and stop seeing friends.	Allow myself no more than 1 hour of worry a day (usually from 4 P.M.–5 P.M.). Do at least two enjoyable things a day to take my mind off my worries.
I could start thinking that the devil is trying to tell me something.	Remember what my pastor said about the devil. Remind myself that the devil in the Bible doesn't talk like the voice I sometimes hear.
I could start dwelling on the past and thinking of all the problems I had as a young mother.	Look at the coping card I wrote with my doctor. Tell myself "I did the best I could. I am a good person and a good mother."
I could have another new grandbaby, or even a niece or a nephew. This could start my problem up again.	Use the coping methods I learned for voices. Begin seeing the doctor more frequently if I need to. Consider an increase in medication.

apy sessions when needed. Of course, collaboration among the patient, therapist, and family is critical to success when family sessions are incorporated in the treatment planning and maintenance phases of therapy. Some specific areas where family members can help bolster the treatment plan include the following: 1) assist with medication adherence by helping to load a weekly pill container; 2) agree to back off on placing too much pressure on a person with pronounced negative symptoms, but to provide support for increased socialization at a pace suggested by the patient and therapist; 3) at the patient's request be a sounding board for checking out the validity of possible delusional perceptions; and 4) participate with the patient in developing a symptom summary worksheet for signs of potential relapse in bipolar disorder and work together in building a relapse prevention plan.

Use Rehearsal Techniques

If a component of a relapse prevention plan involves carrying out a challenging task or applying a skill that the patient may not have fully mastered, time spent on rehearsal can pay significant dividends. For example, Mary had made significant progress in reducing depression and was nearing completion of the acute phase of her treatment. She and Dr. Wright worked on a transition to brief monthly rather than weekly sessions. Although her marriage seemed to be going much better, she and Dr. Wright were concerned that marital conflict could lead to setbacks.

One of the strategies they used was to rehearse methods for coping with criticism from her husband. Dr. Wright asked her to imagine such a scene in order to evoke the thoughts and feelings that could occur. A thought record was used to spot cognitive errors and generate rational alternatives. Mary and Dr. Wright also developed a written list of self-affirming cognitions, assertive responses, and cooperative efforts that might help her deal effectively with future marital difficulties. These strategies were rehearsed in session using imagery and role-playing methods.

The worst-case scenario method is another strategy for preparing patients to manage stressful events by eliciting their catastrophic thinking about future events. The preparation teaches effective coping strategies even if the feared outcome doesn't actually occur. Some examples of potential worst-case scenarios that we have helped our patients manage include "My wife admits that she is having an affair, and she leaves me"; "The diagnosis will be confirmed as multiple sclerosis"; and "Even though I hope she will do OK, my daughter will fail out of school." In each of these situations, the therapist used methods similar to those described above for Mary. In doing so, the therapist spent time showing empathic concern for the patient's projected calamity, and coping methods were developed to match the level of possible injury and distress.

Cognitive rehearsal can also be valuable for behavioral components of relapse prevention plans. For example, Brenda said that she would restrict her worrying to only 1 hour a day and would engage in at least two enjoyable activities daily. Although these ideas sound great, could Brenda follow through with her plans? Obviously, Dr. Turkington couldn't rehearse the actual worry time of 1 hour or the actual participation in the pleasurable activities—but he could ask Brenda to imagine what it would be like to set aside an hour for worry: What would she do to begin the period of worry? How would she organize her time? What topics would she cover? Would there be any topics she would avoid? Would she spend the entire hour worrying or would she allow herself to watch TV, read magazines, cook dinner, or do other activities? How would she end the period of worry? What if worries popped into her head later in the day? After working on answers to these questions, Dr. Turkington and Brenda could simulate the worry hour by having Brenda spend 5 minutes on worry in the session. Then she could try to shut off the worries and move on to another topic.

Reinforce Learning With Notebooks, Coping Cards, and Other Aids

Written materials that summarize the procedures for cognitive and behavioral interventions are invaluable in CBT. These might include a therapy notebook; a folder with handouts used during CBT sessions, such as thought records; or index cards that summarize main points. Patients can refer back to this information when sessions have stopped or are reduced in frequency. For patients who have difficulty with reading or writing, the therapist should inquire about strategies used in the past to recall other important information. What methods has the patient found most useful?

The degree to which patients can collect and use information from therapy sessions will vary with their level of symptoms, cognitive capacity, and degree of engagement and motivation. Yet, even patients who remain quite psychotic or have significant thought disorder may benefit from having a few key concepts recorded on a reminder sheet, a coping card, an audiotape, or a CD. Therapists can reinforce the value of holding on to this information by making comments such as "You have worked hard to develop these coping strategies for voices. Can we think of a way to make a record of our efforts so that you can always remember to use these tools?"

Use CBT Adherence Methods

Perhaps the most important element of a relapse prevention strategy for severe mental disorders is to use the CBT methods for adherence described in Chapter 12 ("Promoting Adherence"). Therapists may assume patients are taking medication reliably when they are not, especially if medication adherence is not a comfortable discussion topic for either party. Also, in longer-term treatment, therapists may forget to check for adherence and may find out later, much to their surprise, that patients have stopped medications, have acted on their own to lower doses, or are taking unreported herbal remedies or other medications.

This type of problem is illustrated by the case of a patient with bipolar disorder who had been visiting her psychiatrist monthly for brief visits for over 4 years, throughout which she had lithium levels in the therapeutic range. The clinician had not asked about medication adherence for over 2 years because the patient was doing well, had not relapsed, and always appeared to be pleased with treatment. This lack of attention to adherence was a mistake. The patient had been harboring cognitions such as "I'm sick and tired of taking medication all the time"; "It was so long ago when I got put in the hospital, maybe I don't have bipolar disorder"; and "I'm not sure it's safe to keep taking these drugs." As could be expected with these types of beliefs, she stopped the medication. Unfortunately, she did not tell her psychiatrist until almost 2 months had gone by. At that point, depressive symptoms had returned, and the patient was struggling to get back on track.

Patients do not usually call their psychiatrists between visits to discuss discontinuing medication unless there has been a preparatory conversation about this possibility. Rather than forbidding patients to discontinue their medications without permission, psychiatrists and therapists should encourage honest conversation about medication adherence, attitudes toward medication, and the pros and cons of continuing to use medications when symptoms are under control. A request can be made that patients call their doctor before making any changes in their regimens if it accompanies a promise by therapists to consider patients' thoughts and feelings and respectfully discuss the options.

> **Learning Exercise 13–1.**   Developing a Relapse
> Prevention Plan
>
> 1. Identify a patient in your practice who may have a significant risk for relapse or symptom worsening. If you don't have such a case, or are not currently seeing patients, use the case of Majir, Daniel, or one of the other persons in this book for the exercise. Imagine that this patient has had a substantial amount of recovery and is now in the maintenance phase of treatment.
>
> 2. Think of possible triggers or an escalation of symptoms that could signal an impending relapse.
>
> 3. Now design a plan to reduce the risk of relapse. Include both cognitive and behavioral interventions if possible.

Methods for Continuation and Maintenance CBT

Patients with severe mental disorders often see their psychiatrists and therapists for very long periods of time. The authors of this book have had many patients in their practices for 10 or more years. In research studies on CBT for schizophrenia, bipolar disorder, and treatment-resistant depression, a defined number of sessions (usually 12–20) is typically delivered over a specific period of time (usually 3–9 months). The long-term results are assessed 1–3 years posttreatment. Although this form of treatment delivery fits well with research designs, it may not offer the best possible method for management of chronic and recurrent conditions. We offer some ideas here for longer-term treatment strategies for severe mental disorders.

Integrating Therapy Efforts

There are many possible scenarios for delivering ongoing treatment for severe mental disorders. Some of these options are listed in Table 13–3. The first item on this list—a psychiatrist is fully trained in CBT and pharmacotherapy and provides both treatments—can be an ideal situation for some patients, because the two forms of therapy can be delivered as a comprehensive treatment package and there are no communication problems between therapists. Another advantage of this approach is that psychiatrists often continue to see patients for medication management many years after the completion of the acute phase of psychotherapy, and thus are in a good position to use CBT methods when needed for crises, signs of a potential relapse, or to help manage other potentially destabilizing stresses. A growing number of psychiatrists are being trained in this approach and are using CBT in clinical practice. However, models 3 and 4 in Table 13–3 are currently being used more frequently in most countries. Also, a comprehensive approach, as exemplified in model 5, may be especially useful for patients with schizophrenia or other conditions that may require extensive therapy resources for long durations of treatment.

Models 1–4 are most commonly used in maintenance therapy of patients with severe, recurrent depression and bipolar disorder, whereas model 5 is more typically used in treatment of schizophrenia and other chronic psychoses. In any of the situations where more than one therapist is involved, it can be very helpful for therapists to work together in developing and implementing the treatment plan. A joint effort to communicate and coordinate efforts can prevent conflicting messages to patients

Table 13–3. Models of treatment delivery

1. A psychiatrist is the sole therapist. This clinician is fully trained in CBT and provides both pharmacotherapy and CBT.

2. A psychiatrist is the sole therapist. This clinician has basic knowledge of CBT but is not highly experienced in this approach. Combined pharmacotherapy and a hybrid of supportive and CBT methods are provided.

3. A psychiatrist and nonphysician cognitive-behavior therapist work as a team in delivering combined pharmacotherapy and CBT. They communicate regularly and have a shared model for treatment.

4. A psychiatrist (or primary care physician) and nonphysician cognitive-behavior therapist provide pharmacotherapy and CBT respectively, but communicate rarely if at all.

5. Any of the first four models are combined with day treatment, rehabilitation groups, social skills training programs, case management, or other mental health services.

and families and promote an overall collaborative tone to the therapy. Because CBT is based on collaborative empiricism, it is important for the various therapists who are working with the patient to follow this same method in their relationships with one another. Some recommended steps for forging effective teams of therapists are shown in Table 13–4.

Booster Sessions

One useful model for delivering CBT for severe mental disorders is to front-load the therapy by providing acute phase treatment as in typical research studies, but then to offer additional sessions as needed. For example, a patient with severe, treatment-resistant depression might receive 12–16 sessions in the first 6 months, followed by 4–8 booster sessions over the next year. Then additional sessions could be arranged if needed after that time. Jarrett and coworkers (2001) have systemized this type of approach in their work in continuation therapy for major depression. This research team has shown a significant reduction in relapse rates in depressed patients who receive additional sessions after the completion of acute phase therapy (Jarrett et al. 2001).

In clinical practice, the spacing of booster sessions can be customized to fit the needs of the patient and the type of therapy being delivered. If a psychiatrist is the sole therapist, booster work can be integrated with pharmacotherapy in brief sessions after symptoms have been stabilized in

---

Table 13–4. Promoting an integrated treatment approach

Work together regularly.

Use a shared cognitive-behavioral-biological-sociocultural model and formulation to plan treatment.

Place medication and psychosocial issues on session agendas in both pharmacotherapy and CBT—thus giving credence to the importance of both types of topics.

Link pharmacotherapy and psychotherapy by having the clinicians inquire about how the other treatment is going.

Pharmacotherapists and cognitive-behavior therapists should become familiar with the approach used by the other therapist and offer full support for the other treatment in sessions with patients.

Communicate regularly, especially if there are new problems or relapses.

If the cognitive-behavior therapist is ending treatment, the transition to seeing only the psychiatrist should be planned carefully.

---

acute phase treatment. If a psychologist or social worker is the primary cognitive-behavior therapist, several booster sessions can be planned for 6 months or longer after acute phase treatment. If the patient is doing well and appears to have gained as much as possible from CBT from the nonphysician therapist, responsibility for all of the treatment can then be transitioned to the psychiatrist.

Long-Term Combined CBT and Pharmacotherapy

For patients who have schizophrenia, bipolar disorder, or recurrent depression, long-term or indefinite maintenance pharmacotherapy is usually a key part of the treatment plan. The use of CBT for periods longer than typical acute phase treatment has received very little study (for example, see Blackburn and Moore 1997; Jarrett et al. 2001), but we have found in our clinical practices that CBT methods, integrated with pharmacotherapy, offer pragmatic tools for helping patients maintain, and sometimes expand, the gains from acute phase treatment.

The therapeutic approach used to treat Kenyatta, a 54-year-old woman with schizoaffective disorder, illustrates this type of longer-term treatment. Kenyatta was first seen by her psychiatrist, a person who was trained in CBT, 5 years previously when she was admitted to a hospital with intense paranoid delusions, depressed mood, and suicidal ideation. The psychiatrist enlisted the help of a licensed, clinical social worker to be the primary cognitive-behavior therapist during this hospitalization and to follow the patient after discharge. During the 3-week hospital stay, the psychiatrist saw Kenyatta daily except weekends for visits of about 20 minutes each, and used basic CBT methods that were integrated with the social worker's sessions (also about 20 minutes each). The psychiatrist also helped organize an overall effort of the inpatient staff to use CBT for paranoia (see Chapter 5, "Delusions"), and depression and suicidality (see Chapter 7, "Depression") while Kenyatta was hospitalized. Thus, from the beginning of this treatment, the psychiatrist, the social worker, and others were part of a team providing comprehensive therapy with CBT and medication.

After the patient improved to a level allowing discharge, sessions were arranged with the social worker for about 30–45 minutes weekly and with the psychiatrist for 20–25 minutes every 2 weeks for three sessions, then every month. Kenyatta also attended a day treatment program for about 1 year. Sessions with the social worker continued weekly for about 10 weeks, and then were tapered to every 2 weeks. After about 9 months, Kenyatta was much less paranoid, was not expressing any depressive symptoms, and was functioning at a considerably higher level. For example, she was babysitting for children in the neighborhood and was participating with a group of women to construct a quilt for a community project. At this point, the social worker was able to stop his sessions with Kenyatta. The psychiatrist continued to see Kenyatta monthly for 20- to 25-minute sessions, which included medication management, reinforcement of CBT methods, work on residual issues, and troubleshooting of any new difficulties.

Examples of some of the work done in these brief sessions over years 2–5 of Kenyatta's treatment were 1) coping with increased paranoia when her boyfriend had a heart attack and was hospitalized (she had trouble trusting doctors, test results, and treatment suggestions); 2) dealing with adherence problems after a 2-year period of relative wellness (Kenyatta wondered if she actually had an illness or needed continued pharmacotherapy); and 3) targeting a previously obscured symptom (Kenyatta revealed that she had agoraphobic symptoms that hadn't been reported before—she was avoiding movie theaters, sporting events, and large stores where there were "lots of strangers," although her boyfriend really wanted her to go with him to these places). The latest problem appeared to be a result of mild, residual paranoia plus a typical agoraphobic pattern of an unrealistic fear of situations coupled with persistent avoidance.

Because the psychiatrist had a strong and long-lasting therapeutic relationship with Kenyatta and was able to deliver efficient CBT interventions, the psychiatrist was able to address the types of problems noted above within the confines of the maintenance therapy. An illustration of this work comes from their efforts to help Kenyatta cope with the aftermath of her boyfriend's heart attack:

Kenyatta: They keep telling us that he has to lose weight and exercise.... There's no way he could lose weight. He's tried everything. And they put him on some really strong drugs. What are they trying to do to us? I think they are just picking on us because we have so many problems.

Psychiatrist: I know that it has been real tough for you and your boyfriend. I'm sorry that you have had to face this problem.

Kenyatta: Yeah, it has been a really hard time for us.

Psychiatrist: Do you remember that in the past we've worked on coping with problems by trying to be as realistic as possible about the situation? If you start with finding out the facts, you usually can figure out a way to deal with things.

Kenyatta: Sure, I know you always want me to check things out before I get too worked up.

Psychiatrist: So, how could we find out about this advice from the doctors? Is there any way we could learn what is usually recommended for heart problems like your boyfriend has?

Kenyatta: They gave me some pamphlets, but I was too upset to read them. I think they were from the American Heart Association.

Psychiatrist: Well, that sounds like a good resource for information. What do you think?

Kenyatta: I suppose I should take a look at them.

The discussion went on for a few more minutes and ended with a plan to 1) read the pamphlets; 2) check the American Heart Association Web site; 3) talk with a cousin who is a nurse about the heart doctors' recommendations; and 4) write down a brief examining-the-evidence exercise for the idea that the doctors were "picking" on them and that the recommendations should be ignored.

They then discussed her fears about her boyfriend further, reviewed the medication regimen, refilled prescriptions, and planned for the next session. Because Kenyatta was having a crisis and needed to cope better with her boyfriend's heart attack, they moved up the next session to 2 weeks instead of continuing with the regular regimen of monthly visits. At the next session they reviewed the homework, discussed ways that Kenyatta could communicate better with the heart doctors and their staff, and worked on ideas for assisting her boyfriend in his rehabilitation efforts. Her mild paranoia subsided quickly, and she was able to focus on efforts to cope instead of being preoccupied with fear, anger, and distrust. After one extra session, they were able to resume the plan of monthly visits.

This case illustration demonstrates a typical scenario for long-term management of severe mental disorders in the clinical practices of the physician authors of this book. After a more intensive period of CBT in the early part of treatment, most patients are able to transition to a less intense form of treatment that may be carried out over very long intervals. If the psychiatrist is not versed in CBT, or the pharmacotherapy is being provided by a primary care physician, plans can be made for referral back to a nonphysician cognitive-behavior therapist for crises or relapses. Also, occasional visits at quarterly, or even yearly, intervals to the nonphysician therapist can sometimes be helpful in maintaining treatment gains.

Group Therapy for Long-Term Treatment of Psychotic Disorders

Several acute phase treatment trials have used a group format for delivery of CBT for psychotic disorders and have generally found favorable results (Kingsep et al. 2003; Wykes et al. 2005). However, most research on CBT for psychoses has examined the effects of individual therapy. Research on long-term group methods for CBT remains to be done, but our clinical experience suggests that this method may offer an efficient and useful alternative for providing continued treatment to patients with schizophrenia and other psychoses.

Although group therapy has been shown to be useful in mild to moderate depression (see review by Lockwood et al. 2004), it has not been studied for chronic or treatment-resistant depression. Limited studies of acute phase treatment of bipolar disorder (Patelis-Siotis et al. 2001; Weiss et al. 2007) have shown some utility of group CBT for this condition. Nevertheless, we find that most patients with mood disorders are not interested in long-term group therapy during the maintenance phase of treatment.

Some of the positive features of group settings for long-term care of psychotic disorders are 1) universality, 2) normalization of illness, 3) mutual support, 4) learning coping strategies from others, and 5) promotion of treatment adherence. To give an illustration of group CBT methods for maintenance treatment, we will draw on our experiences in providing this type of service to patients with long-standing, severe symptoms of psychoses. Dr. Wright has performed continuous therapy for over 25 years with a group of persons with schizophrenia and schizoaffective disorders. The group includes members who have been attending since the first meeting and some who have joined in the last 2–3 years. All members were referred to the group because of chronicity, severe residual symptoms, and repeated hospitalizations, despite having received aggressive courses of pharmacotherapy. The average duration of treatment in the group is about 15 years. Meetings are held twice monthly for 90 minutes. The typical attendance is 10 persons out of 18 on the group roll— some patients only attend once a month or once every 6 weeks. A group discussion is held for about 60 minutes and then patients briefly meet individually with the psychiatrist to review symptoms and medication regimens. Many of the patients are taking clozapine and/or combinations of antipsychotic medications because they have not responded to monotherapy with antipsychotics.

Sessions are organized in a straightforward way. A specific agenda is not set, but each person reports, in turn, on how he is doing and has the opportunity to discuss issues that concern him. Typically in each meeting, two or three individuals bring up topics that lend themselves readily to CBT interventions. For example, a patient might report that she is experiencing increased voices because her father is quite ill with cancer. Another patient may note that he is having trouble following through with a plan (i.e., graded exposure) to overcome agoraphobic symptoms or that he wants help in stopping smoking. And still another patient may note that she has been upset by arguments with a mother-in-law, and this problem is interfering with her job selling newspapers. In each of these instances, the therapist involves both the patient and the group in developing CBT-oriented coping strategies. Frequently, these strategies are written on a whiteboard so that all group members can see the actions being considered and can offer input. Also, attempts are made by the therapist to generalize the intervention so that all group members can see some relevance to their situation.

For those patients not bringing up specific problems, the group process usually involves their giving an update on activities, making supportive comments to others, and discussing practical concerns. Examples might include making a decision about attending a community college, getting feedback on ideas for volunteer work, and asking other group members for ideas on coping with sedation from an antipsychotic medication.

Over the years that this group has been meeting, several basic attitudes about treatment have been encouraged by the therapist and have been largely endorsed by the group members as operating principles:

1. People with schizophrenia and related conditions can live a full and meaningful life.
2. Everyone in the group deserves respect, support, and concern.
3. It is a good thing to have enjoyable and pleasing activities to look forward to every day.
4. A sense of humor helps people cope.
5. Collaborating to find the right medication that gives the most help with the fewest side effects, and taking the medication regularly, keeps people well and out of the hospital.
6. CBT offers valuable skills for managing symptoms.

Adherence to medication appears to be very high in persons who attend this group. Most report that they take every dose, every day. There have been two relapses requiring hospitalization in the past 10 years. One occurred in a person who had an exacerbation of psychosis after the death of a loved one. The other relapse occurred after an insurance plan changed, and the patient was no longer able to continue taking a medication that had stabilized his symptoms. Fortunately, we were able to find a way to obtain the medication.

We present our experience with this type of group CBT to give readers a possible alternative to individual visits in longer-term maintenance therapy. Because this method has not been studied in controlled research, nothing is known about the relative merits of individual versus group maintenance, or for that matter, of the efficacy of very long-term maintenance CBT of any type for severe mental disorders. Yet, we believe that ongoing CBT of at least a minimal nature helps patients with psychoses stick with their pharmacotherapy regimens, learn more about managing their symptoms, and continue work toward meeting their goals.

Finding Meaning: Existential Issues in Long-Term Treatment

Another important element of long-term treatment of severe mental disorders is helping patients accept their illnesses while still finding a rich sense of meaning and purpose in life. To a large extent, this process starts in the earlier phases of therapy with the engaging, normalizing, and educating elements of CBT. However, as the therapy relationship matures and a deeper bond is formed, therapists have opportunities for useful discussions with patients about the significance and impact of the illness on their lives. For many patients, having a severe mental disorder has led to relationship breakups; job losses or unemployment; failure at school; loss or reduction of previous abilities (e.g., playing the piano, being an athlete, having good social skills, being thin and in good shape); financial problems; and disability.

An important principle that we have learned in our work with persons with severe mental disorders is that these types of impairments and losses do not necessarily interfere with living a highly meaningful and satisfying life. In fact, many of our patients with severe mental disorders seem to value their daily existence to a greater degree than persons who have faced much less misfortune. Of course, there are tragic outcomes of persons with severe mental disorders who suffer so much that they cannot continue to exist. One of us recalls a young woman with schizophrenia who had to drop out of college because of psychosis. Although the positive symptoms were in good control, she believed that she would never get back to her previous level of functioning. She had returned home to live with her parents. During her first year after having a psychotic episode, all of her older brothers and sisters returned home for the New Year's holiday. They were bubbling with energy and vitality. One older sister had just had her first baby, and her brother had gotten a fine job as an attorney. This should have been a happy time for the family, but the patient was found dead from a self-inflicted gunshot wound on New Year's Eve.

This very sad outcome underscores the need to assist patients with carving out a meaningful life in the face of having a serious illness. Fortunately, many other patients have been very successful at doing this. For example, David is a 60-year-old man with chronic schizophrenia who has lost two marriages because of psychosis and has been disabled for over 35 years. He lives on a very marginal income. Despite these problems, David has a great sense of well-being. He fully accepts his illness and is grateful for the benefits of clozapine, which has freed him of hallucinations and delusions. David finds special meaning in several activities that are very important to him—a close relationship with his children, visiting a nursing home 3 days a week to spend time with an old friend who lives there, and cooking interesting meals. When he attends his maintenance therapy group, he goes out of his way to offer supportive comments to others and frequently ends his remarks by saying, "Life is good."

The contrasts between these two cases are obviously quite dramatic. Both were treated by the senior author. One is a searing reminder of a failed effort at treatment. The other is a testimony to the resilience and profound capacities of our patients. In trying to help patients accept their illness and find meaning in life, the lessons taught by Victor Frankl offer special guidance and hope. In his book *Man's Search for Meaning*, Frankl (1992) talked about his experiences in a World War II concentration camp and noted that it was possible to find meaning and purpose even in the worst circumstances imaginable.

Frankl observed that it does not work for therapists to tell patients what can be meaningful. But they can ask questions that help patients find a path to a meaningful and purposeful life. Some of the areas where he recommends we help our patients search for meaning are in loving and giving, facing an illness or coping with a loss, finding meaning in everyday things, and creating something or doing a deed (Wright and Basco 2002). If we look at David's adjustment to his illness, he is finding meaning in all of these areas.

One of Frankl's main points is that meaning does not have to be attached to great accomplishments or enormous sacrifices. Instead, most people find it in the ordinary things in life—treasuring and committing to a valued relationship, coping with troubles, enjoying activities, working on projects that have a purpose to the individual. These types of involvements should be within the reach of most of our patients. Helping them achieve this level of adjustment can be a valuable long-range goal for CBT of severe mental illness.

Summary

Key Points for Clinicians

- Studies of long-term results of CBT for depression have shown positive effects on relapse prevention. Studies of bipolar disorder and schizophrenia have yielded mixed results. These studies have typically examined the long-term effects of acute phase treatment instead of assessing treatment methods for providing continuation or maintenance therapy.
- In addition to building basic CBT skills, methods recommended for relapse prevention include 1) identification of potential triggers for symptom worsening, 2) development of specific relapse prevention plans, 3) rehearsal of these plans, 4) use of coping cards and other aides to reinforce learning, and 5) implementation of CBT adherence strategies.
- Long-term continuation or maintenance therapy is recommended for patients with severe mental disorders.
- Long-term therapy can be provided in an efficient manner with booster sessions, monthly or quarterly visits with a psychiatrist (ideally trained in CBT), group therapies, or combinations of these approaches.
- The patient's acceptance of a severe mental disorder, while finding meaning and purpose in daily life, is an important long-term goal of CBT.

Concepts and Skills for Patients to Learn

- There are many skills that can be learned in CBT to help people lower the risk of symptoms coming back or getting worse.
- It is useful to think ahead to possible triggers for relapse. Spotting these potential stresses can lead to effective coping plans.
- Practicing coping strategies in therapy sessions and at home can help strengthen skills for staying well and fighting against symptom return.
- It is also important for patients and families not to catastrophize. Just because there is a reemergence of symptoms (e.g., sleep disturbance

or voices), it does not mean that relapse is inevitable or that life has to be put completely on hold.

- People who have had severe or recurrent symptoms of psychiatric disorders may have the best outcome if they see their psychiatrist and/or therapist on a routine basis for long periods of time. Even if symptoms are in good control, a regular visit several times a year can help maintain the good effects of treatment.
- One of the things that helps people with significant mental disorders to do well over the years is to find meaning and purpose in their lives.

References

Ball JR, Mitchell PB, Corry JC, et al: A randomized controlled trial of cognitive therapy for bipolar disorder: focus on long-term change. J Clin Psychiatry 67:277–286, 2006

Blackburn IM, Moore RG: Controlled acute and follow-up trial of cognitive therapy and pharmacotherapy in outpatients with recurrent depression. Br J Psychiatry 171:328–334, 1997

Bockting CL, Schene AH, Spinhoven P, et al: Preventing relapse/recurrence in recurrent depression with cognitive therapy: a randomized controlled trial. J Consult Clin Psychol 73:647–657, 2005

Fava GA, Bartolucci G, Rafanelli C, et al: Cognitive-behavioral management of patients with bipolar disorder who relapsed while on lithium prophylaxis. J Clin Psychiatry 62:556–559, 2001

Frankl VE: Man's Search for Meaning. Boston, Beacon Press, 1992

Grawe RW, Falloon IRH, Widen JH, et al: Two years of continued early treatment for schizophrenia: a randomized controlled study. Acta Psychiatr Scand 114:328–336, 2006

Gumley A, O'Grady M, McNay L, et al: Early intervention for relapse in schizophrenia: results of a 12-month randomized controlled trial of cognitive behavioural therapy. Psychol Med 33:419–431, 2003

Hollon SD, DeRubeis RJ, Evans MD, et al: Cognitive therapy and pharmacotherapy for depression: singly and in combination. Arch Gen Psychiatry 49:774–782, 1992a

Hollon SD, DeRubeis RJ, Seligman MEP: Cognitive therapy and the prevention of depression. Appl Prev Psychol 1:89–95, 1992b

Hollon SD, DeRubeis RJ, Shelton RC, et al: Prevention of relapse following cognitive therapy vs medications in moderate to severe depression. Arch Gen Psychiatry 62:417–422, 2005

Jarrett RB, Kraft D, Doyle J, et al: Preventing recurrent depression using cognitive therapy with and without a continuation phase: a randomized clinical trial. Arch Gen Psychiatry 58:381–388, 2001

Kingsep P, Nathan P, Castle D: Cognitive-behavioral group treatment for social anxiety in schizophrenia. Schizophr Res 63:121–129, 2003

Kovacs M, Rush AJ, Beck AT, et al: Depressed outpatients treated with cognitive therapy or pharmacotherapy. Arch Gen Psychiatry 38:33–39, 1981

Lam DH, Bright J, Jones S, et al: Cognitive therapy for bipolar illness—a pilot study of relapse prevention. Cognit Ther Res 24:503–520, 2000

Lam DH, Watkins ER, Hayward P, et al: A randomized controlled study of cognitive therapy for relapse prevention for bipolar affective disorder: outcome of the first year. Arch Gen Psychiatry 60:145–152, 2003

Lockwood C, Page T, Conroy-Hiller T: Comparing the effectiveness of cognitive-behavioral therapy using individual or group therapy in the treatment of depression. International Journal of Evidence-Based Healthcare 2:185–206, 2004

Patelis-Siotis I, Young T, Robb JC, et al: Group cognitive behavioral therapy for bipolar disorder: a feasibility and effectiveness study. J Affect Disord 6:145–153, 2001

Scott J, Garland A, Moorhead S: A pilot study of cognitive therapy in bipolar disorders. Psychol Med 31:459–467, 2001

Scott J, Paykel E, Morriss R, et al: Cognitive-behavioural therapy for severe and recurrent bipolar disorders: randomized controlled trial. Br J Psychiatry 188:313–320, 2006

Tarrier N, Wykes T: Is there evidence that cognitive behavior therapy is an effective treatment for schizophrenia? A cautious or cautionary tale? Behav Res Ther 42:1377–1401, 2004

Turkington D, Kingdon D, Rathod S, et al: Outcomes of an effectiveness trial of cognitive-behavioural intervention by mental health nurses in schizophrenia. Br J Psychiatry 189:36–40, 2006

Turkington D, Sensky T, Scott J, et al: A randomized controlled trial of cognitive-behavior therapy for persistent symptoms in schizophrenia: a five-year follow-up. Schizophr Res 98:1–7, 2008

Weiss RD, Griffin ML, Kolodziej ME, et al: A randomized trial of integrated group therapy versus group drug counseling for patients with bipolar disorder and substance dependence. Am J Psychiatry 164:100–107, 2007

Wright JH, Basco MR: Getting Your Life Back: The Complete Guide to Recovery From Depression. New York, Free Press, 2002

Wright JH, Thase ME, Beck AT: Cognitive therapy, in The American Psychiatric Publishing Textbook of Psychiatry, 5th Edition. Edited by Hales RE, Yudofsky SC, Gabbard GO. Washington, DC, American Psychiatric Publishing, 2008, pp 1211–1256

Wykes T, Hayward P, Thomas N, et al: What are the effects of group cognitive behavior therapy for voices? A randomized controlled trial. Schizophr Res 77:201–210, 2005

Appendix 1

Worksheets and Checklists

Contents

Cognitive-Behavior Therapy Case Formulation Worksheet[a] 316
Psychotic Symptom Rating Scales (PSYRATS) 317
What's Happening to Me? A Voice Hearing Pamphlet[a] 321
List of 60 Coping Strategies for Hallucinations[a]. 323
Thought Change Record[a]. 325
Weekly Activity Schedule[a]. 326
Schema Inventory[a]. 327

Cognitive-Behavior Therapy Case Formulation Worksheet and Weekly Activity Schedule: Reprinted from Wright JH, Basco MR, Thase ME: *Learning Cognitive-Behavior Therapy: An Illustrated Guide.* Washington, DC, American Psychiatric Publishing, 2006. Used with permission. Copyright © 2006 American Psychiatric Publishing.

Psychotic Symptom Rating Scales (PSYRATS): From Haddock G, McCarron J, Tarrier N, et al: "Scales to Measure Dimensions of Hallucinations and Delusions: The Psychotic Symptom Rating Scales (PSYRATS)." *Psychological Medicine* 29:879–889, 1999. Reproduced with permission of the lead author, Dr. G. Haddock, and Cambridge University Press.

What's Happening to Me? A Voice Hearing Pamphlet: Adapted with permission from Kingdon DG, Turkington D: *Cognitive Therapy of Schizophrenia.* New York, Guilford, 2005.

Thought Change Record: Adapted from Beck AT, Rush AJ, Shaw BF, et al: *Cognitive Therapy of Depression.* New York, Guilford, 1979, p. 403. Copyright©1979 The Guilford Press. Reprinted with permission of The Guilford Press.

Schema Inventory: Adapted from Wright JH, Wright AS, Beck AT: *Good Days Ahead: The Multimedia Program for Cognitive Therapy.* Louisville, KY, Mindstreet, 2004.

[a]These items are available as a free download in their entirety and in larger format on the American Psychiatric Publishing Web site: www.appi.org/pdf/62321. Permission is granted for readers to use these worksheets and inventories in clinical practice. Items without this footnote are not available for clinical use; please seek permission from the individual rights holder noted.

Cognitive-Behavior Therapy Case Formulation Worksheet

Patient Name:		Date:

Diagnoses/Symptoms:

Formative Influences:

Situational Issues:

Biological, Genetic, and Medical Factors:

Strengths/Assets:

Treatment Goals:

Event 1	Event 2	Event 3
Automatic Thoughts	Automatic Thoughts	Automatic Thoughts
Emotions	Emotions	Emotions
Behaviors	Behaviors	Behaviors

Schemas:

Working Hypothesis:

Treatment Plan:

Note. Available at: www.appi.org/pdf/62321.

Psychotic Symptom Rating Scales (PSYRATS)

A	Auditory hallucinations

1 Frequency

0   Voices not present or present less than once a week.

1   Voices occur for at least once a week.

2   Voices occur at least once a day.

3   Voices occur at least once an hour.

4   Voices occur continuously or almost continuously (i.e., stop for only a few seconds or minutes).

2 Duration

0   Voices not present.

1   Voices last for a few seconds; fleeting voices.

2   Voices last for several minutes.

3   Voices last for at least 1 hour.

4   Voices last for hours at a time.

3 Location

0   No voices present.

1   Voices sound like they are inside head only.

2   Voices outside the head, but close to ears or head. Voices inside the head may also be present.

3   Voices sound like they are inside or close to ears and outside head away from ears.

4   Voices sound like they are from outside the head only.

4 Loudness

0   Voices not present.

1   Quieter than own voice; whispers.

2   About same loudness as own voice.

3   Louder than own voice.

4   Extremely loud; shouting.

5 Beliefs about origin of voices

0   Voices not present.

1   Believes voices to be solely internally generated and related to self.

2   Holds <50% conviction that voices originate from external causes.

3   Holds ~50% conviction (but <100%) that voices originate from external causes.

4   Believes voices are solely due to external causes (100% conviction).

6   Amount of negative content of voices
0   No unpleasant content.
1   Occasional unpleasant content (<10%).
2   Minority of voice content is unpleasant or negative (<50%).
3   Majority of voice content is unpleasant or negative (>50%).
4   All of voice content is unpleasant or negative.

7   Degree of negative content
0   Not unpleasant or negative.
1   Some degree of negative content, but not personal comments relating to self or family (e.g., swear words) or comments not directed to self (e.g., "The milkman's ugly").
2   Personal verbal abuse; comments on behavior (e.g., "shouldn't do that or say that").
3   Personal verbal abuse relating to self-concept (e.g., "You're lazy, ugly, mad, perverted").
4   Personal threats to self (e.g., threats to harm self or family); extreme instructions or commands to harm self or others.

8   Amount of distress
0   Voices not distressing at all.
1   Voices occasionally distressing; majority not distressing (<10%).
2   Minority of voices distressing (<50%).
3   Majority of voices distressing; minority not distressing (~50%).
4   Voices always distressing.

9   Intensity of distress
0   Voices not distressing at all.
1   Voices slightly distressing.
2   Voices are distressing to a moderate degree.
3   Voices are very distressing, although subject could feel worse.
4   Voices are extremely distressing; patient feels the worst he/she could possibly feel.

10   Disruption to life caused by voices
0   No disruption to life; patient able to maintain social and family relationships (if present).
1   Voices cause minimal amount of disruption to life (e.g., interfere with concentration although patient able to maintain daytime activity and social and family relationships and able to maintain independent living without support).

2   Voices cause moderate amount of disruption to life causing some disturbance to daytime activity and/or family or social activities. The patient is not in hospital although may live in supported accommodation or receive additional help with daily living skills.

3   Voices cause severe disruption to life so that hospitalization is usually necessary. The patient is able to maintain some daily activities, self-care, and relationships while in hospital. The patient may also be in supported accommodation but experiencing severe disruption of life in terms of activities, daily living skills, and/or relationships.

4   Voices cause complete disruption of daily life requiring hospitalization. The patient is unable to maintain any daily activities and social relationships. Self-care is also severely disrupted.

11   Controllability of voices

0   Subject believes he can have control over the voices and can always bring on or dismiss them at will.

1   Subject believes she can have some control over the voices on the majority of occasions.

2   Subject believes he can have some control over the voices approximately half of the time.

3   Subject believes she can have some control over the voices but only occasionally. The majority of the time the subject experiences voices that are uncontrollable.

4   Subject has no control over when the voices occur and cannot dismiss or bring them on at all.

B	**Delusions**

1   Amount of preoccupation with delusions

0   No delusions, or delusions that the subject thinks about less than once a week.

1   Subject thinks about beliefs at least once a week.

2   Subject thinks about beliefs at least once a day.

3   Subject thinks about beliefs at least once an hour.

4   Subject thinks about delusions continuously or almost continuously.

2   Duration of preoccupation with delusions

0   No delusions.

1   Thoughts about beliefs last for a few seconds; fleeting thoughts.

2   Thoughts about delusions last for several minutes.

3   Thoughts about delusions last for at least 1 hour.

4   Thoughts about delusions usually last for hours at a time.

3   Conviction
0   No conviction at all.
1   Very little conviction in reality of beliefs, <10%.
2   Some doubts relating to conviction in beliefs, between 10% and 49%.
3   Conviction in belief is very strong, between 50% and 99%.
4   Conviction is 100%.

4   Amount of distress
0   Beliefs never cause distress.
1   Beliefs cause distress on the minority of occasions.
2   Beliefs cause distress on <50% of occasions.
3   Beliefs cause distress on the majority of occasions when they
      occur between 50% and 99% of time.
4   Beliefs always cause distress when they occur.

5   Intensity of distress
0   No distress.
1   Beliefs cause slight distress.
2   Beliefs cause moderate distress.
3   Beliefs cause marked distress.
4   Beliefs cause extreme distress, could not be worse.

6   Disruption to life caused by beliefs
0   No disruption to life, able to maintain independent living with no
      problems in daily living skills. Able to maintain social and family
      relationships (if present).
1   Beliefs cause minimal amount of disruption to life (e.g., interferes
      with concentration although patient able to maintain daytime
      activity and social and family relationships and able to maintain
      independent living without support).
2   Beliefs cause moderate amount of disruption to life causing some
      disturbance to daytime activity and/or family or social activities.
      The patient is not in hospital although may live in supported
      accommodation or receive additional help with daily living skills.
3   Beliefs cause severe disruption to life so that hospitalization is
      usually necessary. The patient is able to maintain some daily
      activities, self-care, and relationships while in hospital. The
      patient may be also be in supported accommodation but
      experiencing severe disruption of life in terms of activities, daily
      living skills, and/or relationships.
4   Beliefs cause complete disruption of daily life requiring
      hospitalization. The patient is unable to maintain any daily activities
      and social relationships. Self-care is also severely disrupted.

What's Happening to Me?

A Voice Hearing Pamphlet

The difficulties you have been having may be related to the stresses you have been facing. You may be having strange experiences that frighten or excite you. There may be problems with your family or at your work. You may be thinking that neither your family nor anybody else understands.

When someone is under stress, it can affect him or her in all sorts of ways. Sometimes the very fact that others don't believe or understand can seem to be part of the problem.

Perhaps you are having trouble sleeping—lack of sleep can make you vulnerable. As an example, some people can start to hear people talking when nobody is around, or else the talking seems to come from places or directions where nobody seems to be. The conversation you hear might be about you, discussing or even criticizing you. There might even be commands telling you to do things—often things that you don't want to do. The voices that you hear may be quite abusive and rude.

At some time or other, many people hear voices or see things when nobody's around them. Surveys suggest that voice hearing can occur in one in six people at some time, and in even more people when put under certain sorts of stress. So voice hearing is not uncommon, but it can be very worrying, particularly if it keeps happening.

What Can I Do About It?

First, are you sure that nobody else can hear what is being said? Sometimes people speaking from outside a room, or machinery (for example, air conditioning), can be deceiving. If you need to, check with someone you trust—maybe a member of your family, a close friend, or the doctor, nurse, or psychologist whom you are seeing—whether they can hear the voices that you are hearing.

If they can't hear the voices, you need to consider why that could be. Do you think there is some special method by which the voices are being transmitted to you? It is difficult to imagine what method there could be, but talk with your therapist about any ideas you have.

Finally, it might be worth considering the possibility that pressures you have been under have stimulated the voices and that your mind is "deceiving" you. These pressures might have occurred recently or been around at

Note. Available at: www.appi.org/pdf/62321.

the time when you first heard the voices. Voices, or hallucinations, can come on when you are not sleeping properly or when you have been very isolated. They can occur when people are put in solitary confinement or held hostage. Very emotional events—like being in an accident or being assaulted—can produce images and sounds that are very vivid. These images and sounds can come on as flashbacks. These types of experiences can also occur during drug taking and after drugs have been abused. Some people have described hallucinating as being just like "dreaming awake." Voice hearing and other hallucinations can happen with severe depression, schizophrenia, or nervous breakdowns.

What Can Help With Coping?

When voices seem to be caused by other people or agencies, it can be very frightening. Being able to understand them better can reduce some of that fear and can make the voices less intense and worrying.

Fortunately, there is also medication that can be useful. You will probably be offered medication by your doctor. Medication will be able to help you with sleeping—if that is a problem—and in more complex ways, help with worries and hallucinations. If you have any concerns about the medication you are taking, or are offered, ask your doctor or therapist. There is good information available about how medication works and what it does.

Sometimes when people are hearing voices, they find that developing ways of coping can help, like listening to the radio or to some music. Others have found assistance from physical exercise, such as going for a walk, or chatting with friends or family. If the voices persist, it is worth trying to work out ways to help you cope.

But most of all, find someone you can trust and let them know how you feel. Ask about the problems and worries you have. There are likely to be ways of helping you deal with the problems you are experiencing.

Note. Available at: www.appi.org/pdf/62321.

List of 60 Coping Strategies for Hallucinations

Distraction

1. Hum
2. Talk to yourself
3. Listen to modern music
4. Listen to classical music
5. Prayer
6. Meditation
7. Use a mantra
8. Painting
9. Imagery
10. Walk in the fresh air
11. Phone a friend
12. Exercise
13. Use a relaxation tape
14. Yoga
15. Take a warm bath
16. Call your mental health professional
17. Attend the day center/drop in
18. Watch TV
19. Do a crossword or other puzzle
20. Play a computer game
21. Try a new hobby

Focusing

1. Correct the cognitive distortions in the voices
2. Respond rationally to voice content
3. Use subvocalization
4. Dismiss the voices
5. Remind yourself that no one else can hear the voice
6. Phone a voice buddy and tell him or her the voice is active
7. Remember to take antipsychotic medication
8. Demonstrate controllability by bringing the voices on
9. Give the voices a 10-minute slot at a specific time each day
10. Play a cognitive therapy tape discussing voice control
11. Use a normalizing explanation
12. Use rational responses to reduce anger
13. List the evidence in favor of the voice content
14. List the evidence against the voice content

Note. Available at: www.appi.org/pdf/62321.

15. Use guided imagery to practice coping with the voices differently
16. Role-play for and against the voices
17. Remind yourself that voices are not actions and need not be viewed that way
18. Remind yourself that the voices don't seem to know much
19. Remind yourself that you don't need to obey the voices
20. Talk to someone you trust about the voice content
21. Use rational responses to reduce shame
22. Use rational responses to reduce anxiety
23. Use a diary to manage stress
24. Use a diary to manage your time
25. Plan your daily activities the night before
26. Use a voice diary in a scientific manner
27. Mindfulness
28. Try an earplug (right ear first if right-handed)

Meta-cognitive Methods

1. Use schema-focused techniques
2. Acceptance
3. Assertiveness
4. Use a biological model
5. Consider shamanistic views of voice hearing
6. Consider cultural aspects of voice hearing
7. Keep a list of daily behaviors to prove that you are not as bad as the voices say
8. Use a continuum relating your own worth to that of other people
9. List your positive experiences in life
10. List your achievements, friendships, etc.
11. Act against the voices (show them that you are better than they say)

Note.   Available at: www.appi.org/pdf/62321.

Thought Change Record

Situation	Automatic thought(s)	Emotion(s)	Rational response	Outcome
Describe a. Actual event leading to unpleasant emotion *or* b. Stream of thoughts leading to unpleasant emotion *or* c. Unpleasant physiological sensations.	a. *Write* automatic thought(s) that preceded emotion(s). b. *Rate* belief in automatic thought(s), 0%–100%.	a. *Specify* sad, anxious, angry, etc. b. *Rate* degree of emotion, 1%–100%.	a. *Identify* cognitive errors. b. *Write* rational response to automatic thought(s). c. *Rate* belief in rational response, 0%–100%.	a. *Specify and rate* subsequent emotion(s), 0%–100%. b. *Describe* changes in behavior.

Note. Available at: www.appi.org/pdf/62321.

Weekly Activity Schedule

Instructions: Write down your activities for each hour and then rate them on a scale of 0–10 for mastery (**m**) or degree of accomplishment and for pleasure (**p**) or amount of enjoyment you experienced. A rating of 0 would mean that you had no sense of mastery or pleasure. A rating of 10 would mean that you experienced maximum mastery or pleasure.

	Sunday	Monday	Tuesday	Wednesday	Thursday	Friday	Saturday
8:00 A.M.							
9:00 A.M.							
10:00 A.M.							
11:00 A.M.							
12:00 P.M.							
1:00 P.M.							
2:00 P.M.							
3:00 P.M.							
4:00 P.M.							
5:00 P.M.							
6:00 P.M.							
7:00 P.M.							
8:00 P.M.							
9:00 P.M.							

Note.   Available at: www.appi.org/pdf/62321.

Schema Inventory

Instructions: Use this checklist to search for possible underlying rules of thinking. Place a check mark beside each schema that you think you may have.

Healthy Schemas

___No matter what happens, I can manage somehow.

___If I work hard at something, I can master it.

___I'm a survivor.

___Others trust me.

___I'm a solid person.

___People respect me.

___They can knock me down, but they can't knock me out.

___I care about other people.

___If I prepare in advance, I usually do better.

___I deserve to be respected.

___I like to be challenged.

___There's not much that can scare me.

___I'm intelligent.

___I can figure things out.

___I'm friendly.

___I can handle stress.

___The tougher the problem, the tougher I become.

___I can learn from my mistakes and be a better person.

___I'm a good spouse (and/or parent, child, friend, lover).

___Everything will work out all right.

Dysfunctional Schemas

___I must be perfect to be accepted.

___I'm invincible.

___I'm stupid.

___Without a woman (man), I'm nothing.

___I'm a fake.

___I always know the best way.

___I'm unlovable.

___I'm useless.

___I'll never be comfortable around others.

___I'm damaged.

___No matter what I do, I won't succeed.

___The world is too frightening for me.

___Others can't be trusted.

___I must always be in control.

___I'm unattractive.

___Never show your emotions.

___Other people will take advantage of me.

___I'm lazy.

___If people really knew me, they wouldn't like me.

___To be accepted, I must always please others.

Note. Available at: www.appi.org/pdf/62321.

Appendix 2

Cognitive-Behavior Therapy Resources

Books for Patients and Families

Basco MR: Never Good Enough: How to Use Perfectionism to Your Advantage Without Letting It Ruin Your Life. New York, Free Press, 1999

Basco MR: The Bipolar Workbook: Tools for Controlling Your Mood Swings. New York, Guilford, 2006

Beck AT, Greenberg RC, Beck J: Coping With Depression (booklet). Bala Cynwyd, PA, The Beck Institute, 1995

Burns DD: Feeling Good: The New Mood Therapy, Revised Edition. New York, Avon, 1999

Greenberger D, Padesky CA: Mind Over Mood: Change How You Feel by Changing the Way You Think. New York, Guilford, 1996

Miklowitz DJ: The Bipolar Survival Guide: What You and Your Family Need to Know. New York, Guilford, 2002

Mueser KT, Gingerich S: The Complete Family Guide to Schizophrenia. New York, Guilford, 2006

Romme M, Escher S: Understanding Voices: Coping With Auditory Hallucinations and Confusing Realities. London, Handsell, 1996

Turkington D, Rathod S, Wilcock S, et al: Back to Life, Back to Normality: Cognitive Therapy, Recovery and Psychosis. Cambridge, England, Cambridge University Press, 2008

Wright JH, Basco MR: Getting Your Life Back: The Complete Guide to Recovery From Depression. New York, Free Press, 2002

Personal Accounts of Mental Illness

Duke P: Brilliant Madness: Living With Manic Depressive Illness. New York, Bantam Books, 1992

Jamison K: An Unquiet Mind. New York, Knopf, 1995

Nasar SA: A Beautiful Mind (biography). New York, Touchstone, 1998

Note. Appendix 2 is available at: www.appi.org/pdf/62321.

Shields B: Down Came the Rain. New York, Hyperion, 2005
Styron W: Darkness Visible: A Memoir of Madness. New York, Random House, 1990

Computer Programs

Beating the Blues (www.thewellnessshop.co.uk/products/beatingtheblues)
Good Days Ahead (www.mindstreet.com)

Web Sites With Educational Information for Patients and Families

Academy of Cognitive Therapy (www.academyofct.org): How to find a cognitive therapist, recommended reading, new research
Depression and Bipolar Support Alliance (www.dbsalliance.org): An advocacy and support group
Gloucestershire Hearing Voices and Recovery Groups (www.hearingvoices.org.uk/info_resources11.htm): Over 20 examples of good advice on coping with voice hearing
Good Days Ahead (www.gooddaysahead.com): General information on CBT, demonstration of computer program for CBT for depression and anxiety
Making Common Sense of Voices (www.peter-lehmann-publishing.com/articles/others/klafki_making.htm): A normalizing essay on the subject of voice hearing that could be used as a homework exercise
Mind (www.mind.org.uk/Information/Booklets/Other/The+voice+inside.htm): A practical guide to understanding voice hearing, written by the Hearing Voices Network
Mood Gym (http://moodgym.anu.edu.au): Self-help program for CBT of depression and anxiety
National Alliance on Mental Illness (NAMI; www.nami.org): Education on severe mental disorders, support for patients and families, advocacy
National Institute of Mental Health (www.nimh.nih.gov): General information on research and treatment of severe mental disorders
Paranoid Thoughts (www.iop.kcl.ac.uk/apps/paranoidthoughts/default.html): Helpful advice on coping with paranoia; based on the book *Overcoming Paranoid and Suspicious Thoughts* by Freeman, Freeman, and Garety (see Recommended Readings later in this Appendix)
University of Louisville Depression Center (http://louisville.edu/depression): Depression screening, educational programs with focus on CBT, general information on depression
University of Michigan Depression Center (www.med.umich.edu/depression): Depression screening, educational programs, general information on depression

Professional Organizations With Special Interest in CBT

Academy of Cognitive Therapy (www.academyofct.org)

Association for Behavioral and Cognitive Therapies (www.aabt.org)

British Association for Behavioural and Cognitive Psychotherapies (www.babcp.com)

European Association for Behavioural and Cognitive Therapies (www.eabct.com)

French Association for Behavior and Cognitive Therapy (Association Française de Thérapie Comportementale et Cognitive; www.aftcc.org)

International Association for Cognitive Psychotherapy (IACP; www.cognitivetherapyassociation.org)

Recommended Readings

Barrowclough C, Haddock G, Tarrier N, et al: Randomized controlled trial of motivational interviewing, cognitive behavior therapy, and family intervention for patients with comorbid schizophrenia and substance use disorders. Am J Psychiatry 158:1706–1713, 2001

Basco MR, Rush AJ: Cognitive-Behavioral Therapy for Bipolar Disorder, 2nd Edition. New York, Guilford, 2005

Baucom DH, Epstein NB: Cognitive Behavioral Marital Therapy. New York, Brunner/Mazel, 1990

Beck AT: Love Is Never Enough: How Couples Can Overcome Misunderstandings, Resolve Conflicts, and Solve Relationship Problems Through Cognitive Therapy. New York, Harper & Row, 1988

Beck AT, Rush AJ, Shaw BF, et al: Cognitive Therapy of Depression. New York, Guilford, 1979

Beck AT, Emery GD, Greenberg RL: Anxiety Disorders and Phobias: A Cognitive Perspective. New York, Basic Books, 1985

Beck AT, Wright FD, Newman CF, et al: Cognitive Therapy for Substance Abuse. New York, Guilford, 1993

Beck AT, Freeman A, Davis DD, et al: Cognitive Therapy of Personality Disorders, 2nd Edition. New York, Guilford, 2003

Beck JS: Cognitive Therapy: Basics and Beyond. New York, Guilford, 1995

Carroll KM, Onken LS: Behavioral therapies for drug abuse. Am J Psychiatry 162:1452–1460, 2005

Chadwick P: Person-Based Cognitive Therapy for Distressing Psychosis. Chichester, England, Wiley, 2006

Clark DA, Beck AT, Alford BA: Scientific Foundations of Cognitive Theory and Therapy of Depression. New York, Wiley, 1999

Dattilio FM, Padesky CA: Cognitive Therapy With Couples. Sarasota, FL, Professional Resource Exchange, 1990

Epstein NB, Baucom DH: Enhanced Cognitive Behavioral Therapy for Couples: A Contextual Approach. Washington, DC, American Psychological Association, 2002

Epstein NB, Schlesinger SE, Dryden W: Cognitive-Behavior Therapy With Families. New York, Brunner/Mazel, 1988

Frank E: Treating Bipolar Disorder: A Clinician's Guide to Interpersonal and Social Rhythm Therapy. New York, Guilford, 2005

Frankl VE: Man's Search for Meaning: An Introduction to Logotherapy, 4th Edition. Boston, Beacon Press, 1992

Freeman D, Freeman J, Garety P: Overcoming Paranoid and Suspicious Thoughts. London, Robinson, 2006

Garner DM, Vitousek KM, Pike KM: Cognitive behavioral therapy for anorexia nervosa, in Handbook of Treatment for Eating Disorders, 2nd Edition. Edited by Garner DM, Garfinkel PE. New York, Guilford, 1997, pp 94–144

Gumley A, Schwannauer M: Staying Well After Psychosis: A Cognitive Interpersonal Approach to Recovery and Relapse Prevention. Chichester, England, Wiley, 2006

Haddock G, Slade PD (eds): Cognitive Behavioral Interventions With Psychotic Disorders. London, Routledge, 1996

Kabat-Zinn J: Full Catastrophe Living: Using the Wisdom of Your Body to Fight Stress, Pain, and Illness. New York, Hyperion, 1990

Kingdon DG, Turkington D: A Case Study Guide to Cognitive Therapy of Psychosis. Chichester, England, Wiley, 2002

Kingdon DG, Turkington D: Cognitive Therapy of Schizophrenia. New York, Guilford, 2005

Linehan MM: Cognitive-Behavioral Treatment of Borderline Personality Disorder. New York, Guilford, 1993

McCullough JP Jr: Treatment for Chronic Depression: Cognitive Behavioral Analysis System of Psychotherapy. New York, Guilford, 2000

Morrison AP: A Casebook of Cognitive Therapy for Psychosis. New York, Brunner-Routledge, 2002

Morrison AP: Cognitive Therapy for Psychosis: A Formulation-Based Approach. New York, Brunner-Routledge, 2002

Naeem F, Kingdon D, Turkington D: Cognitive behavior therapy for schizophrenia in patients with mild to moderate substance misuse problems. Cogn Behav Ther 35:207–215, 2005

Nelson HE: Cognitive Behavioural Therapy With Schizophrenia: A Practice Manual. Cheltenham, England, Stanley Thornes, 2005

Romme M, Escher S: Accepting Voices: A New Approach to Voice-Hearing Outside the Illness Model. London, Mind, 1993

Romme M, Escher S: Making Sense of Voices: A Guide for Professionals Who Work With Voice Hearers. London, Mind, 2000

Safran J, Segal Z: Interpersonal Processes in Cognitive Therapy. New York, Basic Books, 1990

Segal Z, Williams JMG, Teasdale JD: Mindfulness-Based Cognitive Therapy for Depression: A New Approach to Preventing Relapse. New York, Guilford, 2002

Wakefield PJ, Williams RE, Yost EB, et al: Couple Therapy for Alcoholism: A Cognitive-Behavioral Treatment Manual. New York, Guilford, 1996

Weiss RD: Treatment of patients with bipolar disorder and substance dependence: lessons learned. J Subst Abuse Treat 27:307–312, 2007

White JR, Freeman AS (eds): Cognitive-Behavioral Group Therapy for Specific Problems and Populations. Washington DC, American Psychological Association, 2000

Williams M, Teasdale J, Segal Z, et al: The Mindful Way Through Depression: Freeing Yourself From Chronic Unhappiness. New York, Guilford, 2007

Wright JH (ed): Cognitive-Behavior Therapy (Review of Psychiatry Series, Vol 23; Oldham JM, Riba MB, series eds). Washington DC, American Psychiatric Publishing, 2004

Wright JH, Thase ME, Beck AT, et al (eds): Cognitive Therapy With Inpatients: Developing a Cognitive Milieu. New York, Guilford, 1993

Wright JH, Basco MR, Thase ME: Learning Cognitive-Behavior Therapy: An Illustrated Guide. Washington, DC, American Psychiatric Publishing, 2006

Appendix 3

DVD Guide

Instructions

Place the DVD in a DVD player or a computer with a DVD drive. A title page will be displayed. Select **Menu** to view the Menu screens, or wait a few seconds until the Menu screens automatically appear. Select individual videos to view as desired.

If you are viewing the DVD on a personal computer, control options such as Menu, Pause, Play, or DVD Properties should be displayed. If they are not displayed, clicking on the right mouse button will often provide control options.

System Requirements for DVD Playback on a Computer

Windows XP or Vista

Windows Media Player 11 fully supports DVD playback as long as a compatible DVD decoder is installed. Most users with computers that have DVD drives have DVD decoders preinstalled by their hardware manufacturers.

When you insert a DVD movie into your DVD drive for the first time, you'll be prompted to play the DVD movie. If you get an error message when trying to play the DVD with Windows Media Player, you need a DVD decoder. If you bought a PC equipped with a DVD drive, check with the computer manufacturer. The manufacturer may have updated Windows XP or Vista DVD decoder drivers available, often for free.

335

For more information on installing a DVD decoder, please visit Microsoft's support Web site at http://support.microsoft.com, and view article 306331. The article can be found by entering "306331" in the "Search" box.

The minimum system requirements for Windows Media Player 11 are as follows:

- One of the following operating systems:
    – Microsoft Windows XP Home Edition Service Pack 2 (SP2), Windows XP Professional SP2, or Windows XP Tablet PC Edition SP2, including the N and KN editions, which do not include Windows Media Player and related technologies
    – Windows XP Media Center Edition 2005 with KB900325 (Update Rollup 2 for Windows XP Media Center Edition 2005) and KB925766 (the October 2006 Update Rollup) installed
    – Any N or KN edition of Windows Vista that does not include Windows Media Player and related technologies
- A 233 megahertz (MHz) processor, such as an Intel Pentium II or Advanced Micro Devices (AMD) processor
- 64 megabytes (MB) RAM
- 200 MB free hard disk space
- DVD drive with compatible DVD decoder software
- 28.8 kilobits per second (Kbps) modem or broadband connection
- 16-bit sound card
- Super VGA (800 x 600) monitor resolution
- Video card with 64 MB of RAM (video RAM or VRAM) and DirectX 9.0b
- Speakers or headphones
- Microsoft Internet Explorer 6 or Netscape 7.1

Mac OSX

The following Macintosh models support DVD drives and can play DVD-video discs: Power Mac G5, eMac, PowerBook G4, iBook, iMac, and Mac mini computers. For the latest version of the DVD playback software, visit the following Web site: www.apple.com/macosx/features/dvdplayer.

Video Illustrations

Number	Title	Time (minutes)
1	Engaging a Patient With Paranoia: Dr. Kingdon and Majir	8:19
2	Engaging a Patient With Bipolar Disorder: Dr. Basco and Angela	7:06
3	Engaging a Patient With Chronic Depression: Dr. Wright and Mary	12:50
4	Normalizing and Educating: Dr. Turkington and Brenda	7:15
5	Tracing the Origins of Paranoia: Dr. Kingdon and Majir	7:32
6	Examining the Evidence for Paranoia: Dr. Kingdon and Majir	9:31
7	Working With a Resistant Delusion: Dr. Kingdon and Majir	9:04
8	Explaining Hallucinations: Dr. Turkington and Brenda	6:54
9	Coping With Hallucinations: Dr. Turkington and Brenda	9:26
10	An Antisuicide Plan: Dr. Wright and Mary	11:26
11	Behavioral Intervention for Anhedonia: Dr. Wright and Mary	8:23
12	Building Self-Esteem: Dr. Wright and Mary	12:10
13	Reducing Grandiosity: Dr. Basco and Angela	12:38
14	Using an Early Warning System: Dr. Basco and Angela	9:05
15	Helping With Thought Disorder: Dr. Turkington and Daniel	7:40
16	Investigating a Delusion: Dr. Turkington and Daniel	2:19
17	Treating Negative Symptoms: Dr. Kingdon and Majir	6:22
18	Promoting Adherence: Dr. Basco and Angela	10:00
Total Time		158:00

Index

*Page numbers printed in **boldface** type refer to tables or figures.*

ABC technique, for delusions, 111
Academy of Cognitive Therapy, 75, 84–85
Acceptance, and adherence with medication, 276–277
Accepting Voices: A New Approach to Voice-Hearing Outside the Illness Model (Romme and Escher 1993), 56, **68**
Action plan, for demotivation in schizophrenia, 262
Activity scheduling
  antisuicide plan and, 157–158
  depression and, 15, 162–163, 165
  mania and daily activities in, **250**
  negative symptoms and, 61, 267, **268**
  prevention plans for mania and, 186–187, **196,** 202
  self-esteem and, 174
Adaptive cognitions, and suicidality, 153
Adherence
  basic CBT methods and, 12, 17–18

cognitive interventions and, 281–286
common reasons and possible solutions, 275–281
efficacy of CBT for enhancing, 273–274
group therapy and, 310
homework assignments and, 281, 290–291
learning exercise for, 289–290
prevention plans for mania and, 182–183, 198
relapse prevention and, 301–302
types of nonadherence, 275
video illustration and, 280–281
written plans for, 286–290
Affective blunting, **61**
Agenda, for therapy, 17, 38–39, 96, 217, 252, **305,** 309
Aggression
  contraindications for CBT and, 48
  engagement process and, 30
A list/B list exercise, and mania, 202
Alogia, **61,** 258, 259

Anger, and nonadherence, 276

Anhedonia, **3, 61,** 163, 258–259. *See also* Low energy and interest

Antipsychotics, 2, 4, 35, 119, 241, 309

adherence and, 56–57, 274

Antisocial personality disorder, 48

Antisuicide plans, 149–160, **150**

Anxiety

interpersonal relationships and, 215

thought disorder in schizophrenia and, 244

Assertiveness training

adherence with medication and, 280

conflict management and, 186

interpersonal relationships and, 218–219, 231

Assessment. *See also* Diagnosis; Evaluation

basic process of, 45–47

delusions and, 99

evaluation of hallucinations and, 127, **129**

schizophrenia diagnosis and, **52, 53, 54, 55**

of vulnerability to severe mental illness, **85**

Attention. *See also* Distraction and distractibility

cognitive dysfunction in depression and, **251**

negative symptoms and deficit of, 258, 259

Auditory hallucinations, 128, **129, 130**. *See also* Hallucinations

Automatic thoughts. *See also* Thought disorder

adherence and, 17–18

assessment and, 47

basic CBT methods and, 12, 14–15

depression and interpersonal relationships, 222–224, **225**

schizophrenia diagnosis and, **52, 55**

self-esteem and, 170

Avoidance, and bipolar disorder, 229

Back to Life, Back to Normality (Turkington et al. 2008), **68**

Beating the Blues (computer program), 252

Beautiful Mind, A (Nasar 1998), **68**

Beck, Aaron, xii, 1, 16, 18, 44, 69, 145, 171

Beck Cognitive Insight Scale, 104

Beck Depression Inventory, 146

Beck Hopelessness Scale (BHS), 146

Befriending, and therapeutic relationship, 13

Behavior(s). *See also* Behavioral interventions and strategies

antisuicide plans and, 153

case formulation and, 77, 84–86

contraindications for CBT and criminal, 48

hallucinations and, **131**

recurrence of mania and, **207**

self-esteem and, 168–171, 174

therapeutic relationship and, 30–32

working model of CBT and, 8–9

Behavioral activation, 160–162

Behavioral interventions and strategies. *See also* Behavior(s)

adherence with treatment and, 17, 278

basic CBT methods and, 12, 15–16

control of mania symptoms and, 200–203

hopelessness in depression and, 148

low energy and lack of interest in depression and, 160–162

negative symptoms and, 266–270

video illustration and, 163

Beliefs, and delusions, 100, 102, 121–122. *See also* Core beliefs

Bereavement and grief
hallucinations and, **130**
interpersonal relationships and,
216–217
Bipolar disorder. *See also* Mania and
hypomania
case study (Angela)
case formulation, 87, 91, **92–
93**, 93
introduction, 10, **10**
video illustrations, 40–41, 204,
206–207, 280–281
efficacy of CBT for, 19–20
engagement process and, 40–42
interpersonal relationships and,
226–233
learning exercise for, 228–229
normalizing of, 62
psychoeducation and, 68–69
relapse prevention and, 296, 298
substance abuse and, 18
*Bipolar Survival Guide: What You and
Your Family Need to Know, The*
(Miklowitz 2002), 69
*Bipolar Workbook: Tools for Controlling
Your Mood Swings, The* (Basco
2006), 69, 203, 248
Books. *See* Reading
Booster sessions, and continuation of
CBT, 304–305
Boundary issues, and interpersonal
relationships, 218–219
Brainstorming
adherence with medication and,
285
for enjoyable activities, 268
in learning exercises for
examining the evidence, 109–
110
mania prevention plan, 207–208
resistant depression and, 163
Brief Core Schema Scales (BCSS), 139
*Brilliant Madness: Living With Manic
Depressive Illness* (Duke 1992),
68

Case formulation, 75–98
delusions and, 100
examples of biopsychosocial, 87–
93
identification of schemas, 86
learning exercise for, 93–94
mini-formulation and, 94–97
obtaining information on current
cognitions and behaviors, 84–
86
Socratic questioning and, 83–84
timelines and, 80–84
treatment planning and, 75–76, 87
working hypothesis for, 86–87
worksheet for development of,
76–80, **88–93**
Case studies and examples
antisuicide plan, for schizophrenia
(Antonio), 156–158, **159**
bipolar disorder (Angela), 10, **10**,
40–41, 87, 91, **92–93**, 93,
204, 206–207, 280–281
boundary issues (Jim), 218–219
chronic depression (Mary),10–11,
11, 44–45, 77, **78–79**, 80,
150–152, 163, 171–172
cognitive rehearsal, in depression
(Thad), 252–253
examining the evidence in
major depression (Roberto),
119–121
schizophrenia (Rhonda), 107–
109
managing symptom triggers
(Mark), 187–189
mini-formulation (Terrance), 96–
97
normalizing negative symptoms
(Martin), 61
paranoia in
schizoaffective disorder
(Kenyatta), 305–307
schizophrenia (Daniel), 243–244,
244–246, 286–290, **288**,
289

Case studies and examples *(continued)*
 paranoia in *(continued)*
  schizophrenia (Majir), 9, **9**, 30,
   87, **90–91,** 104–105, 106–
   107, 115–116, 263–264
  schizophrenia (Rhonda), 107–
   109
  resistant delusions (James), 114–115
  schizophrenia (Brenda), 54–56,
   80, **81,** 82–83, 87, **88–89,**
   132–134
  setting an agenda (Seth), 38–39
Catatonia, and engagement process,
 30–31
Catch—Control—Correct method,
 and mania, 203–204
CBT. *See* Cognitive-behavior therapy
Checklists
 adherence with medication and,
  279
 list of, 315–327
Circadian rhythms, and sleep-wake
 cycle, 167
Clozapine, 309, 311
Coaching techniques
 adherence with medication and,
  284
 chronic depression and, 163,
  164
Cognitive appraisal, and working
 model of CBT, **8,** 8–9
Cognitive Behavioral Analysis System
 of Psychotherapy (CBASP),
 21
Cognitive-behavioral-biological-
 sociocultural model, 4–12, **5**
Cognitive-behavior therapy (CBT). *See
 also* Adherence; Case formulation;
 Cognitive dysfunctions; Delusions;
 Depression; Engagement;
 Hallucinations; Interpersonal
 relationships; Mania; Negative
 symptoms; Normalizing and
 destigmatizing; Psychoeducation;
 Therapeutic relationship

 assessment for, 45–47
 cognitive-behavioral-biological-
  sociocultural model of, 4–12
 computer-assisted forms of, 252
 continuation and maintenance of,
  303–312
 efficacy of for severe mental
  disorders, 19–21
 guide to resources on, 329–333
 indications for, 47–48
 origins and development of, 1
 overview of treatment methods,
  12–19
 phases of patients learning about,
  71
 rationale for use in severe mental
  disorders, 2–4
 relapse prevention and, 3–4, **12,**
  18–19, 295–302
 targets for in severe mental illness,
  3
 worksheets and checklists for,
  315–327
Cognitive-Behavior Therapy Case
 Formulation Worksheet, 315,
 316
*Cognitive-Behavioural Therapy of
 Schizophrenia* (Kingdon and
 Turkington 1994), **68**
Cognitive dysfunctions. *See also*
 Attention; Automatic thoughts;
 Beliefs; Cognitive interventions
 antisuicide plans and, 153
 basic CBT methods and, 12, 16–
  17
 case formulation and, 77, 84–86
 cognitive appraisal and, **8,** 8–9
 depression and, 251–254, **255**
 engagement process and, **31,** 32,
  43
 in mania and hypomania, 247–251
 recurrence of mania and, **207**
 self-esteem and, 168–171
 thought disorder in schizophrenia
  and, 238–247

Cognitive interventions. *See also*
   Cognitive dysfunctions;
   Cognitive restructuring
   adherence with medication and,
      281–286
   depression and, **255**
   for improving energy and interest
      in depression, 165–166
   interpersonal relationships and,
      219
   prevention plans for mania and,
      203–204
   self-esteem and, 171–174
   sleep management and, 185
Cognitive restructuring. *See also*
   Cognitive interventions
   adherence with medication and,
      281–282
   engagement process in bipolar
      disorder and, 41–42
   hopelessness in depression and, 149
Collaborative empiricism, 127
Collaborative medication
   management, 274
Combined treatment, with CBT and
   pharmacotherapy, 4, 305–308
Command hallucinations, 125, 126,
   140
Compliance, use of term, 274. *See
   also* Adherence
Comprehensive biopsychosocial
   approach, to CBT, 4, 6–7
Computer-assisted CBT, 252, 330.
   See also Web sites
Concentration. *See* Cognitive
   dysfunctions
Concrete thinking, and
   schizophrenia, 239
Confidentiality, and use of
   interpreters, 34
Conflict
   bipolar disorder and interpersonal
      relationships, 227–231
   stress and prevention plans for
      mania, 185–186

Continuation, of CBT, 303–312
Contraindications, for CBT, 48
Coping cards
   adherence with medication and,
      281–282, **283**
   building self-esteem and, **175**
   hallucinations and, 140, **141**
   interpersonal relationships and,
      216
   relapse prevention and, 301
Coping With Depression (Beck et al.
   1995), 69
Coping strategies. *See also* Coping
   cards
   antisuicide plan and, 158
   behavioral methods and, 15
   hallucinations and, 135–139
   hopelessness and suicidality, 155–
      156
   interpersonal relationships and,
      217, 229–230, 231
   mini-formulation and, 96–97
   relapse prevention plans and, **299**
Coping Strategies for Hallucinations
   (checklist), 136, **323–324**
Core beliefs. *See also* Beliefs; Schemas
   adherence and, 17–18
   basic CBT methods and, 12, 16
   delusions and discussion of, 113
Countertransference, and suicidality, 43
Court-ordered treatment, and
   medication, 277
Cross-sectional formulation, 85–86
Cultural issues
   assessment and, 47
   delusions and, 102
   engagement process and, 33–34

Daily activities, mania and
   organization of, **250**. *See also*
   Activity scheduling
*Darkness Visible: A Memoir of
   Madness* (Styron 1990), **63**
Debriefing, and role-playing for social
   skills development, 213, 214

Decatastrophizing methods, for conflict management, 186

Decentering approach, to hallucinations, 130

Decision making, and cognitive issues in mania, **249**

Delusions
  assessment and, 46, 103–104
  basic CBT processes for treatment of, 99–101
  definition of, 102–104
  discussion of, 104–105
  learning exercise for, 109–110
  methods for modification of, 106–113
  mood disorders and treatment of, 117–122
  normalizing of schizophrenia and, 58–59
  resistant forms of, 114–117
  video illustrations and, 115–116, 245–246

Denial, and nonadherence with medication, 276, 277

Dependency, and engagement process for depression, 44

Depression
  case study (Mary)
    case formulation, 77, **78–79**, 80
    introduction, 10–11, **11**
    video illustrations, 44–45 150–152, 163, 171–172
  cognitive functioning and, 251–254, **255**
  delusions and, 117–121
  efficacy of CBT for, 4, 6, 20–21
  engagement process and, 42–45
  hallucinations and, **130**
  hopelessness and, 146–149
  interpersonal relationships and, 222–226
  learning exercises for, 159–160, 167, 175–176
  low energy and lack of interest, 160–168

negative symptoms and secondary, 269

nonadherence with medication and, 276

normalizing of, 62–63

principle forms of CBT for chronic, 145

psychoeducation and, 69–70

self-esteem and, 168–176

suicidality and, 149–160

Depression and Bipolar Support Alliance, **63**

Derailment, and thought disorder in schizophrenia, 241–242, 243

Diagnosis, and normalizing of schizophrenia, **52, 54, 55.** See also Assessment; Evaluation

Differential relaxation, and bipolar disorder, 230

Discharge plan, and negative symptoms, 268–269

Disclosure
  interpersonal relationships and, 220–222
  therapeutic relationship and, 63, 64

Disorganization and disorganized thoughts. See also Thought disorder
  depression and, **251**
  mania and, **247**
  nonadherence with medication and, **276**, 278

Distancing methods, for negative automatic thoughts in depression, 223

Distraction and distractibility. See also Attention
  coping strategies for hallucinations and, **136**, 136–137
  depression and, **251**
  mania and, **247**, 247–251

Down Came the Rain (Shields 2005), **63**

Drug-related psychosis, 234
DSM-IV, and delusions, 102

Education. *See* Psychoeducation
Efficacy, of CBT
    for adherence, 273–274
    for bipolar disorder, 19–20
    for depression, 4, 6, 21
    for relapse prevention, 296
    for schizophrenia, 19
    for suicidality, 146
Emotion(s). *See also* Emotion-focused
    interventions
    case formulation and, 77
    mania and distress from,
        205–206
    responses to and working model of
        CBT, 8
Emotion-focused interventions, for
    mania, 204–206
Empathy, and therapeutic
    relationship, 148, 285, 286
Engagement. *See also* Therapeutic
    relationship
    delusions and, 99
    factors facilitating, **35**
    guidelines for, 37–45
    hallucinations and, 127
    importance of, 29
    patient characteristics and, 35–36
    personal circumstances and, 32–
        33
    service issues and, 34–35
    sociocultural issues in, 33–34
    symptomatic and behavioral issues
        in, 30–32
    video illustration and, 30
Environmental events, and working
    model of CBT, 8
Euphoria, and mania, 205
Evaluation, of hallucinations, 127,
    129. *See also* Assessment;
    Diagnosis
Examining the evidence, 14, 16, 18,
    52, 71, 278, 296

case examples of
    major depression (Roberto),
        119–121
    schizophrenia (Rhonda), 107–
        109
for cognitions in
    depression, **79**, 149, 165
    mania, **93**, 204
for delusions, 106–113, 119
    learning exercise, 109–110
    video illustration, 106–107
for hallucinations, **89**, 129, 132,
    139, 142
self-esteem and, 171, 172, **173**
Existential issues, and finding of
    meaning in long-term treatment,
    310–312
Explanations, for hallucinations, 129–
    130, **131**, 132–134

Family. *See also* Interpersonal
    relationships
    adherence with treatment and,
        277–278, 279–280
    assessment and, 47
    control of mania and, 203
    cultural issues in engagement and,
        34
    long-term treatment planning and,
        298–300
    nonadherence with medication
        and, **276**
    recommended reading for, 329–
        330
    of schizophrenia patients and
        guilt, 261
    social skills and, 212
    Web sites with information for,
        330
Feedback
    cognitive issues in depression and,
        224, **255**
    social skills and, 213
    thought disorder in schizophrenia
        and, 242

Financial constraints
  engagement process and, 34
  nonadherence with medication
    and, **276,** 278
Focusing, and coping strategies for
  hallucinations, **136,** 137–139
Forgetfulness, and nonadherence with
  medication, **276,** 278
*Full Catastrophe Living: Using the
  Wisdom of Your Body to Fight
  Stress, Pain, and Illness* (Kabat-
  Zinn 1990), 166
Fusion, and thought disorder in
  schizophrenia, 242
Future, and meaning of illness and
  treatment, **282**

*Getting Your Life Back: The Complete
  Guide to Recovery From
  Depression* (Wright and Basco
  2002), 69–70
Goals, setting with patients, **147,**
  148, 173–174, 223, 241, 259–
  263, **263.** *See also* Case
  formulation
Good Days Ahead (computer
  program), 252
Graded exposure, and hallucinations,
  139–140
Graded task assignments
  depression and, 15, 164, 165, 269
  negative symptoms and, 269
  self-esteem and, 174
Grandiosity
  engagement process and, **31**
  mania and, 204, **247**
Grief
  in bereavement and hallucinations,
    130
  and interpersonal relationships,
    216–217
Group therapy
  building self-esteem in
    schizophrenia and, 176

long-term treatment of psychotic
    disorders and, 308–310
Guided discovery, and mini-
    formulation, 96–97
Guidelines, for engagement process,
    37–45
Guilt, and families or caregivers of
    schizophrenia patients, 261

Hallucinations
  assessment and, 46
  CBT approach to, 127–132
  engagement process and, 31
  impact of, 125–127
  learning exercises for, 126–127,
    141
  mini-formulation and, 96–97
  normalizing of schizophrenia and,
    54–58
  specific CBT techniques for, 132–
    142
  video illustration and, 132–134
Helplessness, and adherence with
    medication, 282–284
Homework assignments
  adherence with medication and,
    281, 290–291
  cognitive dysfunction in
    depression and, 253, **255**
  hallucinations and, 128, 133
  normalization process for
    delusions and, 59
  self-esteem and, 175
  thought disorder in schizophrenia
    and, 244, **245**
Hope, CBT methods for building,
    147
Hopelessness
  adherence with medication and,
    284–285
  coping strategies for, 155–156
  delusions and, 118
  depression and, 146–149, **251**
  engagement process and, 31, 42

Hospitalization
  adherence with medication and, 287
  engagement process and, 34
Hostility, and engagement process, 30, **31**
Hypnagogic hallucinations, 64

Impaired judgment, and mania, 227, **247**, 248
Impulsivity, and engagement process, **31**
Indications, for CBT, 47–48
Inference chaining, and delusions, 115
Insight, **31**, 47
Insomnia. *See also* Sleep and sleep disruption
  depression and, 166–167
  mania and, 198–199
Integrated treatment approach, 303–304, **305**
Interpersonal relationships. *See also* Family
  adherence with medication and, 279–280
  bipolar disorder and, 226–233
  boundary issues and, 218–219
  common difficulties in, 211–212
  depression and, 222–226
  disclosure of disorder and, 220–222
  engagement process and preexisting problems with, **31**, 32
  learning exercises for, 215, 228–229
  loss and, 216–217
  nonadherence with medication and, **276**
  schizophrenia and, 233–235
  social skills and, 212–215
  social support and, 219–220
  symptom intrusions and, 215–216
Interviews, and engagement process, 38–40
Irritability, and interpersonal relationships, 215–216, 227–231

Knight's move thinking, and thought disorder in schizophrenia, 241, **242,** 243, 244

Language, and engagement process, 37. *See also* Confidentiality; Word salad
Learning, from experience of mania, 206–207. *See also* Learning exercises; Psychoeducation
Learning Cognitive-Behavior Therapy: An Illustrated Guide (Wright et al. 2006), 149, 162
Learning exercises
  advantages and disadvantages of assertive communication, 215
  case formulation, 93–94
  coping with hallucinations, 141
  developing an adherence plan, 289–290
  developing an antisuicide plan, 159–160
  developing a mania prevention plan, 207–208
  developing a relapse prevention plan, 302
  emotion intensity scale, 228–229
  examining the evidence, 109–110
  identifying and managing barriers to collaborative therapeutic relationships, 36
  impact of voices, 126–127
  low energy and anhedonia, using CBT for, 167
  modifying delusions, 116–117
  modifying schemas to improve self-esteem, 175–176
  normalizing the diagnosis of schizophrenia, 53

Learning exercises *(continued)*
  thought disorder, practicing CBT
    methods for, 246–247
  working with negative symptoms,
    269–270
Life events. *See also* Stress
  comprehensive model of CBT
    and, 6–7
  engagement process and, 32–33
  escalation of mania and, **196**
  trauma and, **130**
Lifestyle management
  adherence with medication and,
    288, 290
  prevention plans for mania and,
    182–190
Longitudinal formulation, 85
Loosening of associations, and
  schizophrenia, **239,** 240
Loss, and interpersonal relationships,
  216–217
Low energy and interest. *See also*
  Anhedonia
  CBT for chronic depression and,
    160–167
  engagement process and, **31,** 42, 43
  schizophrenia and, 167–168, **169**

Maintenance, of CBT, 303–312
Major depression, and treatment of
  delusions, 118–121. *See also*
  Depression
*Making Sense of Voices: A Guide for
  Professionals Who Work With
  Voice Hearers* (Romme and
  Escher 2000), 56
Mania and hypomania. *See also*
  Bipolar disorder
  activity managing and, 186–187
  cognitive dysfunctions and, 247–
    251
  factors in recurrence of, **207**
  hallucinations and, 126
  learning from experience of, 206–
    207

lifestyle management and, 182–
    190
  planning ahead for recurrences,
    194, 196–200
  prevention plan for, 182–207
    learning exercise and, 207–208
  primary emphasis of CBT for,
    181–182
  recognizing emergence of
    symptoms, 190–194
  sleep and, 2, **3,** 183–185, 198–
    199, 250
  stress and, 185–186
  substance abuse and, 189–190
  symptoms of, **191**
    triggers of, 15, 187–189
  taking action to control symptoms,
    200–206
  tangential thoughts and, 239
  treating delusions in, 121–122
Man's Search for Meaning (Frankl
  1992), 311
Meaning. *See* Existential issues; Future
Medical conditions, and normalizing,
  52–53
Medication. *See also* Adherence;
  Antipsychotics
  clozapine, 309, 311
  combining CBT with, 4, 305–308
  lifestyle management for
    medication and, 182–183,
    184
  side effects of, 34–35, **276**
  therapeutic relationship and, 34–
    35, 36
Meditation
  chronic depression and, 166
  hallucinations and, 138–139
  sleep management and, 185
Memory, and depression, **255.** *See
  also* Cognitive dysfunctions
Mental retardation, and
  contraindications for CBT, 48
Mental status examination, and
  assessment for CBT, 46–47

Metacognitive approaches, to coping strategies for hallucinations, **136,** 139

Mindfulness. *See* Meditation

Mindful Way Through Depression: Freeing Yourself From Chronic Unhappiness, The (Williams et al. 2007), 166

Mini-formulation, construction and use of, 94–97

Mood, and recurrence of mania, **207.** *See also* Mood disorders; Mood graphs

Mood disorders. *See also* Bipolar disorder; Depression
  long-term group therapy and, 308
  prevalence of, 13, 62
  treatment of delusions in, 117–122

Mood graphs, 192, 194, **195**

Motivation
  methods for building, **263**
  negative symptoms and, **61,** 258, 259
  schizophrenia and demotivation, 260–264

National Institute for Clinical Excellence (U.K.), 2

National Institute of Mental Health, **63**

Negative experiences, with medication, **276,** 278

Negative symptoms. *See also* Symptoms
  assessment and, 46
  behavioral methods for, 266–270
  CBT and conceptualization of, 259–260
  definition of, 258–259
  learning exercise for, 269–270
  normalizing of schizophrenia and, 60–61
  video illustration and, 263–264

Neologisms, 242

Noise, and auditory hallucinations, 130

Nonadherence. *See* Adherence

Normalizing and destigmatizing
  basic CBT methods and, **12,** 13–14
  bipolar disorder and, 62
  delusions and, 100, 101
  depression and, 62–63
  hallucinations and, 128–129
  schizophrenia and, 51–61, 235
  therapeutic relationship and, 63–64
  video illustration and, 54–56

Overcoming Paranoid and Suspicious Thoughts (Freeman et al. 2006), 58, **68**

Overgeneralization hypothesis, and adherence, 278

Overstimulation, and prevention plans for mania, 184, **187**

Paranoia, 6, 96. *See also* Case studies and examples; Schizophrenia
  delusions and, 58–59
  engagement process and, 30, **31,** 99
  interpersonal problems and, 233
  in mania, 122, **191,** 204
  negative symptoms and, 258, 260, **265**
  psychoeducation and, 14, **68,** 101

Paranoid Thoughts Web site, 59

Patient characteristics
  assessment for CBT and identification of strengths or assets, 47
  engagement process and, 35–36

Personality traits, and engagement process for depression, 42, 43–44

Perspective, taking of different
  depression and negative automatic thoughts, 223
  modifying delusions by, 110–111

Pharmacotherapy. *See* Medication

Pillboxes, and adherence with medication, 279

Planning and plans. *See* Antisuicide plans; Prevention plan; Treatment planning; Written plans

Positive imagery, and hallucinations, 138

Positive reinforcement, and social skills, 213

Practice, and building of self-esteem, 174–175

Prevalence
    of comorbid substance abuse in severe mental illness, 18
    of mood disorders, 13, 62
    of nonadherence with medication, 275

Prevention plan, for mania
    activity management and, 186–187
    example of, **183**
    learning from experience, 206–207
    lifestyle management and, 182–190
    planning ahead for recurrences, 194, 196–200
    recognizing emergence of symptoms, 190–194
    sleep and, 183–185, 198–199
    stress and, 185–186
    substance abuse and, 189–190
    symptom triggers and, 187–189
    taking action to control symptoms, 200–206

Problem list, and hallucinations, 131–132

Problem solving approach
    adherence with medication and, 278, 280–281
    depression and, 162, **255**
    cognitive impairment in mania and, **248**

Procrastination, and depression, 251

Professional organizations, with special interest in CBT, 331

Pseudophilosophical thinking, 238, **239**

Psychoeducation
    adherence with medication and, 277, 280
    basic CBT methods and, 12, 14, 64–65
    bipolar disorder and, 68–69
    delusions and, 100, 101
    depression and, 69–70, 170, 252, **255**
    schizophrenia and, 65–67, **68**
    self-esteem issues and, 170, 172

Psychomotor agitation, and mania, 203

Psychopharmacology. *See* Medication

Psychosis and psychotic disorders. *See also* Schizophrenia
    assessment and, 46
    guidelines for engagement, 37–40
    long-term group therapy for, 308–310
    psychoeducation and treatment of, **66**

Psychotic depression, and hallucinations, 126

Psychotic Symptom Rating Scales (PSYRATS), 103–104, 127, 315, **317–320**

Racing thoughts, and mania, **247,** 247–251

Rating scales, for hallucinations, 127

Rational response, to hallucinations, **138**

Reading, recommended
    for families and patients, 329–330
    for normalizing depression, **63**
    for patients with bipolar disorder, 68–69
    for patients with schizophrenia, 67, **68**

Reality testing, and thought disorder in schizophrenia, 244–245

Reattribution, and suicidality, 154, **155**
Recurrences, of mania, 194, 196–
200, **207**. *See also* Relapse
prevention
Rehearsals
adherence with medication and,
290–291
depression and cognitive, 252–
253, **255**
relapse prevention and, 300–301
role-playing for social skills and, 214
Rejection, of treatment, 277
Relapse prevention. *See also*
Recurrences
basic CBT methods and, **12,** 18–
19, 295–302
as goal of CBT, 3–4
learning exercise for, 302
Relaxation methods
depression and, **255**
mania and, 185
Religion and religiosity
delusions and, 114–115, 121
nonadherence with medication
and, **276**
Reminder strategies, and adherence,
278–279
Repetition, as method to enhance
learning, 65
Response prevention
bipolar disorders and interpersonal
relationships, 230–231, 232–
233
command hallucinations and, 140
Role models, and social skills, 212
Role-playing
adherence with medication and,
281
conflict management and, 186
disclosure of disorder and, 221
social skills and, 212–214

Safety, 30, 153
Scale for the Assessment of Insight,
104

Schema(s). *See also* Core beliefs
case formulation and identification
of, 86
cognitive interventions for
depression and, 165
delusions and modification of,
112–113, 121
depression and modification of,
225–226
self-esteem and links between
behavior and, 170–171
Schema Inventory, 139, 315, **327**
Schematic approaches, to coping
strategies for hallucinations, **136,**
139
Schizoaffective disorder, 305–306
Schizophrenia. *See also* Delusions;
Hallucinations; Negative
symptoms; Psychosis and
psychotic disorders
antisuicide plans and, 156–159
case study (Brenda)
case formulation, 87, **88–89**
introduction, 80, **81,** 82–83
video illustrations, 54–56, 132–
134
case study (Daniel)
adherence, 286–290, **288,**
289
introduction, 243
video illustrations, 243–244,
244–246
case study (Majir)
case formulation, 87, **90–91**
introduction, 9, **9**
video illustrations, 30, 104–
105, 106–107, 115–116,
263–264
demotivation in, 260–264
education on treatment of, 65–67,
68
efficacy of CBT for, 19
existential issues and finding
meaning, 311
group therapy for, 308–310

Schizophrenia *(continued)*
  interpersonal relationships and,
    233–235
  key schemas in, 86
  low energy and anhedonia in,
    167–168, **169**
  medication adherence and, 274
  normalizing of, 51–61
    learning exercise for, 53
  relapse prevention and, 296, 298
  self-esteem and, 176
  socialization and, 264–266
  substance abuse and, 18
  thought disorder in, 238–247
  treatment of delusions in patients
    with, 101
Seasonal changes, in mania, 187
Self, and meaning of illness and
  treatment, **282**
Self-care, and normalizing statements,
  61
Self-esteem
  chronic depression and, 168–176
  core beliefs and, 86
  delusions in major depression and,
    121
  video illustration and, 171–172
Self-monitoring, of bipolar disorder,
  62, 192, 194, 233
Sensory deprivation, and
  hallucinations, **130**
Sequenced Treatment Alternatives to
  Relieve Depression (STAR*D)
  trial, 21
Service delivery
  engagement process, 34–35
  models of, **304**
Setting, and engagement process,
  37
Sex drive, and bipolar disorder, 232–
  233
Side effects, of medication, 34–35,
  276
Sleep and sleep disruption
  depression and, 166–167, **255**

  hallucinations and, **130**
  mania and, 183–185, 198–199
"Slow It, Focus It, Structure It"
  strategy, 248
Social anxiety, 266
Social isolation, and depression, 222,
  223, 224. *See also* Social
  withdrawal
Social relationships. *See* Interpersonal
  relationships
Social rhythms therapy, 167
Social skills and social skills training
  common difficulties in
    interpersonal relationships
    and, 212–215
  for schizophrenia patients, 234,
    264–266
Social support, and interpersonal
  relationships, 219–220, 226
Social withdrawal. *See also* Social
  isolation
  engagement process and, 31–32
  normalizing of negative symptoms
    and, **61**
  schizophrenia patients and, 234,
    264, **265**
Socratic questioning
  adherence with medication and,
    277, 284, 285, 286, 287
  case formulation and, 83–84
  maladaptive schemas in
    depression and, 165
  prevention plans for mania and,
    186, 201, 203
Somatic hallucinations, 126
Stigma. *See also* Normalizing and
  destigmatizing
Stimulus control, and mania, 197,
  202
Stress. *See also* Life events
  prevention plan for mania and,
    185–186
  schizophrenia and, 234
  trauma and hallucinations and,
    130

Substance abuse
  basic CBT methods and, 12, 18
  engagement process and, **31**, 32
  hallucinations and, **130**
  interpersonal relationships for
    schizophrenia patients and,
    234
  nonadherence with medication
    and, **276,** 277, 278
  prevention plans for mania and,
    189–190
Subvocalization, and hallucinations,
  137
Suicidality
  CBT for chronic depression and,
    149–160
  delusions in depression and, 118,
    119–121
  engagement process for depression
    and, 42–43
  hopelessness and, 146
Suspiciousness, and psychosis, **59**
Symptom(s), of severe mental illness.
    See also Negative symptoms;
    Self-monitoring
  interpersonal relationships and
    intrusions of, 215–216
  prevention plans for mania and,
    187–194, 200–206
  relapse prevention and triggers,
    297
  as targets for CBT, 2–3
  therapeutic relationship and, 30–
    32
Symptom summary worksheet, 15,
    192, **193,** 206–208, 216, 297,
    299–300

Talking past the point, and
    schizophrenia, 239
Tangential thoughts
  mania and hypomania, **247**
  schizophrenia and, 239–240
Task-orienting cognitions (TOCs),
    214

Temporal lobe epilepsy, and
    hallucinations, **130**
Therapeutic relationship. *See also*
    Engagement
  assessment and, 47
  delusions and, 100
  hopelessness and, 148
  influences on, 30–36
  learning exercise for, 36
  normalizing and, 63–64
  optimization of, 12–13
  socialization and, 266
Therapy notebooks, and relapse
    prevention, 301
Thought blocking, and schizophrenia,
    239, 240
Thought Change Record, 315,
    325
Thought disorder. *See also* Automatic
    thoughts; Disorganization and
    disorganized thoughts
  basic CBT methods and, 16–17
  engagement process and, **31**
  schizophrenia and
    CBT techniques for, 238–247
    normalizing of, 59–60
  video illustration and, 243–244
Thought linkage, and thought
    disorder in schizophrenia, 244,
    245
Thought records, and delusions, 111–
    112
Timeline, and case formulation, 80–
    83, **83**
Trauma and traumatic events
  hallucinations and, **130**
  interpersonal relationships and
    schizophrenia, 234
Treatment planning
  adherence with medication and
    alternatives, **285**
  case formulation and, 75–76, 77,
    80, 87
  family and long-term, 298–300
  relapse prevention and, 297–298

24-hour rule, and bipolar disorder, 232, 233

Understanding Voices: Coping With Auditory Hallucinations and Confusing Realities (Romme and Escher 1996), 56
University of Louisville Depression Center, **63**
University of Michigan Depression Center, **63**
Unquiet Mind, An (Jamison 1995), 14, 68

Video illustrations
   antisuicide plan, 150–152
   behavioral intervention for anhedonia, 163
   building self-esteem, 171–172
   coping with and explaining hallucinations, 132–134
   DVD guide, 335–337
   early warning system, 206–207
   engaging patient with bipolar disorder, 40–41
   engaging patient with chronic depression, 44–45
   engaging patient with paranoia, 30
   examining evidence for paranoia, 106–107
   helping with thought disorder, 243–244
   investigating a delusion, 244–246
   normalizing and educating, 54–56
   promoting adherence, 280–281
   reducing grandiosity, 204
   tracing the origins of paranoia, 104–105
   treating negative symptoms, 263–264
   working with a resistant delusion, 115–116

Voice diaries, and hallucinations, 134–135

Web sites
   delusions and, 59
   depression and, **63**
   hallucinations and, **56**
   information for families and patients, 330
Weekly Activity Schedule (worksheet), 315, **326**
What's Happening to Me? A Voice Hearing Pamphlet (Kingdon and Turkington 2005), 55, 315, 321–322
Wooliness of thought, and schizophrenia, 238, **239**
Word salad, 59–60, 242
Work, and disclosure of disorder, 220, 222
Working hypothesis, for case formulation, **76,** 86–87
Working model, for CBT interventions, 7–12
Worksheets
   for development of case formulation, 76–80, **88–93**
   list of, 315–327
   for symptom recognition in mania, 190, **191,** 192, **193,** 216
Worst-case scenario method, and relapse prevention, 300
Worthlessness, and adherence with medication, 285–286
Written plans
   adherence with medication and, 286–290
   antisuicide and, 156

Disclosures of Interests

Dr. Wright receives book royalties from Simon and Schuster, Guilford Press, and American Psychiatric Publishing. Dr. Turkington and Dr. Kingdon receive book royalties from Guilford Press, American Psychiatric Publishing, Cambridge University Press, and Wiley. Dr. Kingdon also receives book royalties from Routledge Press. Dr. Basco receives book royalties from Simon and Schuster, Guilford Press, and American Psychiatric Publishing.

Additional disclosures are noted below:

Jesse H. Wright, M.D., Ph.D.
I may receive royalties and other payments from Mindstreet for sales of software (authored by J. Wright, A. Wright, and A. Beck) for computer-assisted cognitive-behavior therapy. I am also currently on speaker panels for Pfizer and Bristol-Meyers Squibb.

Douglas Turkington, M.D.
I have received lecture fees from Astra Zeneca, Bristol-Meyers Squibb, and Janssen but have never presented any data related to antipsychotic medication.

David G. Kingdon, M.D.
I have received lecture fees from Lilly, Astra Zeneca, Bristol-Meyers Squibb, and Janssen but have never presented any data related to antipsychotic medication.

Monica Ramirez Basco, Ph.D.
No other interests to disclose.